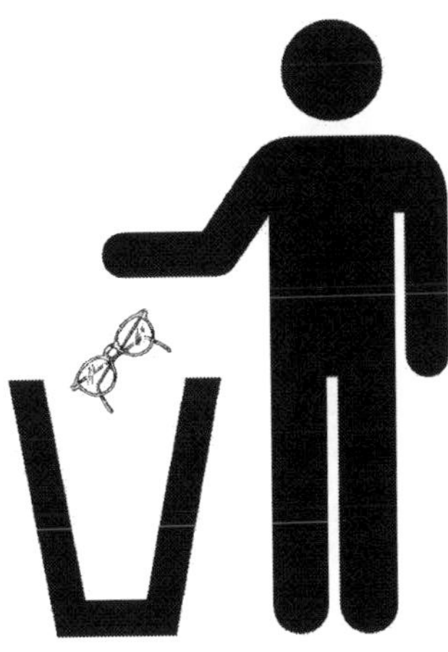

Give Up Your Glasses for Good: Holistic Eye Care for the 21st Century

Third Edition

Second Edition - 2015
First Edition - 2014

ISBN: 978-0-9863953-2-1
Published by The Naked Eye Publishing Co.
North Carolina, USA

Nathan T. Oxenfeld
Certified Bates Method Teacher
Certified Yoga Teacher
Founder & Owner of
Integral Eyesight Improvement LLC
www.integraleyesight.com

Legal Disclaimer:

The content of this book is intended for educational purposes only. It is not, in any sense, diagnosing or advising any medical treatment for any pathological condition and is not a replacement for advice or care from a qualified health care professional.

Dedication

This book is dedicated to my vision teacher, mentor, and founder of the Vision Training Institute in El Cajon, California, Dr. Jerriann J. Taber PhD, for helping me give up my glasses for good and for training me to become the teacher that I am today.

Case Histories & Testimonials

"This is by FAR the best natural eyesight improvement book I came across (I read more than 5 different ones)! Nathan writes with clarity and such eloquence. You will not leave any chapter confused or wondering what if... or will this work. I am savoring this book while taking a class with him and in only 10 days I see sharper images and get flashes after gentle blinks (used to take a good squeeze to get a flash). If you are just starting your Bates program or you are stuck along your journey of recovering your birthright of clear vision get this book!" ***–Vesna M.***

"I had a vision exam today. I am happy that in less than one year my vision has improved from 20/70 to 20/30. The Optometric Physician almost fell off his chair as he told me my astigmatism is completely gone. He told me that he has never seen that before. Thanks again for all your help. I hope to write you again as my vision continues to improve." ***-Andre S.***

[UPDATE] "I passed the motor vehicle 20/30 vision test for the first time in 30+ years. Good-bye to 'corrective lenses driving restrictions'. Now I am working toward 20/20 vision. Thanks again for your good vision training and coaching." ***-Andre S.***

"So in amazement today, I can actually see things. Stuff goes in and out but it feels so freeing in my eyes and my brain. My eyesight did something in sleep and I woke up seeing trees, flowers, details, and sharp edges. In comes in and out but I can't even remember when I could actually see... was wearing glasses at age 7. Bates Method class with Nathan gave me a huge boost to my efforts of 20 years. Now the world looks amazing. No one can ever appreciate who has lost then regained his or her eyesight. I plan to keep going for 20/20 this year." ***–Patrick C.***

"I've known for years about the possibility of vision improvement. I'd read books, bought gadgets, and made halfhearted attempts to free myself from the glasses I've worn since second grade — to no avail. But by working with Nathan, I have absolute belief that I can see clearly without glasses! My nearsightedness is noticeably improving, thanks to Nathan's encouragement and the clear practices he's taught. His manner is gentle and unhurried while firmly committed to my progress. It is a pleasure to learn from him and to achieve such concrete results in improving my vision." ***-Michele D.***

"Nathan presented a great workshop today. He is very knowledgeable about improving your eyesight. I knew it was a sign that I was to take his classes when my eyeglasses dropped on the floor a couple of days ago and I could not find one of the lenses. I am looking forward to better eyesight!" ***-Dawn W.***

"I highly recommend Nathan as your holistic alternative to regain your eyesight. He's knowledgeable and passionate about vision and has a simple, yet comprehensive step-by-step program for you to follow. What adds even more credibility is the fact that it has so dramatically helped his own vision as well." ***-Tony B.***

"Nathan is an excellent, accomplished instructor who inspired confidence every step of the way. The course went beyond anything I could have imagined to touch every area of my life – a profound and enlightening experience – what joy." ***–Carol W.***

"The vision lesson I had with Nathan was extremely helpful in improving my eyesight. I literally went into his class barely able to see the top line of the eye chart and am seeing much more clearly now with ease. I can say with confidence that my vision fluctuates between 20/20, 20/25, and 20/30. He is very knowledgeable, patient, and easy to understand in his approach to people's vision challenges. I am truly thankful to have him as my vision teacher and highly recommend him to anyone with a desire to improve their eyesight." ***-Rickey D.***

"I had many flashes of clear vision on my walk yesterday. So magical! I definitely notice that vision is better when I'm outdoors. I also noticed that things look more 3D than they did with glasses/contacts. I'm working on allowing and believing in this miracle of clear vision, rather than being afraid of or denying it. Really an amazing process." ***-Mara V.***

"I took Nathan's group class and then did a series of individual lessons with him. I find I always learn something when I have a lesson, sometimes subtle, sometimes quite remarkable. Nathan has been a good guide for me and I will continue to make use of my sessions with him. After about 10 lessons I made my vision practice my own. One month later I was able to easily pass my Driver's License Vision Test so now after 15 years I no longer need to wear glasses when I drive! ***-Nancy P.***

"This course was excellent. Nathan teaches in ways that are engaging and helpful. Each class was well paced with ample time to learn and practice the new material. The handouts were excellent, in content and professional design. Nathan's dedication to teaching the Bates Method comes across in a style that is clear and confident. Highly recommended." ***–Michael R***

*"When I started the course, I had tried learning and implementing the Bates method for about a year and a half on my own starting at a -5.75 prescription with minor improvements. I was looking to dive deeper and get more insight on the process and how to speed up the improvements I had already seen. Nathan's way of teaching the Bates Method is clear and concise making it easy to understand week by week as new practices are introduced. Taking the course introduced accountability to the process and I was driven to do the practices every day as new videos came out every week. The biggest take away from the course was that being consistent and doing the various practices everyday is key. After about a month I was noticing details in my vision without glasses or contacts I hadn't seen before. The course provides a great foundation and the tools needed to continue the practices long after the course ends to continue the success as much as you put into it. I will continue to use the knowledge I learned as I keep improving my vision and for the rest of my life." **–Stephen C.***

*"Just came back from the eye doctor... with my old pair of glasses, this July my eye sight was 2/10 (20/100) on my left eye and 7/10 (20/30) on my right eye. Now with the same glasses, it is left 5/10 (20/40) and 9/10 (20/25) on the right. WOOOHOOOO! I am so excited. It's good to know that this is working! During the eye exam, instead of squinting to try to see clearer, I just take a deep breath and relax; somehow I get micro seconds of clarity where the letters are revealed to me. Can't wait to learn more and practice more" **-Bao N.***

*"Nathan's understanding and interpretation of the Bates Method gives me much hope and confidence in my own journey to clearer vision. Since studying with him, my vision has improved from 20/400+ to 20/150. Just as any true healing of the body, this requires time and dedication to achieve the results we are reaching for. I can feel I am towards the end of having to use corrective lenses. Allow Nathan show you the path to a clearer and brighter future." - **Kevin M.***

*"Thank you so much Nathan for the vision lesson on Friday. My eyes were so tense and scratchy. I had been working on my computer too much and knew I needed some help. After you worked with me and we did swinging, palming, and more, my eyes have felt so much better. I can see more clearly too! Plus I have started to incorporate some of the tips you shared with me. Thanks again! I look forward to working with you again!" **-Alicia S.***

Table of Contents

Relaxed Reading *inspired by Aldous Huxley & Dr. William H. Bates OD*

If you follow some of these relaxing warm-ups before reading and simple techniques while reading without wearing glasses, you will begin to experience flashes of clearer sight of the print on the page. There are many more reading techniques described in Chapter 7, but as you make your way through the Introduction and Chapters 1 through 6, see if you can make the following changes to the way you read:

1. Before reading, **'eat a sun sandwich'** (sun your eyes, palm your eyes, and sun your eyes again), and **'eat another sun sandwich'** anytime you need to during reading. Read in bright light. *(Sunning and Palming instructions in Chapters 3 and 4)*
2. Before reading, **give your eyes a 'microprint massage'** and anytime during reading. Do not try to read the microprint, just hold it a few inches from your face and **let your eyes scan through the white spaces** for a few seconds keeping them relaxed. After exploring the microprint, regular size print will seem much larger and easier in comparison. *(Microprint on next page)*
3. **Hold the print between the edge of clarity and edge of blur.** The words must be easily readable, but not 100% clear, so you can tell when you get a **clear flash.**
4. Try **Thin White Line Reading** by nose-drawing an imaginary white line from the left margin to the right margin right beneath the foot of the letters as you read.
5. At the end of every 1 to 3 sentences, **close your eyes** and **remember the last word and punctuation mark** you just read for 1 to 3 seconds in your mind. Then **open your eyes back up and look at the remembered word.** Does it look the same? Does it look clearer? Repeat at the end of the next sentence and try again.
6. **Incorporate your memory and imagination into reading** by closing your eyes often, clearly visualizing **one letter from the last word** you just read, or imagine the **white space that surrounds that letter,** or imagine **two tiny black dots** to the left and right of the letter, or above and below the letter, and shift back and forth between the two dots **mentally with eyes closed** and **physically with eyes open.** How does the letter or word look when you open your eyes after activating your memory and imagination? Try each one of the above techniques in 5 & 6 for **a few seconds with your eyes closed** and then **a few seconds with your eyes open,** then keep on reading.

7. At the end of every 1 to 3 pages, **palm your eyes for 10 to 30 seconds or more** to rest them before reading the next 1 to 3 pages and **taking another short palming break.** How does the print look right after palming? Does it look the same? Does it look clearer? Keep blinking and breathing as you continue reading.
8. Whenever you turn a page, **gaze up at a distant object,** like an eye chart, a wall calendar, or out a window to **look far away** with interest and engagement to **stretch your focus out** and **break the stare.**
9. **Do not hold your breath** while you read. **Breathe rhythmically and deeply.**
10. **Do not stare** while you read. **Blink softly and gently several times per sentence** as you slide swiftly across the **imaginary thin white line underlining words.**
11. **Do not try to see a whole sentence or phrase equally clearly all at once** or diffuse your focus out to too large of an area. **Centralize your focus & attention** to just the part of the page you are looking directly at, **one part of the white page.** Allow the rest of the page to seem less bright white.
12. **Do not squint, strain, or frown** while you read. Catch your facial muscles straining and **consciously relax them**, especially your eyes, eyebrows, and forehead. Check your posture.
13. **Do not read through half closed eyelids. Use a slot reader** instead so you can keep your eyes open normally. Cut a narrow rectangular slot out of a piece of black construction paper to allow you to read only one or two sentences on the page at a time. (See below for an example)

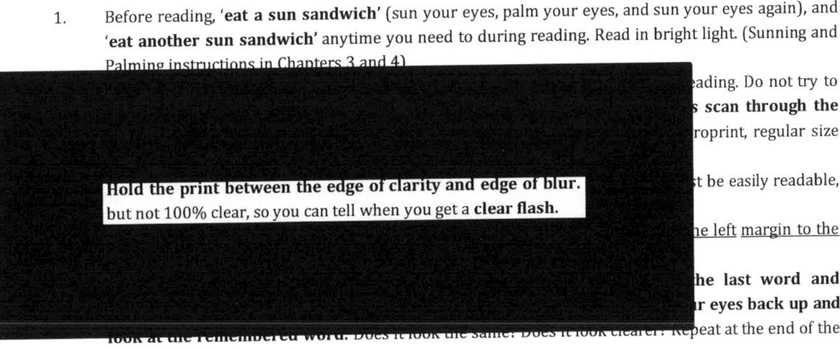

1. Before reading, **'eat a sun sandwich'** (sun your eyes, palm your eyes, and sun your eyes again), and **'eat another sun sandwich'** anytime you need to during reading. Read in bright light. (Sunning and Palming instructions in Chapters 3 and 4)

ading. Do not try to
s scan through the
roprint, regular size

Hold the print between the edge of clarity and edge of blur.
but not 100% clear, so you can tell when you get a **clear flash.**

t be easily readable,

e left margin to the

he last word and
r eyes back up and
epeat at the end of the
next sentence and try again.

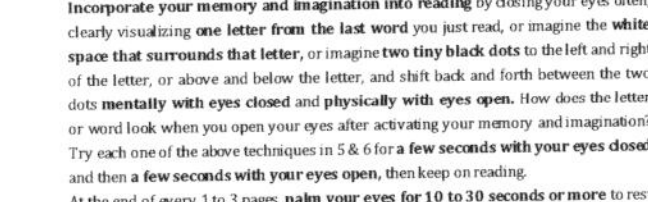

6. **Incorporate your memory and imagination into reading** by closing your eyes often, clearly visualizing **one letter from the last word** you just read, or imagine the **white space that surrounds that letter,** or imagine **two tiny black dots** to the left and right of the letter, or above and below the letter, and shift back and forth between the two dots **mentally with eyes closed** and **physically with eyes open.** How does the letter or word look when you open your eyes after activating your memory and imagination? Try each one of the above techniques in 5 & 6 for **a few seconds with your eyes closed** and then **a few seconds with your eyes open,** then keep on reading.
7. At the end of every 1 to 3 pages, **palm your eyes for 10 to 30 seconds or more** to rest them before reading the next 1 to 3 pages and **taking another short palming break.** How does the print look right after palming? Does it look the same? Does it look clearer? Keep blinking and breathing as you continue reading.
8. Whenever you turn a page, **gaze up at a distant object,** like an eye chart, a wall calendar, or out a window to **look far away** with interest and engagement to **stretch your focus out** and **break the stare.**

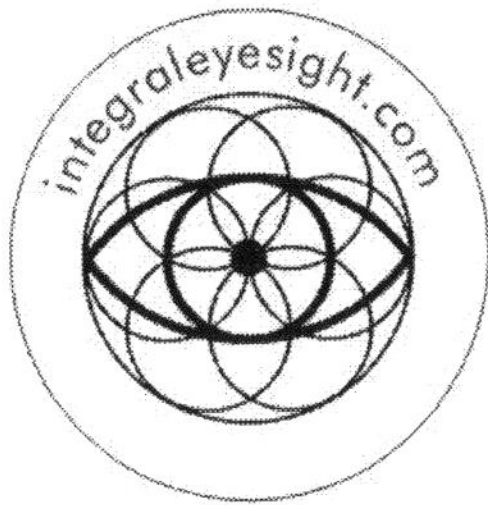

9. **Do not hold your breath** while you read. **Breathe rhythmically and deeply.**
10. **Do not stare** while you read. **Blink softly and gently several times per sentence** as you slide swiftly across the **imaginary thin white line underlining words.**
11. **Do not try to see a whole sentence or phrase equally clearly all at once** or diffuse your focus out to too large of an area. **Centralize your focus & attention** to just the part of the page you are looking directly at, **one part of the white page.** Allow the rest of the page to seem less bright white.
12. **Do not squint, strain, or frown** while you read. Catch your facial muscles straining and **consciously relax them**, especially your eyes, eyebrows, and forehead. Check your posture.
13. **Do not read through half closed eyelids. Use a slot reader** instead so you can keep your eyes open normally. Cut a narrow rectangular slot out of a piece of black construction paper to allow you to read only one or two sentences on the page at a time. See below for an example.

My Story

I wore artificial lenses for nearly 15 years before learning that there were other options. Like many other children, I was prescribed my first pair of glasses in elementary school. When I noticed it becoming harder to read the board in the front of the classroom I was taken to an eye doctor and fitted for glasses. The glasses helped me see the board better, but they did not truly address the root cause of my blur; the physical and mental strains that I wouldn't become aware of until a decade later. Through the years, I became more and more dependent on the glasses and my vision became blurrier and blurrier without them. In middle school I switched to contacts and wore them most days of the week. The pattern of higher dependency and blurrier vision continued throughout high school and college, to the point of approaching -4.00 for myopia and -2.00 for astigmatism.

It was during my senior year of college that I first learned about the Bates Method from a fellow classmate I met while studying abroad at Solheimar Ecovillage in Iceland. He was in the process of improving his own vision using the Bates Method so he shared several of the ideas and practices with me, which I implemented into my daily routine for several months. The first step I took, based on his suggestion, was to switch from contacts to glasses because it was much easier to take off and put on glasses as needed throughout the day as opposed to the daylong commitment of contacts. I quickly realized that not wearing glasses at all was a big part of the process too. Luckily, I was living in a small self-sustainable community in a foreign country so I found copious opportunities to go without my glasses. For example, I did not have to drive since transportation was provided. Not to mention the expansive and tree-less emptiness of Iceland that served as a healthy landscape to rest my eyes on and stretch my vision far off into the distance.

Not only did I witness physical eyesight improvement, but I also developed a new inner vision and worldview while in Iceland. The topics my classmates and I studied varied from renewable energies and sustainable societies to intentional communities and voluntary simplicity. I began seeing the world in a different way – in a more optimistic and interconnected way. Learning how to peacefully coexist with the earth and with each other made me look forward to a brighter future, not the doom-and-gloom attitudes I often encountered at the time in the United States. Natural vision improvement fit right in with the topic of sustainability. My desire to give up my glasses for good came from a desire to take responsibility for my own health and to become less dependent on artificial lenses, which are costly and unsustainable for the environment. I was no longer interested in funding the 95 billion dollar a year optical industry.

Returning from Iceland, however, I fell out of my regular vision practice and began using my glasses more while concentrating on graduating from college and catching up to the fast-paced lifestyle of the United States. Upon graduation, I was able to refocus on my vision practice and I stopped wearing my glasses again while working outdoors for the summer. That fall I went through a one-month residential yoga teacher-training program at Satchidananda Ashram (Yogaville) in Virginia. During that month, I established my own daily yoga practice and become a certified yoga instructor, but also developed major improvements in my vision. This was partly due to the daily routine of yoga, meditation, vegetarian/vegan diet, natural sleep cycles and rhythms, replacing screen time with outdoor time, and abstaining from sugar, caffeine, alcohol, and drugs. I also went without my glasses for the majority of the month, which helped prove to myself that the more I wore my glasses the worse my vision became, and the less I wore them the better my vision became. Seeing how much clearer my vision became after yoga or meditation helped me understand that vision is so much more than just physical eyesight, and that there really may be something I could do to make my eyes healthier and keep them that way.

After becoming a certified yoga instructor, I moved to Asheville, North Carolina to begin teaching. I went back to the eye doctor because my glasses were starting to feel too strong since my vision was beginning to improve. To my delight, my eyes tested at -2.0 for myopia (previously -3.50) and -0.50 for astigmatism (previously -1.50). This gave me an objective indication that there was something to this vision practice, but I wanted it to go faster. I had been practicing it on and off for two years and was ready to take it to the next level.

After extensive research online, I decided to get help from a Bates Method teacher named Dr. Jerriann J. Taber in El Cajon, California. I chose to work with her because she is in direct teaching lineage of the method's founder, Dr. William H. Bates, and she has over 40 years of teaching experience. She told me exactly what I needed to do, when I needed to do it, and for how long. She made sure I was performing all of the practices correctly and made me accountable for doing my homework. I noticed a significant difference in my vision once I began working with a teacher who had already gone through the process herself. It took me two years to drop from -3.50 to -2.00 working alone, but it took me less than a year to drop from -2.00 to 0.00 with Dr. Taber's help. That demonstrated how people could achieve much greater success by working with a coach as opposed to doing it alone.

My profound success using the Bates Method motivated me to share it with others by becoming a certified Bates Method teacher. This idea fully aligned with my newly realized purpose of becoming a holistic practitioner and also presented an opportunity to combine my passion with my profession. So I enrolled in an online Bates Method teacher training program under the tutelage of Dr. Taber, who taught the practice handed down originally from Dr. William H. Bates and Margaret D. Corbett to her. This training required two years of intensive work and over 200 hours of hands-on experience with willing volunteers. To complete this phase, I worked with family, friends, and acquaintances to gain the experience I needed to become a proficient teacher. One of my very first practice students was able to drop down from her -4.25 glasses to -2.00 glasses within a few months of weekly lessons. Another practice student regained her ability to read magazines and do cross stitching without her reading glasses. Yet another one went on to pass his vision test with 20/30 vision without glasses in order to remove the restriction from his driver's license. Once I became a certified Bates Method teacher I began hosting workshops, leading group class series, and working with more private students within the local community and online from across the world, which enabled me to help even more people overcome their vision-related issues.

I am living, breathing, seeing proof of the efficacy and potency of the Bates Method when practiced properly. I act as a beacon of hope for people who always instinctively knew there was something they could do to take better care of their eyes. I hope to open a dialogue about holistic eye care and create a community of visionaries keen on improving their own vision. My goal is to spearhead the resurgence of the original Bates Method in the 21st century and facilitate the passing on of the material to the next generation of children growing up in a vision-intensive culture. I feel blessed to have stumbled upon this material so early on in my life and only wish I had learned about it earlier.

Writing this book has been a goal of mine for a long time and to see it come into fruition is deeply satisfying. However, my true passion is to actually to teach the material in this book to vision students in person or online. This entire book was written to accompany the material covered in private one-on-one vision coaching lessons or my online vision courses.

When I first heard about natural vision improvement and the Bates Method, I did not know that working with a vision teacher to help me accomplish my goals was even an option. I went at it alone initially with lots of doubts and limited success. Working with my vision teacher enabled me to fully reach my goal of normal vision in a much shorter time than it would have taken me by myself. She was my vision coach: guiding me, instructing me, motivating me, and making sure I was doing all the practices perfectly. She set me up for success and I succeeded. She opened the door and I walked through it. And that is what I wish to do for you. I want to make it easier for you to get your own eyes working again.

Therefore, I encourage you to explore the option of in-person or online vision training lessons with me, or a certified Bates Method teacher in your area, to jumpstart your vision improvement practice and get your eyesight back on track. I look forward to *seeing* you soon. Good luck!

-Nathan T. Oxenfeld

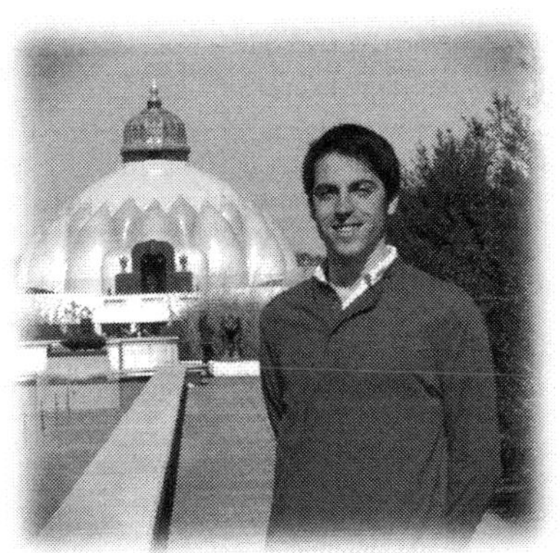

About This Book

The information conveyed in this book is the original method that was developed by Dr. William H. Bates in the early 20th century, furthered by Margaret D. Corbett in the 1930s, and passed down through a direct line of Bates Method teachers to me. I founded Integral Eyesight Improvement LLC in Asheville, North Carolina in 2013. This holistic vision approach helps bring balance and equilibrium back into the visual system and allows the eyes to return to their normal shape and function through relaxation, as taught by ophthalmologist Dr. William H. Bates.

The Bates Method is the major platform I use in my teaching. Additionally, as a certified Integral Yoga teacher I also draw from the ancient wisdom of various other self-healing methods like yoga, meditation, breath work, Chinese medicine, diet, nutrition, supplementation and more. In addition to the time-honored practices above, I include the most current scientific research and vision training techniques in my teaching as well. We live in a different world today than when Dr. Bates was helping people take better care of their eyes a century ago. Lifestyles have evolved, technology has advanced, and time has *sped up* to accommodate a faster pace of life with seemingly more stress than ever before. At the same time, more and more people are starting to take healing into their own hands by taking more responsibility for the prevention of problems and long-term maintenance.

Even though a century has passed since it was developed, proper and regular application of the original Bates Method remains as effective as ever in producing successful results in increasing overall eye health and preventing and eliminating vision problems by addressing the root causes of those problems rather than treating the symptoms.

The practices outlined in this book can produce measurable results in a short amount of time when performed regularly and with conviction. It is an extremely empowering process to give up your glasses for good and continue to watch your own eyesight get better and better as opposed to watching your eyesight get worse and worse by wearing glasses and doing nothing to prevent deterioration. Additionally, reclaiming your natural eyesight can save you a significant amount of money in the future by eliminating the need to buy a new supply of contacts every year, pay for stronger prescriptions as you age or new frames as they break, or paying thousands of dollars for risky and impermanent laser eye surgeries. Congratulate yourself for taking the first steps toward a lifetime of clarity.

As you will discover, the eyes are a very unique entry point for healing and relaxation. The eyes are extensions of your brain and, in fact, are made up of brain tissue. When you bring more awareness and relaxation into your eyes, it enters directly into your brain, travels down your spinal cord, emanates through your whole nervous system, and spreads throughout your entire body. The way your eyes feel influences the way you feel. This simple way to calm down your visual system and nervous system produces profound improvements not only in the quality of your vision but in the quality of your entire life. I am excited for you to find out how powerful this practice can truly be.

I originally created this book to accompany either a series of private one-on-one vision training lessons with me in person or online to be used as a reference in between lessons, or to accompany one of my online courses to provide a written companion to the instructional videos and audios contained in those courses. If you wish to explore the various options of working with me in some capacity as your vision teacher or vision coach, please consider scheduling an initial vision consultation with me online so I can get your complete vision history, explain my holistic approach to eye care, answer your specific questions, and overview my different vision coaching options to figure out what the best custom plan will be for you. It is possible to just use this book by itself to go quite far through the vision training process on your own, but people always tend to get better and more efficient results when working under the supervision and guidance of a professional. It's like comparing learning how to play the piano out of a book rather than taking piano lessons with a music teacher. Just using the book by itself may leave some room for errors or may leave you with some unanswered questions.

To schedule an initial vision consultation with me, visit
www.integraleyesight.com/schedule
or to learn about my online Holistic Vision Program, see Page 295

How to Use This Book: 3 Phases of Vision Training

This book begins with an **Introduction** to holistic eye care that covers the history of the Bates Method, the anatomy and physiology of the eyes, the underlying root causes of most vision problems, how the practices in this book can help slow down and even reverse vision loss, how to gradually wean off prescription glasses, and some important mindsets to adopt in preparation for this transformative process.

Chapter 1 provides a bird's eye view of the vision improvement process, listed in accordance to ten of the most common vision problems. If you know what types of vision problems you wish to prevent or the ones you may already have, skimming through the first chapter will give you a glimpse of what is typically required to prevent and reverse. If you have a less common vision problem that is not mentioned, the Bates Method has historically helped in nearly all cases of defective vision. Don't worry if you don't fully understand everything at the beginning of the book, for it is all explained in the subsequent chapters. You will find a list of positive affirmations and confirmations for you to write down, repeat mentally, and say out loud in order to assist the healing process within on a more subconscious level for more permanent improvements by changing the way you think about your eyes and the way you use your eyes every single day from here on out.

Chapter 2 zooms you in from the bird's eye view of the vision improvement process directly into the process of exploring ways to address and release your own unique underlying root causes of your vision problems, which is the first step in truly healing holistically. Simply doing physical 'eye exercises' is not enough. See if you can expand your understanding of vision to go beyond just eyesight and identify some deeper psychological and emotional connections to your past, present, and future vision.

Chapter 3 begins the first phase of vision training called Relaxation Foundations, which is all about replacing the bad vision habit of strain with the good vision habit of relaxation. You will learn your first Bates Method practices and begin to implement a short daily vision routine that repeats the first simple relaxation techniques to deeply relax your eyes and mind.

Chapter 4 continues the first Relaxation Foundations phase of vision training with a series of movement practices designed to break the bad vision habit of staring and encourage the good vision habits of breathing, blinking, and shifting.

Chapter 5 concludes the first Relaxation Foundations phase of vision training with the fundamental principle of the Bates Method, called central fixation or centralization, which helps you map out your visual field (central vs. peripheral) and teaches you the correct way to use your eyes and look at the world all day long. Centralization is a habit, not a practice.

Chapter 6 moves into the second phase of vision training called Fusion Warm Ups, which is all about balancing your left and right brain hemispheres, balancing your left and right eyes, and getting your two eyes to work together as a team by building the valuable skills of eye teaming, tracking, converging, diverging, and fusing.

Chapter 7 moves into the third phase of vision training called Vision Building, which is all about developing your visual acuity. Vision Building Near explores techniques to make blurry text up close appear clearer. Vision Building Far explores techniques to make blurry text far away appear clearer. Vision Building tools include reading cards and eye charts that are used to practice achieving 'clear flashes' with, which are temporary moments of clarity without glasses that will become more permanent with time and repetition. Eventually, you will learn how to take your vision building techniques out into the real world with you and apply them to three dimensional objects at all different distances. Your world can become your fun vision playground that stimulates good vision habits and effortless auto-focus.

Chapter 8 takes a detour from the Bates Method and focuses more on Yoga, which can be a complimentary approach to heal your vision problems. You will learn yoga poses, breathing practices, meditation techniques, eye movements, how yoga philosophy can enlighten your vision practice, and the importance of diet, nutrition, and supplementation for your eye hygiene. You will also have a chance to go even deeper into exploring the emotional realms of your root causes than you did in the first chapter by balancing the energies of your seven chakras, with special attention on the third eye chakra.

The **Conclusion** wraps things up with a few parting sentiments, explains the best strategies to structure your vision routine and continue advancing your vision practice into the future, provides you with options for getting additional help from a certified Bates Method teacher, and leaves you with a list of recommended resources and references.

At the very end of the book you will find a collection of Vision Tools like eye charts and reading cards that you can either remove or scan and reprint. If you do not want to take them out of the book, you can also visit *www.integraleyesight.com/visiontools* to download the PDF versions of all the vision tools and print them out on your own.

The vision practices in this book are introduced in a workbook style covering:

- the purpose and benefits of each practice,
- step-by-step instructions to perform the practice,
- a suggested amount of time and frequency for the practice,
- photographs or diagrams demonstrating the practice,
- and a commentary describing the practice in depth.

The end of each chapter includes a new Mental Focus Practice and a Daily Practice Checklist. The mental focus practice is something for you to think about, remember, imagine, or visualize when your eyes are closed or while you are palming your eyes, which is the best way to work on your insight, instead of just working on your eyesight. The daily checklists are designed to help you stay accountable and to keep track of your practice and progress. As you get farther in the book, more practices get added to your checklists. This does not necessarily mean that you are expected to do every single practice every single day. **Do not overwhelm yourself with the amount of practices contained in this book.** Remember that relaxation is paramount, and it is more important to do short practice sessions more frequently than it is to do long practice sessions more sporadically. In short: quality over quantity.

I organize my vision training into three main phases. Phase One is called Relaxation Foundations, and consists of the practices found in Chapters 2, 3, and 4. Phase Two is called Fusion Warm Ups, and consists of the practices found in Chapter 5. Phase Three is called Vision Building, and consists of the practices found in Chapter 6. The first phase of vision training for everyone is always to learn how to recognize strain and replace it with relaxation. Once your eyes and mind are feeling more relaxed, then you will be more prepared to move into the second phase of vision training and begin warming up your eyes with some fusion practices involving eye coordination, convergence, and divergence. Once your eyes and mind are feeling more warmed up, then you will be more prepared to move into the third phase of vision training and begin building your vision near and far.

Do not rush through this book. There are three whole chapters devoted to building your relaxation foundation. If you do not have a solid foundation, you cannot build a solid house on top of it. Therefore, the best way to use this book is to read one chapter per seating and practice what you have learned for at least three full days before reading the next chapter. My recommendation would be to read one chapter per week. Read through Chapter 1 on week 1, Chapter 2 on week 2, Chapter 3 on week 3, etc. That way you will have plenty of time to implement the practices in each chapter before you add any new practices into your routine, and not become overwhelmed. It is not enough to just read this book; you must also perform the practices contained in the book on a daily basis. Although the tendency may be to read through the book all at once, the process of improving eyesight cannot be rushed. The eyes respond much more to a gentle approach and the material tends to sink in deeper when taken in small, frequent doses. If used properly, it will take between five to ten weeks to read this book, if not longer. Take your time and allow the process to unfold gradually.

It is recommended that you keep track of your progress and keep a vision journal to help you better navigate this journey. At the end of each chapter you will find a daily practice checklist that has boxes for you to check once you have completed your vision practices for that day. There is also always blank space for you to write any vision reports, successes, revelations, challenges, thoughts, feelings, or emotions that arise along the way. If your goal is to improve your vision naturally, it is important to write that goal down on paper, tell your friends and family about your goal, and ask them to keep you accountable for achieving it. This will greatly increase your chances of accomplishing your goal of improving your own eyesight naturally. As a natural vision teacher, I also provide a stable source of inspiration and accountability for the vision students I work with 1-on-1.

All of the practices included in this book are to be performed without wearing any type of glasses, contacts, or corrective lenses. The very first step I took in this process was quitting wearing contacts and making the switch back to glasses. I also used weaker prescription glasses as my vision improved naturally over time. Make this a priority in your life and practice a little bit every day. **You do not necessarily have to do every single practice in the book every single day**, but you do need to do at least something every day to achieve permanent results. All the practices are suggestions and can be modified to fit your individual needs and preferences. Starting today, you may set aside 5 to 45 minutes a day for your physical vision practices either all at once or spread out and repeated throughout your day, 1 or 2 minutes here and there, while also infusing good vision habits into your pre-existing routines and activities. The physical vision practices will only take up a limited amount of time of each day. The mental vision habits however, will be ongoing throughout all visual tasks. Any task you use your eyes for, near or far, can be turned into a vision improvement practice of some sort. Once you learn the fundamentals you can begin noticing opportunities to use your eyes correctly all day long. Make your vision practice fun, and something you look forward to each day. Build days off into your weekly schedule.

The physical practices are simply designed to teach your eyes and your mind the underlying principles and habits contained within the practices. Each time you repeat a physical practice, you are reminding your visual system of the correct way to work. The physical practices take time and energy out of your day to perform and are limited to when you are physically performing the practice itself. The good vision habits however, do not take any extra time or energy out of your day to perform because they can be happening in the background while you are performing other activities or tasks. You will only be spending 5 to 45 minutes a day doing physical vision practices like swinging, sunning, palming, visualizing, and reading eye charts, but you will need to learn how to maintain good vision habits like dynamic relaxation, centralization, and accommodation 24/7.

Once you repeat the physical practices enough, your visual system is going to learn and memorize the correct vision habits, thus making the physical practices less important. You will reach a point where you no longer have to continue repeating the practices to remind your visual system how to work correctly because it will already be working correctly, effortlessly, and automatically. Once you clear your vision, it ought to stabilize and you will be able to taper off your daily vision routine. However, I generally do recommend that you keep up some sort of maintenance routine to make sure that the improvements you obtain become long lasting and permanent. There are so many different practices and approaches in this book because everyone responds to vision training differently. The purpose of learning them *all* is to figure out which ones work for you and which ones do not work for you, to help build a custom vision-training plan for yourself based on the immediate feedback you get during and after each practice. All the practices are designed to lead to fairly immediate physical and mental relaxation so pay attention to which practices make you feel most relaxed, or the ones that you naturally gravitate toward. These are the ones you want to repeat. Keep in mind that the results from any given vision practice may appear immediately, a few hours after, or even the next day. If a practice does not make you feel relaxed either modify it to make it more relaxing for you or leave it out of your daily vision routine. Try coming back to it after a few weeks and it may feel more relaxing then. This is your path and it is up to you to make it as fun and relaxing a process as you can.

Overall, Integral Eyesight Improvement teaches a new way to use your eyes in a dynamically relaxed way all day and all night long. Think of it less as a set of eye exercises, and more as a new way of seeing altogether. It boils down to the habits that surround vision and replacing your old, poor vision habits with new, proper vision habits. Below is a simplified table that shows you the bad habits you need to begin noticing and avoiding, as well as the proper habits you ought to begin encouraging right from this very moment, which will all be explained in more detail throughout the book.

Poor Vision Habits	Proper Vision Habits
Over-dependent on Glasses / Contacts to See Clearly	*Independent from Glasses / Contacts, Focusing Using Eyes*
Light Sensitivity / Over-dependent on Sunglasses / Starving Eyes of Sunshine	*Receiving Daily Dose of Sunshine Vitamin D, No Sunglasses Needed*
Squinting / Squeezing Eye Muscles / Half-Closing Eyelids / Scrunched Brow	*Softening / Loosening Eye Muscles / Keeping Eyes Open Normally / Eyebrow Raises*
Straining Eyes / Stressing Mind	*Relaxing the Eyes / Focusing Mind*
Staring / Focusing at One Distance Too Long	*Blinking / Shifting / Moving / Adjusting Focal Distance*
Shallow Chest Breathing	*Abdominal / Diaphragmatic Breathing*
Overworking Eyes	*Resting / Closing / Palming Eyes*
Eccentric Fixation / Diffused Focus	*Central Fixation / Central Focus*
Voluntary Vision / Using Voluntary Eye Muscles	*Involuntary Vision / Using Involuntary Eye Muscles / Nose Drawing*
Only Involving Your Eyes / Eyesight	*Involving Your Mind / Memory / Imagination / Visualization / Insight*
Imbalanced Use of Eye Muscles / Uncoordinated Eye & Head Movement	*Balanced Use of All Eye Muscles / Coordinated Eye & Head Movement*
Convergence Insufficiency / Inability or Difficulty Crossing Eyes	*Easy Convergence / Can Cross Eyes Comfortably*

Fundamentals of Eye Training *by Dr. William H. Bates OD*

1. Vision can be improved by natural methods.
2. Tension causes eyestrain and impairs vision. Relaxation relieves tension.
3. Relaxed eyes are normal eyes. When eyes lose their relaxation and become tense, they strain and stare and the vision becomes poor.
4. Vision can be improved only by education in proper seeing. Proper seeing is relaxed seeing. Normal eyes shift rapidly and continuously. Eyes with defective vision are fixed and staring. When staring eyes learn to shift, vision is improved.
5. The eyeball is like the camera, and changes in focal length. To focus the camera, you must adjust the distance from the negative to the front of the camera.
6. To focus the eye, the distance between the retina at the back and the cornea in the front must be increased for close vision and decreased for the distant view.
7. Six muscles on the outside of the eyeball control its shape;
   four, reaching from front to back, flatten the eye;
   two, belting it around the middle, squeeze it long from front to back.
8. When the eyes are relaxed, these six muscles are flexible and cooperate automatically, adjusting the focal length so eyes may see both near and far.
9. Just as dependence on crutches weakens leg muscles, so dependence on glasses weakens eye muscles by relieving them of responsibility. But muscles can be reeducated to do their duties.
10. Relaxation of the eyes and mind brings relaxation of the entire body. This general relaxation increases circulation and brings improved physical, visual and mental health.
11. **Relaxation is a sensation.**

THOU SHALT NOT STRAIN

The eye records images, the mind interprets and sees. When the mind is tense, the eye is tense; when the mind is relaxed, the eye is relaxed. Perfect memory of any object increases mental relaxation. Mental relaxation results in relaxation of the eyes, and both together result in better vision.

Simplification of Eye Training *by Nathan T. Oxenfeld*

1. Do not overcomplicate this process.

2. Keep it as simple as possible.

3. Training your eyes simply requires achieving better visual hygiene, which involves learning how to do a few things, like how to:

- *a.* **wake up your eyes every morning.**
- *b.* **prepare your eyes for a full day of easy seeing.**
- *c.* **feed your eyes their primary nutrient: light.**
- *d.* **rest your eyes throughout your day as you use them.**
- *e.* **relax your eyes to eventually see better without glasses.**
- *f.* **use your eyes correctly by adopting good vision habits 24/7.**
- *g.* **protect your eyes from computer vision syndrome.**
- *h.* **lubricate your eyes without eyedrops.**
- *i.* **wash your eyes with an eye bath.**

4. Training your eyes requires establishing new physical and mental vision habits all day long.

5. Do not get overwhelmed with the amount of practices.

6. You don't have to do everything every day.

7. Just start by closing your eyes more.

8. Closing your eyes rests your eyes.

9. Try to balance the time you have your eyes open and closed.

10. Close your eyes and take three deep breaths at the end of every page of this book.

(like right now...)

Introduction

Phase 0.1:
Pre-Practice Groundwork
What Is Holistic Eye Care?

"More than thirty years ago, not knowing any better and being guided by the practice of other eye doctors, I recommended patients with imperfect sight to throw away their eyes and see with their glasses. Since that time I have made some valuable discoveries, which have enabled me to cure people without glasses. The slogan now is: 'Throw away your glasses and see with your eyes.'"

-Dr. William H. Bates

"Vision can be improved; the secret is relaxation of the mind and eye. This simple truth is the basis of the system through which Dr. William H. Bates and those who have taught his methods have been so successful in helping men, women, and children to better sight. Efficient seeing in our modern, super-civilized world is a skill and must be developed just like any other skill. Dr. Bates demonstrated that this skill can be developed."

-Margaret D. Corbett

Creating a Starting Point

Before you begin your self-healing journey, it is helpful to establish a starting point in order to better understand the current state of your unaided vision to keep track of your individual progress and improvements over the next several weeks, months, and years. This is not a test and there is no right or wrong answer. The only rule is to not strain. You will record how you see up close and far away without glasses or contacts. You get to choose the distance that you read your charts. Make sure the distance you choose allows you to stay comfortable and relaxed. The purpose of the Near Chart is to see how close you can hold the chart to your nose and still make out what some of the words or letters are, even if they are not clear. The purpose of the Far Chart is to see how far you can stand from the chart and still make out what some of the words and letters are, even if they are not clear. The Near Chart will be more challenging than the far chart if you are farsighted, and the Far Chart will be more challenging than the Near Chart if you are nearsighted. The distance doesn't matter so much, as long as you write it down so you can check at the same distance the next time you measure your vision. The purpose is to create a general baseline measurement that you can compare to in the future *(See progress point charts on Page 227-229).*

Begin by checking your near vision using the *Fundamentals of Eye Training* Near Chart *(Page 323).* Hold the chart at about eye-level with plenty of light on the page, without creating a glare. Without wearing lenses, hold the chart as close as possible (not closer than 6 inches) where at least the top line is readable, even if it appears blurry. If you are nearsighted you may be able to hold the chart at six inches, but if you are farsighted you may need to hold it farther away. Measure that distance with a ruler, or get someone to measure it for you, and write that down next to 'Near Chart distance'. Cover your right eye with your cupped palm or an eye patch and find out what the smallest line of text you can read is at that distance. If you are farsighted, it may only be line 1 or 2. If you are nearsighted, you may be able to easily make it all the way down to line 10 or 11. Write that number down in the 'left eye' column and also describe in as much detail as you can how the text looks, ie. blurry, clear, fuzzy, wavy, shadows, doubles, gray, colors, etc. Repeat the same procedure while covering your left eye with your cupped palm or eye patch and record your results in the 'right eye' column. To finish, look at the Near Chart with both eyes together and record your results in the 'both eye' column. Notice if you saw better with your left eye, your right eye, or with both eyes. You may discover that you have a dominant eye or a weaker eye for up close vision.

Once you record the results of your near vision, you can check your distance vision using the two-page *YES I CAN* eye chart *(Page 325 & 327)*. Attach the two pages together vertically so the text starts large and gets smaller and hang the chart on a sunny surface outdoors or a well-lit surface indoors. It may be convenient to tape the chart to a poster board or foam board to make it more moveable. Without wearing lenses, stand as far as you can (not farther than 20 feet) where at least the top line is readable, even if it appears blurry. If you are farsighted you may be able to stand at 20 feet, but if you are nearsighted you may need to stand closer. Measure the distance from the chart with a tape measurer and write that down next to 'far chart distance'. Cover your right eye with your cupped palm or an eye patch and find out what the smallest line of text you can read is at that distance. If you are nearsighted, it may only be line 1 or 2. If you are farsighted, you may be able to easily make it all the way down to line 8, 9, or 10. Write that number down in the 'left eye' column and also describe in as much detail as you can how the text looks, i.e. blurry, clear, fuzzy, wavy, shadows, doubles, gray, colors, etc. Repeat the same procedure while covering your left eye with your cupped palm or eye patch and record your results in the 'right eye' column. To finish, look at the far chart with both eyes together and record your results in the 'both eyes' column. Notice if you saw better with your left eye, your right eye, or with both eyes. You may discover that you have a dominant eye or a weaker eye for far away vision. Be as descriptive as you can about the quality of the words and letters because sometimes the improvements you achieve can be very subtle at first.

Date: ________	***Near Chart Distance:*** ________	***Far Chart Distance:*** ________
Left Eye:		
Right Eye:		
Both Eyes:		

Lastly, using the *Fundamentals of Eye Training* Near Chart, I want you to determine three distances: the edge of clarity, the edge of blur, and the edge of readability. The edge of clarity is the distance where you can read normal sized text *(line 4 or 5)* the best, or where it feels most comfortable and appears clearest. If you are nearsighted that may be a few inches. If you are farsighted that may be at arm's length. Measure that distance and write it next to 'edge of clarity'. The edge of blur is the distance where that same normal sized text just begins to lose its clarity or focus and become slightly blurry. If you are nearsighted, slowly move the text farther away and stop when it first loses clarity. If you are farsighted, slowly move the text closer and stop when it loses a little clarity. Measure that distance and write it next to 'edge of blur'. The edge of readability is the distance where the normal sized text is too blurry to make out or read. If you are nearsighted, that may be at arm's length or beyond. If you are farsighted, that may be very close to your eyes. Measure that distance and write it next to 'edge of readability'. Once you record these three distances, notice when they begin to change as you improve your vision and either stretch your vision closer in if you are farsighted or stretch your vision farther out if you are nearsighted.

Date: __________________ ***Edge of*** ***Clarity:*** __________________ *(where text seems clearest)*
Edge of ***Blur:*** __________________ *(where text starts to blur)*
Edge of ***Readability:*** ____________ *(where text is too blurry to read)*

Holistic Eye Care

Holism is a Greek word meaning 'whole' or 'total.' In this case, it refers to the interrelation of all the parts of the human body that comprise its entirety. The approach of Integral Eyesight Improvement is holistic in that it is not only about the eyes. All aspects of the human system are taken into account including the physical, mental, emotional, and spiritual.

The physical side of vision deals with the anatomy and physiology of the human eyes. Integral Eyesight Improvement addresses the physical muscle tension held in and around the eyes, which once relieved, allows the eyeball to return to its natural shape and normal functioning. The physical approach is characterized by all the 'open-eyed' practices you will learn in this book that develop your eyesight. The physical human body is an intelligently complex organism with interconnected parts working in harmony to create the being as a whole and no part of the body is separate from another part. Improving physical eyesight is the main reason why most people begin practicing the Bates Method, but I'd like to inform you that this is about more than just physical eyesight and there are other visual components to explore and master first before your visual acuity begins to sharpen up.

The mental side of vision involves the use of the mind through memory, imagination, and visualization to interpret what is seen. For example, it is possible to successfully navigate through your house with all the lights out because you have memorized the layout of your furniture. Mental stress decreases vision, increases heart rate and blood pressure, shortens the breath, compromises posture, constricts blood flow, and interferes with digestion. Mental relaxation has the opposite effects and is, therefore, both desired and achieved through the Bates Method. The mental approach is characterized by all the 'closed-eye' practices you will learn in this book that develop your insight. Dr. Bates taught that vision is 90% mental and only 10% physical, so Integral Eyesight Improvement incorporates many mental focus practices designed to induce mental relaxation and attune the mind to the idea of clear vision. The barrier of preconceived ideas about the eyes and vision must be overcome. This book is full of new ideas and information that may shatter old paradigms or beliefs. By educating yourself about how the eyes work and the correct way to use them, you carve new neural pathways in the brain that allow for the possibility of self-healing and vision improvement. When I first started improving my own vision, I noticed that simply reading books on the topic brought about more visual acuity because I was already improving my mental vision.

The emotional past and present can play a part in vision as well. There is a psychological aspect of vision and often boils down to the repression of fear or anger. Take a moment to reflect upon the time in your life when you first noticed that your vision was declining or when you were first prescribed corrective lenses. Was there something that you weren't ready to see, didn't want to see, or tried to blur out or hide from yourself or others? Times of emotional trauma and life transitions often accompany a change of visual status. Many times, simply confronting or dealing with unprocessed emotions can result in a clearing of both inner and outer vision. There is also a large psychological component of glasses addiction that needs to be adjusted. You must let go of the deeply engrained idea that you need glasses in order to see clearly and you are blind without them. Entertain this new idea that you will one day see more clearly without glasses than with them. Glasses will eventually become a hindrance to your natural clear vision.

There also exists a spiritual aspect of vision improvement. Here, spiritual refers to the level of enjoyment, excitement, or quality of life. Many people find the process of improving their eyesight very exciting and uplifting. They begin to see things more clearly, both on the outside and the inside. Insight or intuition begins to develop as vision improves. This leads to a greater amazement of the human organism and the other beings we share the planet with. Also, almost every single spiritual tradition in the world references the spiritual aspect of light within texts and scriptures, and since the eye organ is the body and mind's receiver of light, it is worth exploring the connection of light, vision, and spiritual enlightenment. Eyesight will improve whether you recognize the spiritual aspect or not. It is up to you.

The origin of Holistic Eye Care can be traced back to an ophthalmologist named Dr. William Horatio Bates, who was one of the first orthodox eye doctors to challenge the conventional approach to eye care and provide alternate solutions to deal with vision problems beyond just treating the symptoms with glasses or surgeries. However, he was not the first person in history to explore natural ways to care for the eyes. Glasses were not invented until the 13th Century, yet we have had eyes and eye issues for much longer. Tribal people and traditional cultures had certain knowledge of how to care for the eyes naturally, accounting for many elders maintaining crystal clear vision late into life. Ancient healing traditions like Yoga, Ayurveda, and Chinese Medicine contain various suggestions for maintaining eye health and healing vision problems. Herbal and folk remedies have existed for thousands of years to help preserve eye health. So, although Dr. Bates was one of the first ophthalmologists to pioneer the field of holistic eye care, when you learn and apply his methods you are actually tapping into much more ancient knowledge.

Positive Side Effects of Holistic Eye Care

- Happier, healthier eyes,
- More relaxed mind, nerves, muscles, and eyes,
- Better vision habits all day and night,
- Increased circulation of blood, lymph, and energy,
- Healthier tear film and less dry eyes,
- Clearer eyesight and greater visual acuity,
- Decreased eyestrain, increased relaxation,
- Calmer nervous system,
- Lower stress levels and better coping mechanisms for stress,
- Improved memory, imagination and visualization,
- Higher level of self-confidence and self-reliance,
- Better quality of sleep with more vivid dreams,
- Heightened bodily awareness,
- Stronger intuition,
- Clearer thoughts and more mental focus,
- Increased productivity and concentration,
- Longer attention span,
- Less fatigue,
- Increased brain activity,
- Heightened senses,
- Longer attention span,
- Strain-free reading and speed reading without fatigue,
- Deeper connection with yourself, others and the environment,
- Easier expression of emotions,
- Reconciliation of the past,
- Clearer view of the future,
- Deeper breathing,
- Better posture and balance,
- Healthier lifestyle,
- Feeling and appearing younger,
- More positive mental outlook and worldview,
- Harmony and joy,
- Youthfulness and longevity.

Dr. Bates' Story: The Renegade Ophthalmologist

Dr. William Horatio Bates lived from 1860 to 1931. Dr. Bates held degrees from Cornell University and the College of Physicians and Surgeons in New York City. He began his career as an orthodox ophthalmologist in New York City, performing eye, ear, nose, and throat surgeries. He was an authority in his field and instructed doctors in ophthalmology in the New York Post-Graduate Medical School and Hospital. After prescribing glasses to countless patients, he began to pick up on a trend that all eye doctors encounter. All his patients kept returning and needing stronger glasses because their vision kept getting worse.

Dr. Bates developed a hunch that the glasses were doing more harm than good. His understanding of a good medicine was one that you must only take for as long as was necessary, until you no longer need the medicine because the problem is gone or has healed. When he considered glasses as medicine for vision problems, he saw the exact opposite. Not only did his patients need continually stronger medicine (stronger glasses), but the medicine was making the problems worse over time. Dr. Bates prophesied, "Glasses are not right; they are but a crutch. Someday we will find a better way."

To find that better way, he left his lucrative and prestigious practice in New York behind and spent five years conducting independent research at Columbia University before presenting his findings to the American Medical Association. It was during this critical time that he made valuable discoveries about the eyes and vision. This was made possible by setting aside his previously held beliefs about vision and approaching vision from an open-minded perspective. Following in his footsteps, I encourage you do to the same as you read this book. Temporarily suspend certain self-limiting beliefs about your eyes and vision that you have absorbed from a combination of personal experiences and what you have heard from authorities.

The discoveries Dr. Bates made challenged what his colleagues were perpetuating. His three main discoveries dealt with:

- uncovering the underlying root cause of almost all vision problems,
- the intimate relationship between the eyes and the mind,
- and the role that the six external eye muscles play in accommodation.

The following pages will dive deeper into each of these discoveries to give you a new understanding of the miracle of clear, natural vision. You are about to learn the root cause of your vision problems and the natural remedy, explore the non-physical realms of your vision, and understand the anatomy and physiology of the eyes and how they are designed to focus naturally. Armed with this new information, you will be one step closer to learning how to slow down the progression of vision problems, stop them in their tracks, and even begin to reverse them through relaxation.

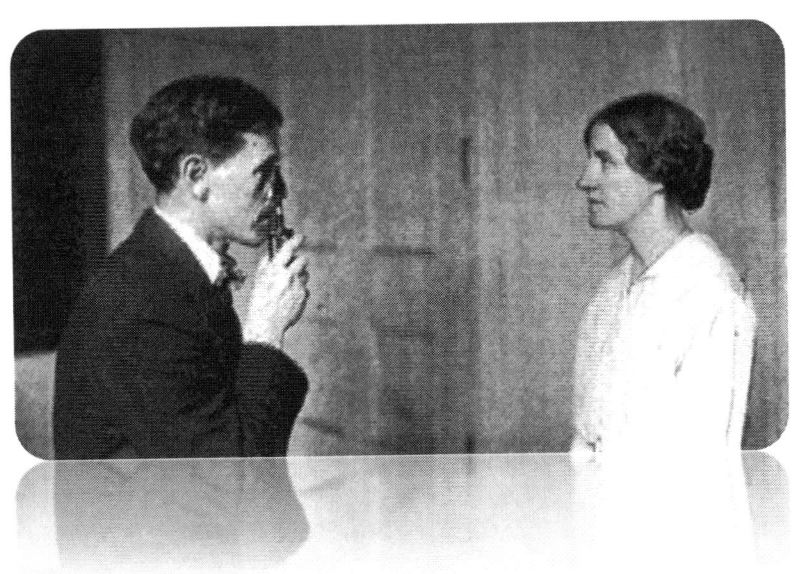

"Dr. Bates' work was with vision – not eyes. When vision becomes better, eye defects tend to disappear. Strain [and] effort... cause defective vision, technically known as refractive error. If we eliminate strain, the refractive error takes care of itself. The orthodox hold the opposite contention that refractive error makes the strain. They treat the refractive error, allowing the strain to continue unattended."

-Margaret D. Corbett

Discovery #1: The Underlying Root Cause

Since Dr. Bates understood that glasses and surgeries were simply covering up the symptoms of vision problems and not addressing the underlying root causes of vision problems, he set out to discover what the underlying root causes could be. To do this, he studied thousands of pairs of eyes belonging to people with all different types of vision problems, as well as people with perfect vision. Rather than examining his patient's eyes while they were sitting still in a chair looking at a flat eye chart, he instead took his ophthalmological instruments out into the field to study his patient's eyes while they were walking, talking, moving, and performing various tasks. This gave Dr. Bates a much different understanding of how the eyes function while in use. Gathering all of this data led Dr. Bates to pick up on the trend that almost all the people with vision problems seemed to exhibit a common trait that the people with perfect vision did not exhibit. The people with perfect vision used their eyes in a more relaxed way, whereas the people with vision problems used their eyes in a more strained way.

Therefore, Dr. Bates discovered that the underlying root cause of almost all vision problems is strain. Strain appears in many forms: mental, physical, and emotional. Any form of strain decreases vision and manifests in eye problems. Not only did Dr. Bates discover the cause of most functional vision problems, but he also recognized a simple yet powerful remedy: *relaxation*. Like its counterpart, relaxation may assume mental, physical, or emotional forms. Any form of relaxation increases vision and is the key to improvement.

The Bates Method in a nutshell is, *'Strain is the cause, and relaxation is the remedy.'*

It's quite simple when you consider the phenomenon of vision to be just like the other four senses of smell, sound, taste, and touch: an effortless and automatic process. You needn't strain to smell, hear, taste, or touch. The same applies to the eyes. Normal eyes are relaxed eyes that move freely about, simply allowing light to enter them and focus automatically. Involuntary systems like the eyes function perfectly in the presence of relaxation and imperfectly in the presence of strain. People with perfect vision are not doing eye exercises to see clearly, they are just using their eyes in a more correct way than people who experience blur. Improving your vision involves learning how to use your eyes like someone who already has perfect vision uses their eyes.

The eye organs, like every other part of the human organism, can heal if given the opportunity, time, and energy. This healing process cannot occur when strain is present. Healing can only happen in a state of relaxation. Instead of focusing by straining, or using 'manual-focus mode,' you must learn how to focus by relaxing, or using 'auto-focus mode.'

Try this analogy: Clench your hands. Do you think you would be able to paint a beautiful picture with a clenched hand? Clench your feet. Do you think you would be able to dance a beautiful waltz with clenched feet? Clench your jaw. Do you think you would be able to sing a beautiful song with a clenched jaw? What must be done to accomplish all the beautiful feats listed above? Relaxation. So, based on the questions above, do you think you will be able to see perfectly with clenched eyes? No. Not only will the vision become imperfect, but tension in and around the eyes, which are simply extensions of the brain, can wreak havoc on the rest of the nervous system and affect much more than just eyesight. Eyestrain, left unchecked, can affect your posture, your performance, your mood, and your mental state. The blur prompts fear, panic, and mental strain, which only contributes to more blur and physical strain, and thus a downward negative spiral begins. It's time to flip that around and turn it into an upward positive spiral.

Most people do not realize that they are continuously and unconsciously clenching their eyes. It may not be as extreme as when you consciously clench them, but even the slightest amount of strain can cause complications and constriction. Sometimes the strain can be physical, as tension in the muscles inside and around the eyes. This can constrict circulation, hold the eyeball out of shape, or prevent it from accommodating or focusing. Other times the strain can be mental, as tension or stress in the mind. This can affect how the brain processes and interprets the images taken in by the eyes. The strain usually originates in the mind and then manifests in the eyes.

In either case of strain, most people resort to placing artificial lenses in front of their eyes or even getting laser eye surgery, but continue to clench their eyes all day and all night long. Would you use a brace or get surgery on your hands, feet, or jaw if they were simply clenched? No! You would just let them go by retraining the muscles how to relax, which is precisely what the Bates Method teaches - how to release eyestrain, how to achieve muscular balance, and how to use your eyes in a strain-free, relaxed way all day, which can all lead to healthier eyes, increased circulation and lymph flow, increased nutrient absorption, decreased pressure, and better visual acuity. According to Dr. Bates, almost all vision problems are rooted in and produced by mental and physical strain, as demonstrated by the 'vision problem tree' diagram on the next page.

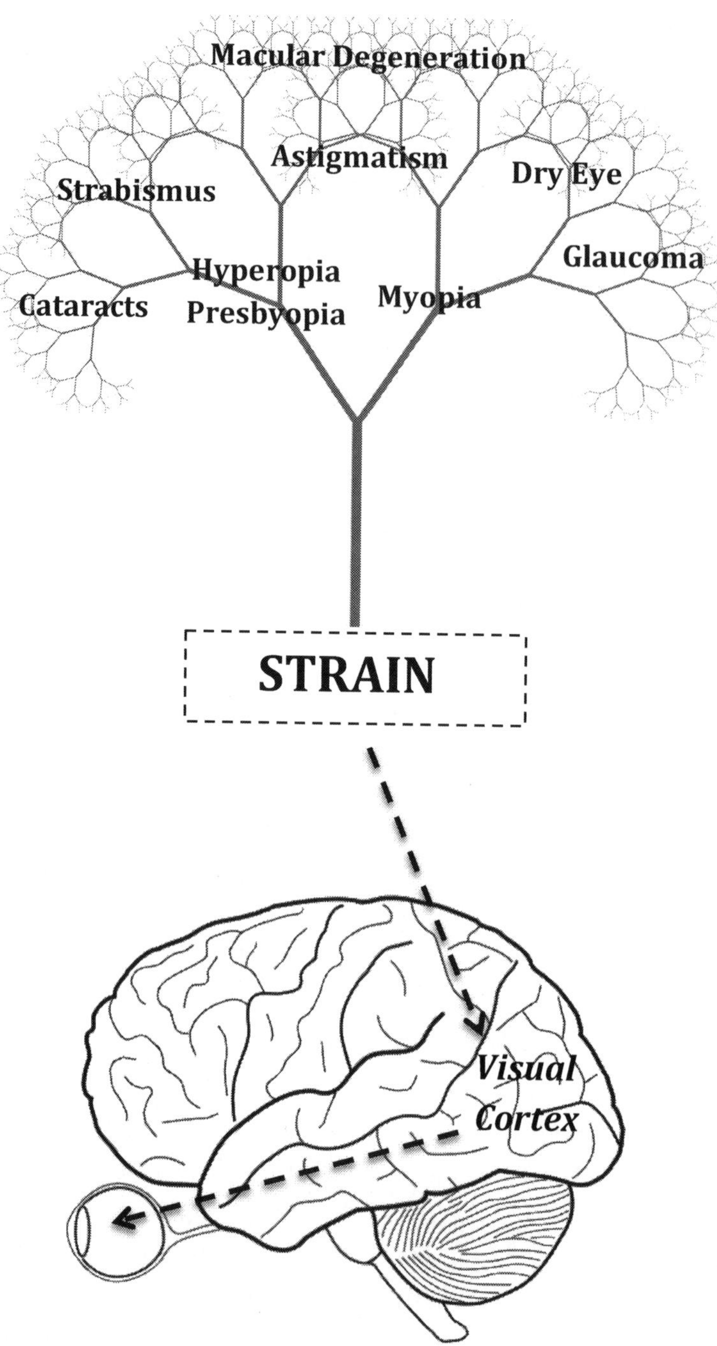

Mental strain and stress in the mind leads to physical strain in the eyes...

Discovery #2: The Eye-Mind Connection

Vision is so much more than just eyesight. Many eye doctors are only interested in testing visual acuity and examining the eyes as if they were purely physical mechanisms isolated from the rest of the body and mind. Dr. Bates did not stop there. He was interested in the mind behind the eyes, the personality, and emotions that contributed to the refractive errors. Dr. Bates understood that vision is not solely a physical phenomenon. On the contrary, he discovered that **vision is 90% mental and only 10% physical**.

That means at any given moment the visual cortex, which constitutes over one third of your brain, is only receiving roughly one tenth of its information from the eye organs. The other nine tenths comes from other areas in the brain, like your memory, imagination, and visualization. So, you do not actually 'see' with your eyes; you see with your mind. Your eyes are simply receivers of light. The light enters your eyes, strikes your retinas, and transmits through your optic nerves all the way through your brain to your visual cortex in the very back of your brain where the signal is processed and your vision is created. If there is any strain or tension in or around your eye organs, it will interfere with your mind's ability to interpret the image.

Out of all the different types of strain that affect vision, Dr. Bates found that mental strain was the biggest culprit in most cases. This is because the mind controls the eyes. Eyes are incredibly tough and resilient organs that can heal from physical wounds, abrasions, and even burns. However, the slightest amount of mental strain can instantly create a measurable error of refraction. It is important to understand that errors of refraction are not permanent. Dr. Bates proved they are temporary and can fluctuate in accordance with what is going on in the mind.

Your thoughts, emotions, and mental state can directly influence your physical sight.

When the eyes and mind are strained, refractive errors appear. When the eyes and mind are relaxed, refractive errors decrease or disappear. Unfortunately, most people get fitted for glasses when they experience a temporary refractive error instead of giving it the time and awareness it needs to normalize. What you see is largely influenced by what you believe, and how you see is largely influenced by the state of your mind. This book is not only focused on improving *eyesight*. It is also focused on improving *insight*. In order to be able to see clearly on the outside, you must first learn how to see clearly on the inside by strengthening your inner vision, including your memory, imagination, and visualization.

Discovery #3: Bates' Theory of Accommodation

The eyeballs are extensions of the brain and are made up of lymph, brain, nerve, and muscle tissue. The eyeballs rest in the *eye orbits*, protective cavities formed by the connection of 7 bones. The *eyelids* consist of skin, muscles, and *conjunctiva*, a membrane that lines the inner lids and part of the eyeball. Blinking is very important in lubricating the eyes and keeping their surfaces clean and refreshed. Surrounding each eyeball are 6 *extraocular muscles*. There are 4 *rectus muscles (plural: recti)*, which attach on the top, bottom, left, and right of each eye and 2 *oblique muscles*, which wrap around the middle of the eyes. These extrinsic muscles are responsible for both voluntarily pointing the eyes in different directions and for involuntarily changing the shape of the eyes for focusing.

The terms* ***rectus* *&* ***recti*** *will both be used interchangeably to refer to the 4 rectus muscles**

The eyeball itself consists of three layers.

1) The outer layer is the external, *fibrous layer* composed of the *sclera* (thick white part of the eye) and the *cornea* (transparent area that allows light to enter the eye).

2) The middle layer is called the *uveal layer* and is composed of the *choroid* (provides oxygen and nourishment to retina), *ciliary body* (responsible for changing the shape of the lens for focusing), and *iris* (colored area that regulates the amount of light that enters the eye).

3) The innermost layer is the *nervous layer* and is composed of the *retina* (where light focuses on the back of the inside of the eye). The *retina* contains light-sensitive cells called *rods* and *cones*. Almost all of the 7 million *cones* are found in the *macula*, specifically in the *fovea centralis*, giving us our central vision. Almost all of the 120 million *rods* are dispersed throughout the entire rest of the *retina*, giving us our peripheral vision.

The inside of the eye is divided by the *crystalline lens* (contracts and flattens to focus at different distances) into the *aqueous chamber* in front of the lens and the *vitreous chamber* behind the lens. These chambers contain *aqueous humour* and *vitreous humour* respectively, which is the transparent, gel-like fluid that fills the inside of the eyes. The electrical signals recorded on the retina get sent via the *optic nerve* to the *visual cortex* in the back of the brain for visual processing and interpretation.

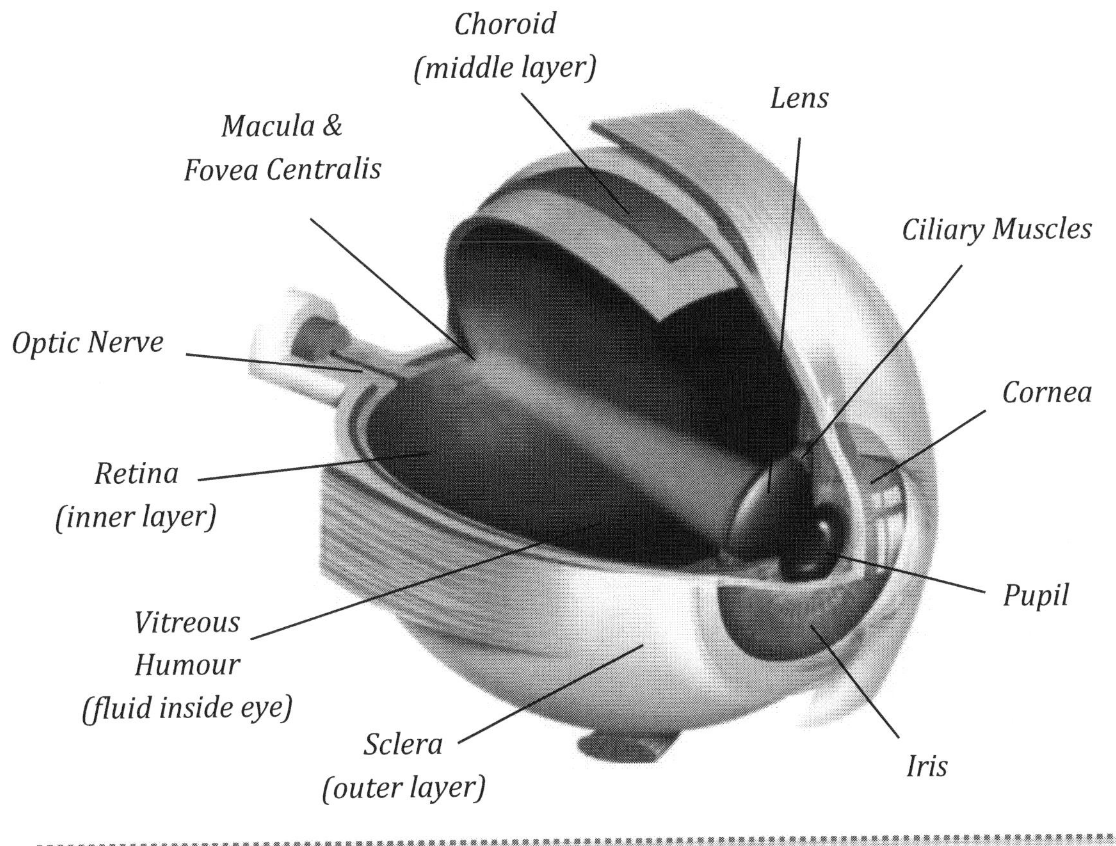
Choroid
(middle layer)
Lens
Macula &
Fovea Centralis
Ciliary Muscles
Optic Nerve
Cornea
Retina
(inner layer)
Pupil
Vitreous
Humour
(fluid inside eye)
Sclera
(outer layer)
Iris

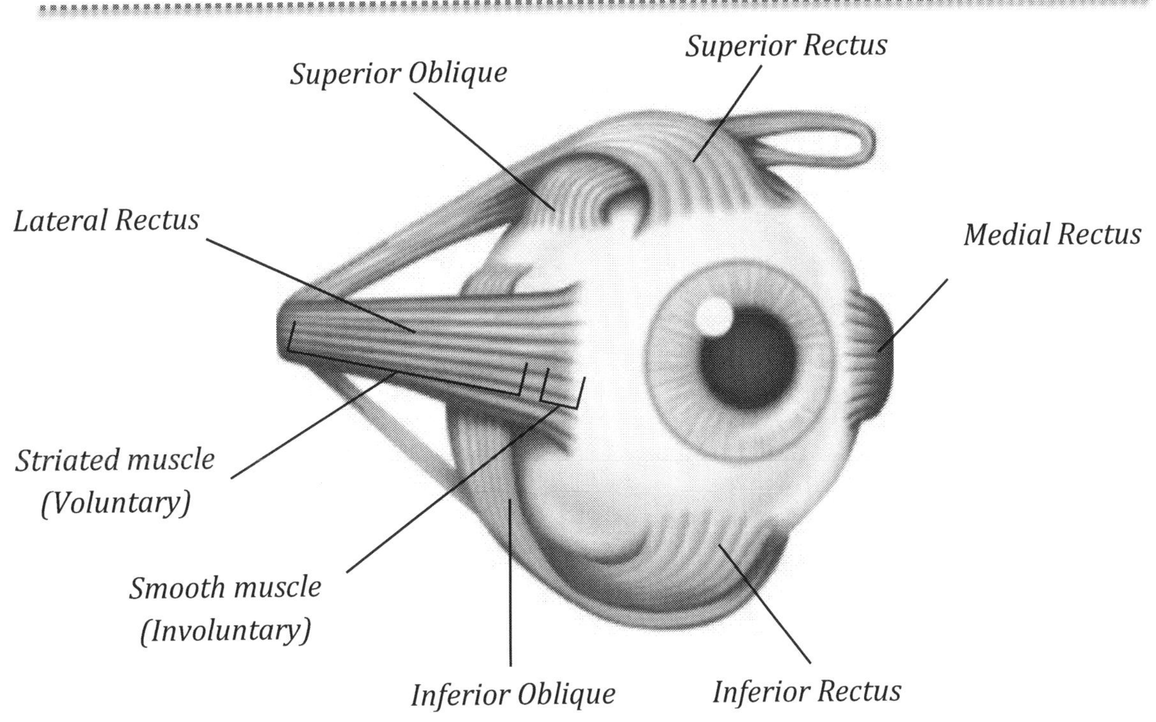
Superior Rectus
Superior Oblique
Lateral Rectus
Medial Rectus
Striated muscle
(Voluntary)
Smooth muscle
(Involuntary)
Inferior Oblique
Inferior Rectus

The Focus: How Eyes Harmonize

Accommodation is the eye's ability to focus on objects at varying distances. The current theory of accommodation that our vision science is built upon to this day has remained relatively unchanged for over 150 years. This theory, called the Helmholtz Theory of Accommodation, states that the lens is the only focusing mechanism of the eye. The involuntary ciliary muscles change the thickness of the lens to focus the light. This theory discredits the idea that the six ocular muscles around each eye play any part in focusing.

However, accepting the Helmholtz theory contradicts the nature of the human body, which is a highly complex and interconnected organism, not a combination of isolated parts that have no influence on neighboring areas. Dr. Bates challenged this old notion and parlayed for an updated theory of accommodation. When Dr. Bates retested Helmholtz's experiments, he kept finding exceptions and anomalies, which led him to develop his own theory of accommodation after years of scientific testing and research.

Bates' Theory of Accommodation states that the six muscles around each eye also play a part in focusing near and far. Those six extraocular muscles can change the focal length of the eyeball by a few millimeters to focus the light. This explanation emphasizes the team effort between the extrinsic eye muscles working in conjunction with the lens, rather than the lens acting on its own. Indeed, the lens has the greatest power of accommodation, but it is not the sole contributor to focusing. The contraction and relaxation of the muscles outside the eye stimulates the contraction and relaxation of the muscles inside the eye and vice versa. Bates' theory also went beyond just the physical mechanisms of accommodation. Bates also believed that non-physical factors and influences from the mental and emotional domains could also affect accommodation.

There are two main types of muscle groups in the body: *striated* and *smooth*. The ocular muscles are unique because they are both. The long section of each eye muscle that stretches back to the optic nerve is striated. Striated muscles are voluntary muscles, like those found in your arms and legs. They can be easily and consciously controlled, which gives you the ability to look around in all directions at will. However, where the muscles attach to the sclera, the white part of the eye, they become smooth, or involuntary, like those found in your lungs, heart, and digestive tract. These muscles cannot be easily and consciously controlled, but rather are more automatic and involuntary. This is the section of the muscle that contributes to accommodation, which means that focusing is meant to be an involuntary and automatic function that requires no effort on your part.

This subtle distinction is what sets the Bates Method apart from 'eye exercises'. Eye exercises only address the striated, voluntary section of the eye muscles, whereas the Bates Method relaxation techniques address the smooth, involuntary section of the eye muscles to encourage effortless focus. The goal of the Bates Method is to relax, not to exercise.

Like all other antagonistic muscle pairs in the body, the agonist must relax while the antagonist contracts. If this teamwork between opposing muscle pairs were out of harmony, movement and function would be greatly compromised. The same applies to the two ocular muscle groups: the 2 oblique muscles and 4 recti muscles.

When looking in the distance 20 feet or further, the eyes diverge (uncross), the lens thins, and the eyeball shortens. This is achieved by the contraction of the 4 recti muscles and the relaxation of the 2 oblique muscles making the eye slightly flatter than a sphere. The *ciliary muscles* relax and allow the lens to thin, which focuses the light entering the eye directly onto the *fovea centralis* in the back of the retina, creating a crystal-clear image. Overall, the eyes are more relaxed looking far into the distance than when focusing near.

When looking at a near object 20 feet or closer, the eyes must converge (cross), the lens thickens, and the eyeball elongates. This is achieved by the contraction of the 2 oblique muscles and the relaxation of the 4 recti muscles making the eyeball slightly longer than a sphere. The *ciliary muscles* contract and the lens thickens like a magnifying glass, which focuses the light entering the eye directly on the *fovea centralis* in the back of the retina. The eyes cross by the medial recti muscles pulling while the lateral recti muscles release, enabling the two eyes to turn in and look at the same point at the same time.

Vision is fluid and eyes are living, breathing organisms that are meant to go back and forth between focusing near and focusing far all day long. The eyes are not rigid and the shape of the eyes is not set in stone. All components of the visual system have to be in harmony for perfect vision to occur. The *recti* and *oblique muscles* must contract and relax to change the overall shape of the eyeball while the *ciliary muscles* simultaneously contract and relax to change the shape of the lens inside the eyeball. The shape of the eye influences the shape of the lens. The convergence and divergence of the eyes signals which set of eye muscles to contract or relax. These micro-movements and focal adjustments are constant, involuntary, and automatic. Normal eyes are set to the 'auto-focus' mode. You may have simply lost touch with your 'auto-focus' function, which is what happens in the case of nearsightedness and farsightedness.

Normal (Relaxed) Eyes

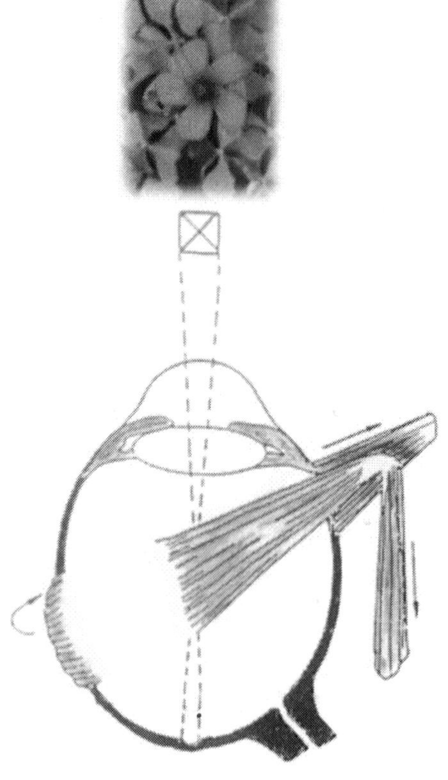

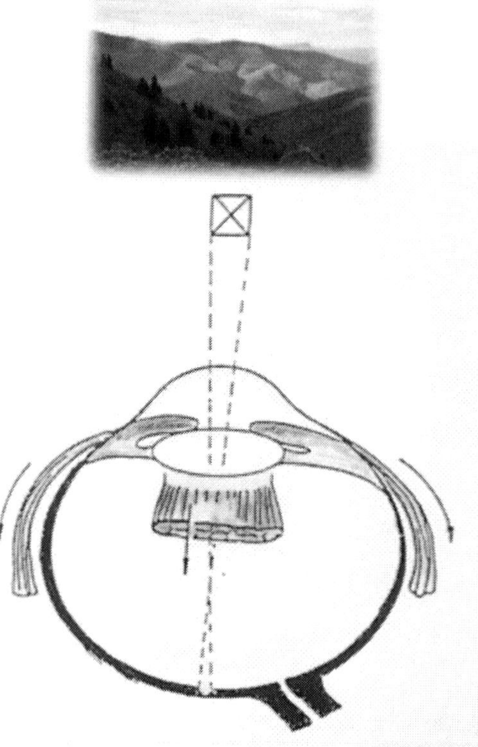

to Focus Near...
Lens becomes thicker
2 Oblique Muscles
Lengthen the Eye

to Focus Far...
Lens becomes thinner
4 Recti Muscles
Flatten the Eye

NEARSIGHTED & FARSIGHTED (STRAINED) EYES

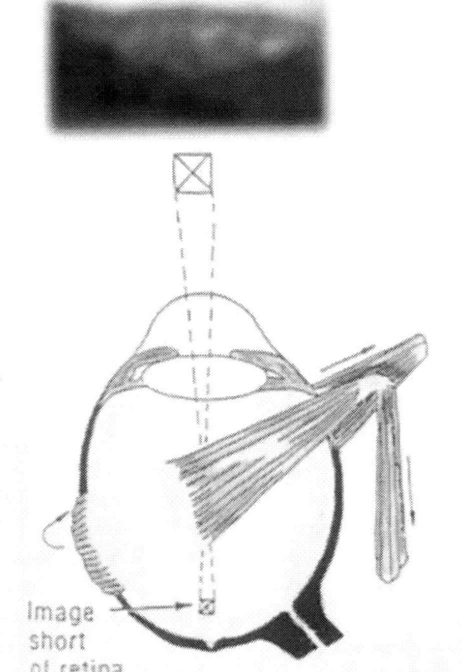

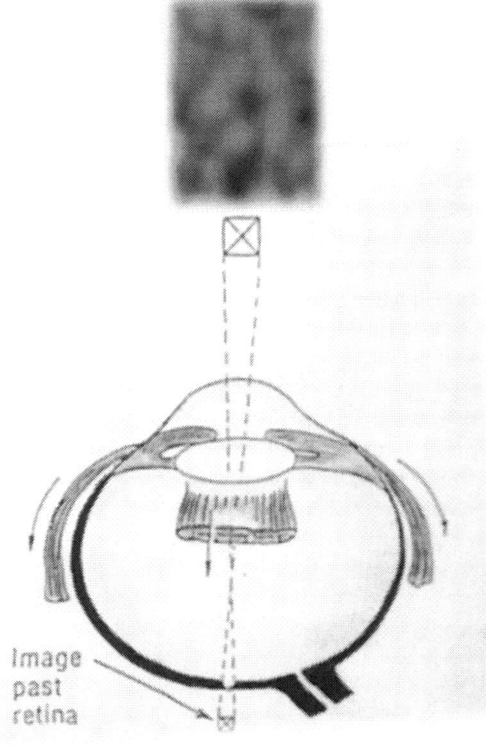

\\\NEARSIGHTEDNESS\\\

BLURRY FAR AWAY BECAUSE
TIGHT OBLIQUE MUSCLES
PREVENT EYES FROM FLATTENING
TO FOCUS FAR

///FARSIGHTEDNESS///

BLURRY UP CLOSE BECAUSE
TIGHT RECTI MUSCLES
PREVENT EYES FROM LENGTHENING
TO FOCUS NEAR

The Blur: When Vision Goes Wrong

A normal eye with perfectly clear vision, and no blur, is said to have *emmetropia*, and is free from any refractive errors. Refractive errors or accommodative errors are errors in the eyes' ability to focus light onto the retina.

So, what happens when the process above falls out of harmony and blur is experienced? When there is muscular imbalance or strain present in the muscles of the eyes we end up with refractive errors. Two of the most common refractive errors or vision problems are nearsightedness *(myopia)* and farsightedness *(hypermetropia/presbyopia)*. These are functional problems because they are caused by the stress and strain from improper use of the eyes on a daily basis. Using the eyes in a strained way over and over eventually leads to nearsightedness or farsightedness. Tense and tight eye muscles hold the eyes out of shape and prevent light from being focused on the retina correctly. The result is a blurry image near or far or both. What makes some people experience nearsightedness and others experience farsightedness? Not only does it have to do with different manifestations of strain, but it is also connected to different personality types, different vision habits, past experiences, and different ways of dealing with strain and stress.

In the case of *myopia*, or nearsightedness, the eyeball is 'stuck' in the elongated shape for near vision so that things are clear near but blurry far. This happens when the 2 oblique muscles hold chronic strain or tension and the 4 recti muscles cannot pull against them to shorten the focal length of the eyeball. The ciliary muscles also lose the coordination to thin the lens in order to focus the light reflecting off distant objects onto the retina. The light actually gets focused in front of the retina, which creates blur in the distance. So, the nearsighted eye remains highly accommodated for near vision even when looking far away into the distance.

In the case of *hypermetropia/presbyopia*, or farsightedness, the opposite happens. The eyeball is 'stuck' in the shortened shape for far vision so that things are clear far but blurry near. This happens when the 4 recti muscles hold chronic strain or tension and the 2 oblique muscles cannot pull against them to flatten the eyeball and lengthen its focal length. The ciliary muscles also lose their ability to thicken the lens in order to focus the light reflecting off near objects onto the retina. The light actually gets focused behind the retina, which creates blur up close. So, the farsighted eye remains accommodated for far vision even when looking up close at something near.

So, if you are nearsighted your eyeball is too long and if you are farsighted your eyeball is too short. You just learned that the reason the eyeball is too long or too short is because the extraocular muscles are chronically straining and squeezing the eye out of shape. Instead of just accepting that your eye is the wrong shape, you are using this book to teach you dozens of ways to retrain and relax your extraocular muscles, to gradually encourage your eyes to reassume a more normal shape and achieve more flexibility and functionality.

In both cases of functional nearsightedness and farsightedness the chronic tension is equal on all sides of the eye so that only general blur is produced. In the case of *astigmatism*, there are unequal forces pulling on the eye and the cornea or lens can become misshapen, which not only leads to blur, but can also lead to overlapping, doubling, tripling, or quadrupling of images. Rather than general blur, astigmatic images are produced when the misshapen surface of the eye focuses the light reflecting off objects onto multiple points on the retina, which creates the illusion of multiples, shadow images, or ghost images.

In the case of *strabismus*, or a crossed eye, one muscle is pulling more than the other resulting in one or both eyes turning in, out, up, down, or diagonally. The lack of muscular coordination prevents the eyes from fixing on the same point at the same time. The double image that is produced is confusing for the mind and the brain often shuts one eye down. In the case of *amblyopia*, or a lazy eye, there is a disconnection between the optic nerve and visual cortex in the brain. One eye may or may not drift off-center, but just like in the case of strabismus, one eye often shuts down and the other one becomes dominant.

In the case of *glaucoma*, or high intraocular pressure, the drainage canals inside the eye that normally allow fluid exchange get constricted or clogged and there is a buildup of pressure inside the eyeball, which can sometimes result in damage to the optic nerve and vision loss. The pressure of the eyes may also rise from external forces from tight eye muscles holding the eye in an incorrect shape and preventing free flexibility.

In the case of *cataracts*, or opacities in the lens, strain constricts circulation to the eye, prevents the lenses from maintaining flexibility, and debris stagnates in between the thin layers of the lens, which leads to a cloudiness that can interfere with light entering the eye and impede central or peripheral vision.

In the case of *dry and wet macular degeneration*, debris called drusen gathers behind the retina, which can cause oxidative stress, inflammation, deprive the retina of oxygen and nutrients, and interfere with the retina's ability to dispose of waste, leading to peripheral or central vision loss.

What is important to understand is how all the above listed vision complications, and even unlisted complications, are mostly rooted in some form of physical, mental, or emotional stress or strain. Yes, certain people are genetically predisposed to certain vision problems and the human body does deteriorate over time, but age and genes are only partly to blame. In order to address these vision problems holistically, you must also take into account the functional aspect of what contributes to the development of these problems. In other words, the way you use your eyes day by day and the precautions you take to care for your eyes, or not care for your eyes, determines how they feel and see tomorrow, and the next day, and next week, and next month, and next year, and so forth.

Another important thing to consider is the fact that the more complicated or advanced eye issues do not usually just appear out of nowhere. People who develop cataracts, glaucoma, and macular degeneration, have usually already been wearing glasses or contacts for a more basic refractive error like myopia or presbyopia for many years. So, the more advanced vision issues arise out of the more basic ones. They are connected, and by addressing the more basic refractive errors, you are actually working on removing the root cause of the more advanced issues.

Taking responsibility for your role in the development of your vision problem is the first step in overcoming it. The conventional explanation of vision problems puts no responsibility on you and your lifestyle, because it says that 'vision problems cause strain', assuming that the vision problem came out of the blue and is more random or by chance. The holistic explanation is the opposite by saying that 'strain causes vision problems'. The fundamental difference between those two explanations is that you cannot do anything about the conventional one, whereas you can do something about the holistic one. You can replace the strain with relaxation. When there is no strain left, there is nothing causing a vision problem anymore, and the vision problem can begin to decrease or disappear. If you go back to your old habits of straining, the vision problem will come back. But the goal of this book is to show you how to permanently replace the bad strain habits with the good relaxation habits for good, so that the vision problem does not come back.

One of the biggest obstacles in that process is the visual crutches you wear on your eyeballs and face: prescription contacts and glasses, which often perpetuate the strain. Therefore, a necessary step in recovering from vision problems is to gently wean off prescription lenses, and eventually become totally independent from them.

How To Improve Your Vision Naturally

The more you realize that the glasses are only treating the symptoms and ignoring the underlying root causes of our vision problems, the more it makes sense that the glasses must be given up in order to improve our vision naturally. The next several pages will explain in detail how to accomplish the goal of breaking your addiction to prescription lenses, both by weaning off with weaker prescription training glasses and by spending time with the naked eye wearing no glasses.

The first day I learned about the Bates Method was the last day I ever wore contact lenses. Once I understood how artificial lenses were negatively influencing my eyes, I had a strong urge to spend more time without them on. I immediately realized glasses are easier to take off and put on throughout the day in different seeing situations compared to contacts, which were more of an all-day commitment. I decided that day to never wear my contacts again and make the switch back to glasses as I worked on improving my vision naturally.

Just the act of spending more time without wearing lenses can lead to your first vision improvements. When I began my vision improvement journey, I honestly could not remember the last time I had spent more than a few hours without looking through prescription lenses. I was so addicted to them that I would put them on immediately upon waking every morning until right before bed every night. I soon realized that after an hour or two without lenses, my vision would actually begin to adjust and if I could stay relaxed without them I could actually see a little better. It turns out that working on the edge of blur can actually improve your vision. If I felt stressed or strained without lenses, that was my signal to put them back on so I could reconnect with my physical and mental relaxation.

Based on my own experience, taking your glasses off and spending time with the naked eye for the first time in a long time can be an extremely humbling experience. You may feel vulnerable, helpless, or scared. Some of your mental worries, fears, anxieties, or stresses that are normally suppressed beneath the surface by your artificial lenses may bubble up to the surface and confront you. This is the first test of the Bates Method. Instead of succumbing to the fear, discomfort, and strain, see if you can stay relaxed and happy in the face of the blur. Relax into the blur. If you are doing an activity that does not require 100% visual acuity, it's okay for things to be blurry. The blur will only be temporary, because the more you learn and apply the good vision habits taught in this book, the blur will transform into clarity before your eyes.

Therefore, in addition to wearing weaker glasses and no glasses, the other necessary ingredient in improving your vision naturally is a form of active vision training, like the Bates Method. Just stopping wearing your glasses is probably not enough to lead to improvement. Combining the reduced-lens method with the Bates Method, and other self-healing approaches like Yoga, Meditation, Breathwork, Diet & Nutrition, and more, is the best way to guarantee that you experience positive growth and development of your vision.

That is the purpose of this book: to show you the best way to learn and apply the practices and principles of holistic eye care into your everyday life, and how to navigate your way down through weaker prescriptions as your vision improves naturally.

You can read this book at your personal edge of blur by wearing a pair of weaker prescription training glasses while you read or by taking your glasses off while you read. That will start the adjustment process. As you read Chapter 1 to get a preview of what your holistic vision routine might look like and Chapter 2 to get clearer about the unique root causes of your vision problems, you are laying the groundwork before beginning your more active vision training. Once you complete Chapters 3, 4, and 5 you will have established a solid relaxation foundation, which is the first phase of the vision training process. By the time you memorize and integrate all the relaxation practices and principles like swinging, sunning, palming, visualizing, shifting, blinking, and centralizing, you will be even more adjusted to your weaker glasses or no glasses. You may experience your first flashes of clearer vision that last for a few seconds. You will feel ready to begin phase two.

Chapter 6 takes you to the next level of vision training with even more active vision training techniques involving fusion, convergence, divergence, and optical illusions. These vision warm ups become more complex, but do not forget about your foundation of relaxation. All the fusion practices need to be performed in the most relaxed way possible without any strain or excess effort. By the time you master all the fusion practices, you will be even more adjusted to your weaker glasses or no glasses. You may experience more flashes of clearer vision that last for a few minutes. You may be ready to drop down to an even weaker pair of training glasses. You will feel ready to begin phase three. Chapter 7 takes you to the pinnacle of vision training with relaxed reading techniques up close for farsightedness and far away for nearsightedness. With the groundwork, the foundation, and the warm ups, you are ready to build your vision. Once you master all the vision building techniques, you will be getting closer and closer to seeing 20/20 and beyond. You may experience even more flashes of clearer vision that last for a few hours. With time and practice, those flashes do not go away, and you have permanently improved your vision.

Breaking Your Addiction to Prescription Lenses

The orthodox treatment for refractive errors is 'vision correction' with prescription lenses or invasive laser surgery. Both options simply change the refraction of the light so it lands on the retina, but neither do anything to address the chronic physical or mental strains that are causing the problem in the first place. Glasses and contacts take away the job of your eyes so the eyes weaken and the muscles atrophy. The more lenses are worn the less responsibility the eyes have, which is why so many people experience a continual decline in visual acuity after lenses are fitted. Laser eye surgeries are risky and temporary. Nearly everyone who gets the procedure experiences negative side effects including increased eyestrain, decreased night vision, halos around lights, light sensitivity, dryness, and difficulty focusing over time. The clarity brought by surgery is not permanent either. It lasts for a few years and then the vision begins to deteriorate again, necessitating either another surgery or going right back to wearing glasses again.

Glasses, contacts, and surgeries 'correct' the vision in that they change where the light lands on the retina to create a clear image. However, none of these 'artificial corrections' do anything to address the underlying root causes of vision problems. They actually perpetuate the problems by simply treating the symptoms on the surface level, which suppresses the root causes even further down. The strain that causes vision problems is still deeply embedded within, so the eyes remain unhealthy and the vision remains truly uncorrected. The Bates Method gives you the tools to permanently correct vision by addressing the underlying root causes of vision problems and replacing them with the natural remedies. The good news is that even if you have already worn glasses or contacts for years or have already had laser eye surgery, there is still hope. Your eyes and mind can still relearn how to see naturally.

Success is highly dependent upon going without corrective lenses as much as possible. Dr. Bates was strict about requiring all his patients to discard glasses immediately and permanently. However, that was a century ago and we now live in a much different world. The pace and demand of your life may not allow you to simply toss away your lenses. If this is the case, it is recommended that you use 'transition lenses' or 'training glasses' as stepping-stones to wean from a life with glasses to a life without glasses. You may either use an old pair of glasses if they are weaker than the ones you use now, or you can request a pair of glasses corrected to 20/40 instead of 20/20 from your eye doctor. There are also some websites that you can order glasses from, if you have no luck in finding an eye doctor who is open to vision training. If you use contacts you will need to switch back to glasses in order to have the freedom to put them on and take them off as needed.

From this point on, go without your glasses as much as you possibly can. When you do need them, try using weaker prescription 'training glasses'.

You may be wondering how you will be able to function without your glasses. Do not fret; you may still use your glasses as tools when you need them. But the first step to getting rid of your glasses for good is breaking your addiction to them, and then beginning to experiment with weaker and weaker prescriptions until eventually no prescription is needed and the glasses can be discarded. You may be surprised to find out how independent you can become from your visual crutches in a short period of time. If you were like me and put your glasses on, or your contacts in, first thing in the morning and wore them all day long until right before going to sleep, this may be a challenge at first.

Think about the longest amount of time you have gone without your lenses. That may be hard for you to remember, especially if you are very dependent on them. See how long you can go in the morning before putting your glasses on. Try going for a walk outside without them to get some fresh air and sunshine. Notice how it makes you feel to be without them. Observe any thoughts, feelings, fears, or emotions that arise while spending time with just your naked eyes. Never squint or strain without glasses. Each morning go a little while longer without your lenses to begin decreasing your dependency upon them. Record how much time you spend without them each day to boost your confidence. Perform all the practices in this book without glasses on. You may be surprised by how many things you can actually do without them, especially when you start experiencing more and more flashes of clarity. It took time for your brain to adjust to the glasses when you first got them, and it will take time for your brain to adjust to not wearing them.

Glasses and contacts can be extremely addictive and habit forming, and you may have a strong physical and psychological dependence on them. You may feel naked without them, or vulnerable if you cannot see clearly without them. Not only do you need to let go of your physical glasses, but you need to let go of your mental glasses too. That means overcoming your psychological dependency upon them and letting go of the idea that you can only see clearly with them and will always see blurry without them. Consider the fact that you may be able to actually see even better without them one day. Just like how weaning off prescription medications can have some uncomfortable withdrawal effects, weaning off prescription lenses can present some uncomfortable withdrawal effects too.

At first, I got headaches and felt uncomfortable without my glasses on and would feel relief when I put them back on. But the longer I went without them and the more I improved my vision naturally, that eventually reversed so that I got headaches and felt uncomfortable the longer I wore them and would feel relief when I took them off. It will not take you very long to realize how free and relaxed you and your eyes feel without having constricting glasses on your face all the time. Vision improvement is a positive feedback system. Once you start seeing clearly again you feel even more free and relaxed and you tap into more energy, vitality, and motivation to keep going.

If you were on crutches because you broke your ankle, your physical therapist would not tell you to throw away your crutches in order to heal your ankle. Instead, you would gradually strengthen your ankle with home stretches and weight bearing exercises as you gradually wean off the crutches. So it goes with glasses. The practices in this book will be used to gradually heal your own eyes as you wean yourself off your glasses.

This approach differs slightly from Dr. Bates' original approach. He often instructed his patients to 'quit cold turkey' and discard their glasses completely from the start. Although that approach is probably the fastest way to improve your vision when done correctly, it is not often realistic in our modern day and age. The world is a much different place now than it was 100 years ago, and simply tossing away glasses is not always an option for students, parents, drivers, or professionals. Although it may take a little bit longer than quitting cold turkey, the training glasses enable you to still function on a daily basis at school or work while in the process of improving your vision over time.

In order to get a pair of training glasses online, you'll need to use a website like Zenni Optical or Eye Buy Direct that allows you to enter your own prescription, and you'll need a copy of your most recent prescription. At first you may not know how to read your prescription, but this may help. OD refers to your right eye and OS refers to your left eye. SPH stands for 'sphere', which refers to the strength of either nearsightedness or farsightedness. Those numbers are called 'diopters' and go in quarter-increments (-0.25, -0.50, -0.75, -1.00, etc.). If the diopters are negative (-) it indicates nearsightedness. If the diopters are positive (+) it indicates farsightedness. The farther the diopter number is from 0, the stronger the lenses are. If it says ADD and then another number, there may be two prescriptions in one lens, like in the case of bifocals or progressive lenses. The CYL stands for 'cylinder', which refers to the strength of astigmatism and also goes in quarter-increments. AXIS refers to the angle of astigmatism and ranges from 0 degrees to 180 degrees. If you do not have astigmatism, the cylinder and axis will either be 0 or left blank.

PD stands for 'pupillary distance', which is the distance in millimeters between your left and right pupils, and averages between 57 and 65 mm. Sometimes the PD is not included on your prescription, so you have to either specifically request it from your eye doctor or try measuring it yourself with the help of a friend using a ruler or tape measurer.

The process of weaning off prescription glasses needs to be gradual, with the first pair being a very slight decrease. This is because your eyes respond to gentle changes at first better than extreme changes. You do not want your training glasses to be too weak; otherwise you may end up straining physically, mentally, or emotionally. Maybe your first pair of training glasses will only be a quarter or half diopter weaker than your full-strength prescription.

Rx #1	SPH	CYL	AXIS	PD
OD (right)	-3.25	-1.0	70	62mm
OS (left)	-3.50	-0.5	110	

Rx #2	SPH	CYL	AXIS	PD
OD (right)	-3.00	0	0	62mm
OS (left)	-3.00	0	0	

In this example, the full prescription has -3.25 myopia with -1.00 astigmatism at a 70-degree angle in the right eye and -3.50 myopia with -0.50 astigmatism at an angle of 110 degrees. The first pair of training glasses has -3.00 myopia with 0 astigmatism in both left and right eyes. This example demonstrates three ideals when it comes to training glasses. The first is to take a little baby step, only decreasing the right eye a quarter diopter and the left eye a half diopter. The second is to have the same strength prescription in both eyes, which was possible in this case because they were originally only a quarter diopter apart. The third is to remove astigmatism correction from the lenses, which was possible in this case because the strength of the astigmatism was below -1.50. As long as there is an astigmatism correction in the lens, it is locking the astigmatism in the eye. Only once it is removed from the lens can it start to unwind from the eye. The pupillary distance will always stay the same.

If you are farsighted and have plus (+) diopters in the SPH (sphere) column, you would do the same exact thing as described above, except replace the minus with plus numbers. You can either order them online or go get +3.00 glasses at a local pharmacy.

At first your training glasses may feel a little too weak, but your eyes and brain ought to adjust in a matter of days or weeks, just like they had to 'get used to' your stronger prescriptions over time. Except now you are simply going in the reverse direction. The training glasses are not meant to make everything 100% clear. Instead of totally taking the job away from the eyes, they simply help the eyes while leaving some room for them to work. You ought to still be able to see well enough through them without having to strain at all. Remember, even when you have glasses on, the number one goal is relaxation. Once you get used to your first pair of training glasses or they start to actually feel normal or too strong, you can drop down to your next weaker pair. You may be ready to take bigger jumps down, like a half diopter, three-quarter diopter, or even a full diopter decrease.

Rx #3	SPH	CYL	AXIS	PD
OD (right)	-2.00	0	0	62mm
OS (left)	-2.00	0	0	

In this example the sphere has decreased a full diopter from -3.00 to -2.00. Start experimenting by using the -2.00s for certain activities and see how your eyes feel and see with them. If they are too weak, you can always go back to your -3.00s, or even your full-strength glasses if needed. Honor yourself and honor the process of healing your eyes by understanding that you may need to use the 'visual crutches' while your eyes are relearning how to work on their own. Try not to deny yourself the clarity or beat yourself up about needing to wear the glasses for certain activities or at certain times. Although the glasses may slow down the improvement, they may not necessarily negate the positive benefits you obtain from your holistic vision practice. After a few weeks or months with the -2.00s you may be ready to either get one more pair of -1.00s as a stepping stone to a glasses-free life or go ahead and take the leap to no glasses.

If you have a higher prescription than the example above, the way you wean off glasses may look different. If your left and right prescriptions vary more, you may need to equalize them more gradually. If your astigmatism is higher than -1.50, you may want to decrease it slowly instead of removing it right away. For example, if your full-strength prescription is:

Rx #1	SPH	CYL	AXIS	PD
OD (right)	-7.00	-2.00	70	62mm
OS (left)	-5.50	-2.50	110	

Your first pair of training glasses might look like:

Rx #2	SPH	CYL	AXIS	PD
OD (right)	-6.50	-1.50	70	62mm
OS (left)	-5.00	-2.00	110	

Instead of equalizing the myopia and eliminating the astigmatism, this example just subtracted -0.50 from all the spheres and cylinders and left the axis the same. This is because the original spheres were a diopter and a half apart, which might make it uncomfortable to get the same strength in both eyes since one is considerably weaker than the other. Since the astigmatism is a little higher than in the first example, it may be better to slowly eliminate it instead of removing it altogether at first. So, it's essentially the same as the full-strength, except a little bit weaker. Once those feel comfortable or too strong, then the second pair of training glasses might look like:

Rx #3	SPH	CYL	AXIS	PD
OD (right)	-5.50	-0.75	70	62mm
OS (left)	-4.50	-1.00	110	

The spheres are still not the same, but they are getting closer to each other. The left sphere dropped a half diopter and the right sphere dropped a full diopter. So now instead of a diopter and a half apart, they are only a diopter apart. In this case the cylinder was cut in half, from -1.50 to -0.75 in the right and from -2.00 to -1.00 in the left. The axis remains the same. After accustoming yourself to these training glasses and continuing to perform the vision improvement practices, you may be ready to drop down more considerably:

Rx #4	SPH	CYL	AXIS	PD
OD (right)	-4.00	0	0	62mm
OS (left)	-4.00	0	0	

Now the left and right eyes have the same strength correction for myopia and no correction for astigmatism. Over time you could gradually wean down to -3.00s, -2.00s, and -1.00s, until no prescription is needed. Be patient with this process and make the changes to your prescription that feels right for your eyes.

When ordering glasses online, you can usually leave out all the extra 'bells and whistles' they ask you to add on like high index lenses or UV coating, unless you want them. When I ordered my training glasses online, the only thing I included was the anti-reflective coating, which cuts down glare when driving or working on the computer. Since light sensitivity is one thing you will learn how to overcome in this book, it is not advised to get the transition lenses that automatically darken when you go outside.

If you are farsighted, the process of obtaining training glasses is usually a lot easier. Distance glasses can only be obtained through an eye doctor or online, whereas reading glasses can be found at almost any drug store, pharmacy, book store, or even dollar store. That way, you can actually try on the different strengths to see what the most comfortable next step down will be. Let's say you're currently using +2.75 reading glasses. Your first step down might be +2.50. From there you could try dropping down to +2.00. You can keep making your way down, a quarter, a half, or full diopter at a time.

If you are both nearsighted and farsighted and have one pair of glasses correcting for both, like bifocals, progressive lenses, or trifocals, your best bet is to separate the prescriptions into two different pairs. You can order one pair of distance glasses online with a minus diopter, and buy a pair of reading glasses at a store with a plus diopter. It may be inconvenient at first to have to switch back and forth from reading glasses to distance glasses, but it will help you wean off your prescriptions easier by separating them.

Please be safe and smart about going without glasses, especially when your safety or the safety of others is involved. If you find yourself physically squinting, staring, or straining then that is a sign you ought to put your glasses on. If you find yourself mentally straining or stressing then that is a sign you ought to put your glasses on. Do not let going without glasses take you away from your primary goal of achieving the sensation of relaxation. Only go without your glasses when you are able to stay physically and mentally relaxed. Straining without your glasses on can make your vision worse, whereas relaxing without your glasses on can make your vision better.

One of the most helpful tools that helped me break my addiction to prescription glasses was a glasses strap that attached to the arms of my glasses so I could hang them around my neck like a necklace. That way I could spend as much time as possible without my glasses, but whenever I needed them they were right there on my chest. Then when I no longer needed them I could take them back off and let them hang on my chest. I never had to worry about losing them or misplacing them.

Visit www.integraleyesight.com/shop to buy glasses straps and more.

*"**MEDICUS CURAT, NATURA SANAT**—the doctor treats, nature heals. The old aphorism sums up the whole scope and purpose of medicine, which is to provide sick organisms with the internal and external conditions most favourable to the exercise of their own self-regulative and restorative powers... When conditions are favourable, sick organisms tend to recover through their own inherent powers of self-healing. If they do not recover, it means either that the case is hopeless, or that the conditions are not favourable—in other words, that the medical treatment being applied is failing to achieve what an adequate treatment ought to achieve...*

*In the light of these general principles let us consider the current medical treatment of defects of vision. In the great majority of cases the only treatment consists in fitting the patient with artificial lenses, designed to correct the particular error of refraction which is held to be responsible for the defect. **Medicus curat**; and in most cases the patient is rewarded by an immediate improvement in vision. But in the meanwhile, what about Nature and her healing process? Do glasses eliminate the causes of defective vision? Do the organs of sight tend to revert to normal functioning as the result of the treatment with artificial lenses? The answer to these questions is, No. Artificial lenses neutralize the symptoms, but do not get rid of the causes of defective vision. And so far from improving, eyes fitted with these devices tend to grow progressively weaker and to require progressively stronger lenses for the correction of their symptoms. In a word, **medicus curat, natura NON sanat**."*

–Aldous Huxley

Giving Up Your Glasses

Create two lists. The first list includes activities that you absolutely need your glasses for. These may include driving, working on a computer, social gatherings, meetings, etc. The second list includes activities that you do not necessarily need your glasses for. These may include exercising, doing the dishes, cleaning, doing yoga, spending time with friends or family, etc. The purpose of putting these activities down on paper is that it brings more awareness to how and when you depend on glasses. It also makes you more accountable for yourself if you catch yourself wearing glasses during a time when you don't necessarily need them. This is the first step to becoming more independent and free from artificial lenses and proves to you that life without lenses is indeed possible. An ongoing goal for you is to cross items off the left list and add them to the right list.

I absolutely need my lenses when...	*I do not necessarily need my lenses when...*

Has anyone every asked you how you use your eyes? Copy some of the activities from both sides of the last table into the left side of the next table and analyze *how* you use your eyes while performing those activities. Are your eyes strained? Are your eyes relaxed? How do your eyes feel before, during, and after each activity? Start paying more attention to how your eyes feel throughout your day.

Activities I use my eyes for:	***How I use my eyes during this activity:***

Scientific Evidence

Despite the Bates Method's long history of success, it has not yet been fully embraced by the medical community. Dr. Bates was considered a 'renegade ophthalmologist' and was ostracized from the field of vision science. He was not taken seriously and great efforts were made by the behemoth optical industry to silence him. His findings may have been viewed as a threat to the survival of the optical industry because if more people knew how to improve their own eyesight, less people would need to wear glasses, and a lot of opticians would be out of the job. Not only that, but much of what Dr. Bates discovered and taught contradicted the worldview that optical professionals spent a large amount of time, money, and energy adopting.

Even to this day, the Bates Method remains controversial and you can find articles, studies, and opinions discounting its efficacy. However, I had already gone down the 'normal' path that the optical industry considers correct and I was not pleased with the negative effect it had on my eyes and vision. I am not one who requires hard, concrete scientific evidence to convince me to try something out for myself. If I were, I'd still have blurry vision. Instead, I am more of an experiential learner and I suspect that you are too. Nevertheless, modern science is slowly catching up to and validating many of the findings that Dr. Bates put forth a century ago. The most notable advancements have been in the emerging field of neuroplasticity. Neuroplasticity, or the plasticity of the brain, refutes previously held claims that the brain is a fixed, static organ that does not change throughout adulthood. These new findings are backed up by studies in various topics such as vision rehabilitation, growth of gray matter through yoga and meditation, and successful treatment of learning disabilities at any age.[1] See Page 279 to learn the tenants of neuroplasticity, and how they apply to your vision.

The myth that your brain becomes set in stone once you pass a 'critical period' is rapidly being disproven by people like Dr. Susan Barry, who corrected her stereoblindness using some of the vision therapy techniques that are found in this book.[2] It used to be thought that after the age of five or six, children with crossed eyes, lazy eyes, or other types of optical disorders could do nothing to regain normal vision. Children's brains are indeed more absorbent and malleable, forming and changing more dramatically with each stimulus. Adult brains can still form and change, but in a more active way. To change an adult brain, you have to become much more self-aware, maintain a deep sense of interest and motivation as you trek down a time and energy consuming path, and learn how to replace deeply engrained habits with new habits.

The Bates Method in particular can be a challenging vision training method to study using materialistic science because each pair of eyes is unique and each mind behind those eyes is even more unique. Everyone responds to the Bates Method differently and everyone achieves results at different rates. The results are not always repeatable and are highly dependent upon the involvement of the student learning and practicing the Bates Method. However, today more studies are being conducted on vision therapy and its effectiveness in improving eye health and function in children and adults. One of the most recent inquiries into the Bates Method was conducted in April 2018 on a randomized group of 16 people in Romania. Only 7 of the 16 participants stuck to the suggested daily routine, but 5 out of those 7 participants who followed the Bates Method protocol as described in this book obtained significant vision improvement in just 28 days with objectively measured decreases in their diopters, particularly those with hypermetropia. Another promising study from Saudi Arabia in 2013 "...revealed a significant improvement of visual acuity in both right and left eyes indicating that eye exercises as vision-therapy based program could improve visual acuity for female adolescents with myopia."[3] Both of these studies sourced specific practices from the Bates Method like palming, swinging, and central fixation, but they only spanned four to six weeks. I have witnessed even more impressive results in students who have gone through several months or several years of vision training.

In the April 2014 edition of *JAMA Ophthalmology*, Dr. Sabel published a research article proving that vision training is a valid rehabilitation treatment option for glaucoma patients due to neuroplasticity of the visual cortex.[4] *The New York Times* published an article in May 2014 about athletes using vision training techniques to improve performance on the field. This specific study introduced the University of Cincinnati baseball team to six weeks of various vision training techniques, which resulted in significant improvement in batting averages.[5] The article also pointed out that professional sports teams, including the Indiana Pacers, Brooklyn Nets, St. Louis Rams, and Pittsburgh Steelers, also utilize vision training. Margaret D. Corbett, Dr. Bates' main protégé, helped hundreds of eager men improve their eyesight to be able to enlist in World War II.

The biggest mountain of scientific evidence supporting the Bates Method though was compiled by Dr. Bates himself in the form of medical articles spanning from 1886 to 1923.[6] Dr. Bates also compiled the essence of his research in to a book titled, *The Cure of Imperfect Sight by Treatment Without Glasses* published in 1920. Revised editions have been made since then and the name was changed to *Better Eyesight Without Glasses*. The original version of the book can be read online for free, and I always advise my students to read his original work.[7]

Eyesight Insights

Below you will find some helpful mindsets to adopt before you dive into your own personal vision-healing journey. Some of these mindsets may challenge some of your previously held beliefs about eyes and vision, and I would encourage you to investigate the source of those beliefs and see if they really are true, or if you have ever put them up to the test before. Sometimes limiting self-beliefs can get in the way of vision improvement, so make sure there is nothing holding you back in your mind.

You'll see it when you believe it

1. Your beliefs and your attitude toward how you approach this vision practice will influence how much you get out of it. If you go into it full of skepticism and doubt, or if you perform the practices in an aimless or unengaged way, the practices may not provide many results. If however, you have faith in the process and you remain fully present and focused while performing each practice, you will achieve a deeper state of relaxation and get much more significant improvement. Try reversing the old saying of 'I'll believe it when I see it' to 'I'll see it when I believe it'. Naturally, once you do start experiencing flashes of clarity and temporary improvements, it will be much easier for you to believe it, but you may need to suspend some disbelief until you start getting your own improvements. Do not underestimate the power of your mind and beliefs in the process of natural vision improvement. You can do anything that you truly put your mind to.

Vision is fluid, not fixed

2. Vision problems are temporary, not permanent. Wearing prescription lenses sets the vision problem more in stone and makes you think that your vision is a static phenomenon. However, right when you begin to take your lenses off you may begin to notice fluctuations in your vision. Sometimes it will appear better, other times it will appear worse. Understand that your vision is a fluid and ever-changing phenomenon. Not only does it change year by year, but also month by month, week by week, day by day, hour by hour, minute by minute, and even second by second. You need to allow these fluctuations to happen and start to become aware of any trends of what makes your vision better and what makes your vision worse.

Work with the blur

3. The only difficult part of improving your own eyesight is keeping up with the daily practices required and resisting the temptation to wear your glasses. The first few weeks always present the most challenges in your relearning, because you are not wearing glasses as much, and you have not done enough vision training to experience big improvements to help you see better without glasses. This transitional period can be a trying time. It is a time where you must accept the state of your vision regardless of how unfocused it is and work *with* the blur instead of resisting it. The more you resist, the more it persists. Although it can be hard, this time is precious because you are learning about yourself, your body, your mind, and your own healing process. Consider taking a personal retreat to be able to fully dedicate yourself to normalizing your vision.

Don't just blame age or genes

4. Although age and genes can contribute to the development of certain vision problems, they are not the only cause. If you think of vision problems as being more functional in nature, then you begin to realize that the way you use your eyes influences the way they act, feel, and see. Our internal and external environments can determine how well or how poorly we see. On the outside, poor lighting, unpleasant or scary scenes, and stressful situations can shut the vision down. On the inside, mental stress, anxiety, and fear can shut the vision down even more. One of the biggest contributions Bates made to vision science is his discovery of how one's mental state can have an immediate and direct influence on the physical focus, and that the internal environment has much more of an effect on the eyesight than the external environment does. Bad physical and mental vision habits are to blame, and good vision habits are the solution.

A new way to use your eyes

5. Strain is the cause to almost all vision problems, and relaxation is the remedy. No matter what vision problem you may have, relaxation will always be the starting point, and the end goal of most all the practices contained in this book. Dr. Bates said, "All methods of curing errors of refraction are simply different ways of obtaining rest. Patients who do not succeed with any particular method of obtaining rest for their eyes need to abandon it and try something else. The cause of the failure is strain, and it does no good to go on straining." If anything you learn in this book

does not make you feel physically or mentally relaxed, you are either doing it incorrectly or you may want to skip over that practice for the time being. You can always come back to it later once your eyes and mind are more relaxed from your other favorite practices. The purpose of this book is to teach you a totally new way to see and use your eyes that involves no effort, strain, or tension. Let go of the idea that seeing clearly requires effort, or squinting. Dr. Bates said that the number one cause of blurry vision up close was from the strain to try and see clearly up close, and the number one cause of blurry vision far away was from the strain to try and see clearly far away. Even though it might not work right away, realize that eventually you will be able to see clearly near and far effortlessly, without any strain to try and see where you are looking. Remind yourself that your eyes are sensory organs and operate just like your other special senses of sound, smell, taste, and touch. Your eyes, ears, nose, tongue, and skin all have something in common: they all operate automatically, involuntarily, and effortlessly. So stop trying to force your eyes to focus and allow them to figure out how to focus on their own again.

Passive vs. Dynamic Relaxation

6. Did you know there are two types of relaxation? Passive relaxation refers to being able to relax in a state of repose or inactivity. An example of passive relaxation of the eyes is closing the eyes or palming the eyes, because the eye muscles have nothing to look at or focus on, so they may be more inclined to relax. Dynamic relaxation refers to being able to relax in a state of motion or activity. An example of dynamic relaxation of the eyes is opening the eyes and reading an eye chart. When you look at an eye chart without glasses, are you able to stay dynamically relaxed and keep all your eye muscles soft and fluid, or do you automatically tighten, tense, and strain your eye muscles? Passive relaxation is certainly important, however dynamic relaxation is the ultimate key to attaining clearer vision naturally. The more modern explanation of dynamic relaxation is the 'flow state' or being 'in the zone'. Athletes, dancers, and musicians all exemplify this concept perfectly. The muscles in the hands of a concert pianist must be relaxed in order to play every single not perfectly. The muscles in the arms and legs of dancers and athletes must also remain relaxed in order to perform at a high level. If any of those muscles were chronically squeezing or tightening, the music would sound awful, the dancer would fall, and the athlete would fail. Think of your eyes in this same exact way. Tension only impedes your eyes' ability to see and function correctly. Relaxation is the natural state of your eyes, and dynamic relaxation in particular.

Not a set of eye exercises

7. Often when people hear about the Bates Method or natural vision improvement they think of eye exercises, such as rolling the eyes or strengthening the eye muscles. It is important to understand that eye exercises are not a part of the original Bates Method, and were never taught by Dr. Bates. The reason is that exercise is a voluntary activity and usually implies effort. The eyes are involuntary organs and vision ought to be effortless. The problem is not that the eyes are weak and need strengthening, but rather they are overstrained and need relaxing. Eye exercises may actually even perpetuate incorrect vision habits. Only relaxation will allow normal vision to occur.

Replacing bad habits with good habits

8. Instead of calling them exercises, I call them vision practices, and this book contains dozens of them. So you will be learning specific physical techniques to relax and retrain your eyes by using this book. However, the practices are simply there to teach you the underlying principles and good vision habits contained within them so that eventually your eyes and mind will be able to maintain the good vision habits 24/7 without you having to keep remind them by repeating the physical practices. As you build your daily vision routine, your physical practices may only consume between 5 and 45 minutes, either all at once or spread out throughout the day. Your good vision habits however, need to be maintained from the moment you open your eyes upon waking until the moment you close your eyes to go to sleep. And actually, you want your good vision habits to continue overnight while you sleep, because Dr. Bates discovered that some people who strain their eyes in the daytime actually strain their eyes more overnight. *(see Page 24 for a list of bad vs. good vision habits)*

Start caring for your eyes every day

9. I understand that we live in a fast-paced world filled with busy people with a limited amount of free time. That said everyone has enough time to improve their eyesight, because anything you use your eyes for can be turned into a vision improvement practice. At first you must set aside time for your vision practice every single day. Even if you only have five minutes free, it will be more beneficial in the long run to fill 1 to 5 minutes with a practice of your choosing than to not do anything at all. Eventually though, your entire life becomes your vision practice because every single visual activity presents a new opportunity to maintain dynamic relaxation

and avoid eyestrain. Since this is a type of physical therapy for the eyes that rewires the brain through neuroplasticity, frequency and intensity are absolutely crucial in establishing new routines and habits. Once you have established the routines and habits, the practices become more subconscious and self-sustaining. You are learning a new way that you use your eyes 24/7. Think of it as how routine your daily shower is, or brushing your teeth, or. . . putting on those glasses or contacts. You don't question the importance of brushing your teeth every day to maintain your oral hygiene. Start treating your eyes as well or even better than your teeth. Make it a new habit to do your vision practices once or twice a day in order to maintain your visual hygiene.

It's simple and relaxing

10. Improving your own eyesight is not difficult. It simply requires time, dedication, desire, and repetition. None of the practices in this book should ever produce any pain, strain, or discomfort. It is designed to totally relax the entire body, nervous system, and mind. If any of the drills do produce undesirable results, stop at once. Either consult me directly for clarification or leave that drill out of your routine for the time being. Since everyone is unique, everyone's path to clear eyesight looks different. That is why there are so many practices to choose from. The practice that works for one person might not work for another person. Always let comfort be your guide. Listen to and honor your own body as you practice the different drills in order to build your own custom vision training program.

Not a quick fix

11. This is not necessarily a 'quick-fix' solution. Going to the eye doctor and getting fitted for prescription glasses or contacts is a quick solution. Laser eye surgery is another quick solution. Both of these 'band aid solutions' give you artificially clear eyesight immediately. However, they neither address the underlying root cause of the problem, nor do they provide permanent solutions. If you've worn glasses for a while you know that they only make your vision worse and you continue to require stronger glasses over time. If you have gotten a laser eye surgery you may know that the results only last 5, 10, or 15 years before the vision problems begin to reappear. Integral Eyesight Improvement addresses both the cause of the blur and produces long-lasting results. Instead of being given crutches to lean on for life in the form of glasses, you will be given the knowledge and tools to re-train your eyes and mind to see clearly on their own. Even though permanently improving vision typically takes most people months or years, don't rule out the possibility of getting faster results.

A lifelong journey

12. Do not get hung up on how long it will take you to normalize your vision. Often that is one of the first questions people ask me. I cannot give an exact estimate because I cannot tell the future and I also do not want to limit your progress. Since every pair of eyes is unique and every mind behind those eyes is even more unique, no two people will achieve the same results in the same time frame. From experience, I can tell you that those who practice on a regular basis are more likely see improvements faster than those who practice on a less regular basis. Depending on lots of individual factors, this process can take weeks, months, or years. At first this may seem like a lot of time, but it may only a fraction of the amount of time you have already spent wearing glasses or struggling with a vision problem. Maintain that bigger perspective and remember that everyone is unique, so don't be surprised if you see results faster than you expected and don't be hard on yourself if it takes a little longer than you thought it would.

Self-healing program

13. The information presented in this book provides you with a foundation. The real magic begins to appear when you do the work yourself. This is a self-healing program; you are 100% responsible for your own vision improvement. It takes a special kind of person to succeed in improving vision permanently. It requires dedication, discipline, courage, patience, repetition, and non-attachment. The only cases of failure are when the student does not follow through with daily practices or does not continue them for long enough to solidify improvements. So stick with it, and remember that the more you put into the practice the more you will get out of it.

Not a replacement for eye doctors

14. Integral Eyesight Improvement is not a replacement for going to the eye doctors. It is designed to accompany and enhance your normal routine eye doctor visits. The practices outlined in this book will lead to overall healthier eyes, which ought to make your eye doctor happy even if they are not necessarily sympathetic to the Bates Method. Everyone needs to have a medical eye exam every year or two, or anytime a change is noticed in vision. Eye doctors have instruments to examine deep inside the eye to foresee any possibility of developing concerns. Since some eye doctors do not support or subscribe to alternative methods such as the Bates Method, you may, if that is the case, wish to seek out an open-minded eye doctor or behavioral optometrist who is willing to work with you as you go through the process of vision training.

Address your emotional root causes

15. Your eye doctor has probably never asked you about your emotions during an eye exam, so why would you make any connection between your emotions and your vision? Upon deeper investigation, you may discover that your vision problems are rooted in some unresolved emotion or unpleasant past experience, transition, or trauma. Your eyes are not just for seeing; they are also for expressing emotions. When you feel joy and excitement, your eyes light up. When you feel grief or sadness, your eyes cry tears. From my own experience, crying is actually one of the best 'eye exercises' there is because you are expressing your emotions and releasing built up energy.

    The primary emotion associated with nearsightedness is fear and fear of the future. The primary emotion associated with farsightedness is anger and fear of the present. The primary emotion associated with astigmatism is indecisiveness or self-doubt. The primary emotion associated with glaucoma is un-forgiveness or holding onto grudges. The primary emotion associated with cataracts is denial or a bleak outlook of the future. The primary emotion associated with dry eyes is anger or spite.

    By accepting the emotional connection and actively finding ways to express or release these emotions, you may experience a significant improvement in your physical eye health and quality of eyesight. Oftentimes it is not the emotion itself that causes the physical problem, but rather the suppression of the emotion. When you bottle it up and don't let it out, that's when it begins to manifest on the physical level showing up as various types of imbalances or diseases, including vision problems. Only addressing the physical side will not be enough to get full improvement. You must also take into account the non-physical side and address your own unique emotional root causes, which you will learn more about in the second and eighth chapters of this book.

    If your vision problem was represented by a big overgrown bush that you're trying to get rid of, doing the physical practices would be like pruning the bush leaf by leaf or branch by branch from the outer edges, whereas doing the emotional inner-work would be like uprooting the entire bush by the trunk. So, the more you deal with the root causes, the bigger and more permanent improvements you may expect.

Chapter 1

Phase 0.2:
Pre-Practice Groundwork
Customizing Your Own Vision Training Plan

"The art of seeing is not primarily a therapy. It does not, that is to say, aim directly at the cure of pathological conditions of the sensing apparatus. Its purpose is to promote normal and natural functioning of the organs of vision – the sensing eyes and the selecting, perceiving and seeing mind. When normal and natural functioning has been restored, it generally happens that there is a marked improvement in the organic condition of the tissues involved in that functioning. In this particular case, the tissues involved are those of the eyes and the nerves and muscles connected with them. When people have learnt the art of seeing and conscientiously follow its simple rules, their eyes, if these are diseased, tend to get better."

-Aldous Huxley

👁 *Are you still following the 13 Rules of Relaxed Reading from Page 12-13?* 👁

How is your posture? How are the muscles in your face, eyes, and brow? How is your breathing? How is your blinking? Are you stopping at the end of every few sentences to close your eyes and picture the last word you read clearly? Are you looking off into the distance every so often? Can you see an imaginary bright white line underlining the sentences you read? Can you imagine a bright white line underlining these words with your eyes closed?

This chapter will give you an example of what your custom vision training plan might look like, based on the types of vision problems you wish to prevent or reverse. All of the practices taught in this book are designed to benefit all types of vision problems, since almost all vision problems share the identical root cause of strain. Once the root cause of strain is removed and replaced with relaxation, most manifestations of vision complications may begin to decrease and even disappear. However, every pair of eyes is unique and every mind behind those eyes is even more unique. Although everything in this book can be beneficial for you, there are certain ways you can adapt the practices to fit your individual vision and your specific vision goals. The reason there are so many different vision practices is to please all different types of people. One person may love one particular practice, while another person doesn't like it. Therefore, your goal as a vision student is to build your own custom vision-training plan. Read through the sections of this chapter that pertain to you to get a bird's eye view, and then slowly make your way through the rest of the book to learn the practices contained in your custom plan and more.

Like Dr. Bates said, all the various methods and practices to improve vision are simply different ways to obtain almost immediate rest in your eyes and mind. If anything contained in this book does not create a feeling of rest or relaxation in your eyes or mind, and certainly if anything creates the undesired feeling of strain or stress in your eyes or mind, then that particular practice ought to be skipped over and left out of your routine for now. You can always come back to in in the future, but you may not be ready for it yet.

It is still suggested that you try all the practices in order as outlined in this book and see how they make you feel and how they make you see. Despite the different practices having their own unique purposes, there is one purpose that they all share: relaxation. If relaxation is not achieved, that is either an indication that you are not performing the practice correctly, or that it ought not to be included in your custom plan. Through time and repetition you will learn which practices you absolutely love, that make you feel totally relaxed, and allow your eyes feel great. You will also learn which practices you don't care for as much or that don't seem to do much for your vision. Streamline your own vision training plan by spending more time doing the practices that work for you and less time doing the practices that don't work for you.

A good way to tell which practices to incorporate into your plan are the ones that stick naturally, the ones that are effortless and enjoyable to do, and the ones that are very easy to remember without having to reference the book. Another way to customize your vision-training plan is to focus most on the practices that apply to your individual visual situation.

On the following pages you will find some of the most important and beneficial practices for particular vision problems. Keep in mind though, that just because a practice is not listed in that section does not necessarily mean it is to be skipped. They ought to still be performed normally as described in their respective chapters, especially if they seem to produce measurable results for you.

Myopia

Commonly called 'nearsightedness,' myopia is often brought about by a strain or an effort to see something in the distance, rather than the commonly held notion that excessive near work is the cause. The effort of trying to force focus far away leads to a malfunction of the two oblique muscles that squeeze the eye around the middle and keep the eye 'stuck' in the long position for focusing at the near point. Myopic eyes are therefore too long. The lenses inside nearsighted eyes tend to be in a constant state of contraction and lack the ability to relax and get thinner in order to focus light reflecting off far away objects on the retina, making the distance appear blurry.

Even when looking into the distance, they remain long and focused at the near point instead of flat and focused at the far point. Therefore, the distance appears blurry because upon entering the eye, the light reflecting off distant objects focuses in front of the retina. The higher the myopia, the farther forward the light focuses inside the eye. When distance glasses are worn, the light reflecting off distant objects gets shot farther back inside the eye so that it focuses on the retina. This gives a clearer image in the distance, but only exacerbates the tension held in the oblique muscles surrounding the eyes, which is causing the blur in the first place. In other words, the oblique muscles get rewarded for their bad straining habits when glasses are worn and therefore keep on straining.

Distance glasses are meant to help you see in the distance, not up close. If you are nearsighted, you can probably see clearly up close without glasses somewhere between 12 and 3 inches from your eyes. This means that the light is already focusing on your retina correctly at that distance. When you wear distance glasses to focus on up close objects, the light actually focuses behind the retina, which encourages the eyeball to lengthen even more, making the myopia even worse over time. Instead, the plan for reversing myopia is to utilize the clear vision you already have up close by focusing on near objects at a distance where they appear clearly without glasses on, and gradually stretch the vision, imagination, visualization, attention, and focus farther and farther out over time. If you need to, wear your weaker prescription training glasses for near or mid-range activities.

Imagine that a 'myopia bubble' surrounds you. Everything inside your bubble is clear. Everything outside your bubble is blurry. How big is your myopia bubble right now? Where is the edge of your bubble? Improving your vision naturally is expanding your bubble. The bigger your bubble gets, the more things can fit inside of it, and the farther you can focus clearly with the naked eye. Maybe one day your bubble will get so big that it stretches around the whole world and out into space so that you can see the moon and the stars and the cosmos clearly without any effort. Remember that the harder you try to see clear far, the blurrier it becomes. The less you try to see clear far, the clearer it becomes.

On an emotional level, nearsightedness is almost always caused by fear. Fear, or some manifestation of fear, brought about by a traumatic experience or a significant life transition, is usually what prompts us to create those bubbles of protection around us. As a defense mechanism, we hide inside the bubble and try to blur the outside world. Nearsighted people tend to have more introverted personalities. In order to expand your bubble and see the distance clearly again, you must overcome old and new fears that are keeping your vision in a constricted and limited state.

By releasing fears, your eye muscles will become more relaxed. The eye muscles to pay particular attention to are the two oblique muscles that wrap around the middle of the top and bottom of each eye. Once they stop chronically straining, your other four recti eye muscles will be more adept at shortening your eye to focus better far away.

Morning Relaxation: (Chapter 3) Think about tapping and massaging acupressure points as efficient ways to release the oblique muscles. When tensing and releasing, try to feel your oblique muscles squeezing your eye around the middle and then totally letting go when you exhale. Nose draw on a piece of paper 5 to 10 feet away from you or on a big billboard 20 to 50 feet away from you to stretch out your imagination and visualization and get better at picturing clear images at farther distances.

Sunning: (Chapter 3) Think about the warm bright light loosening your tight oblique eye muscles and melting away your mental stresses and fears.

Palming and Visualizing: (Chapter 3) Palming ought to be practiced for several minutes every day. For best results, palm for a few minutes every hour. Let the warm darkness soothe your tight oblique muscles and remind them that they do not need to squeeze your eyes when you palm. While palming, stretch out your imagination and visualize things far away perfectly clearly, even if they are not clear when your eyes are open. For example, imagine a mountain peak far away, the letters of an eye chart far away, or gazing out over the horizon.

Swinging: (Chapter 4) Myopic eyes tend to stare, so break the stare with your long swings, medium swings, and short swings. Try swinging outdoors to notice optional movement far away. Remember that blinking breaks the stare too.

Centralization: (Chapter 5) Practice centralization up close where you can already tell a significant difference between your central and peripheral vision. The better you get a centralizing up close, the better you will get at centralizing far away where you might not notice as much of a difference between central and peripheral yet if they both look blurry. Become more curious about the world around you. Pay more attention to your surroundings. Count lights, pictures, doors, and people when you enter a room. Count trees, leaves, animals, and people when you walk around outside. Pick out particular colors on different days of the week. Do not fear the distance. Give the distance a chance. Even if distant objects lack details, you can still perceive their colors, shapes, and textures. Stop diffusing your focus and stop trying to see too much all at once. Keep your point of focus small and keep your eyes moving from one part of a distant object to another.

Gateposts: (Chapter 6) Even when myopic eyes look into the distance, they stay focused up close. Holding a finger, pen, pencil, or pointer vertically in front of your nose while you look into the distance will make the one near object split into two objects, therefore subconsciously telling your brain that you are not trying to focus up close. This will encourage your eyes to focus farther away on whatever single object falls in between the two 'gateposts', which also happens to be your central vision.

Near to Far Shifting: (Chapter 6) Imagine your far thumb and your distant object perfectly clear when you repeat this practice mentally with your eyes closed, even if they are blurry with your eyes open. Apply the 5-10-15 rule to all near work like reading books and working on computers.

Rope Fusion: (Chapter 6) Use a 10 to 20 foot long rope to track up and down with to help stretch your focus out. Even if the rope gets blurry in the distance, you can still see the V, X, and A shapes the rope makes.

Lens Flexor: (Chapter 6) Start up close and move your flexing object (thumb, pen, alphabet card, etc.) slowly farther away from your nose until you reach the edge of your bubble. Go just beyond the edge so that it becomes a little blurry, and then bring it back inside your bubble so it becomes clear again. Over time your bubble will get bigger and you can flex farther away.

Divergence Games: (Chapter 6) Nearsighted eyes need to learn how to relax and diverge. Since the comfort zone is at the near point, most nearsighted eyes are more comfortable converging since things up close appear clearer. Practice your convergence games beyond the edge of your bubble, where the two objects or letters appear blurry. When you converge them into a third object or letter in the middle, it ought to become clearer. Work on getting better at the divergence version until convergence and divergence are of equal ease and promote the same amount of relaxation.

Thin White Line Reading: (Chapter 7) Hold your reading material just past your 'edge,' right past where the letters switch from clear to blurry. Get little tiny flashes of clarity within arm's length to help get more flashes of clarity farther out on your distance eye chart. Improving near vision helps improve distance vision as well.

Vision Stretching: (Chapter 7) Balance near focusing time with relaxed distance gazing without glasses. Breathe, blink, shift, swing, centralize, and keep visualizing or remembering perfectly clear mental pictures as you relax your eyes in the distance for several minutes at a time. Sometimes it takes up to 7 minutes for your obliques to relax.

Vision Building Far: (Chapter 7) Daily relaxed reading of eye charts is usually the most important practice for helping with myopia. Start at an easy distance, between one and five feet, to practice and repeat the six step chart clearing formula on one line of the chart at a time, with one eye at a time. Each time you play with the chart, move back one or two feet until after a few weeks you are all the way at 20 feet. The vision building phase is when you will experience and observe most of your clear flashes, since the chart acts as an objective measurement tool of your visual acuity. In a matter of time you will be able to read the next smaller line down on the chart that you were not able to see before. Use the letter chart, number chart, and picture chart. Keep clearing the eye charts until you can read all the way down to the very bottom line. Why stop there? Take your chart practice with you out into the real world and apply your vision building techniques on three dimensional objects.

You will reach a point in your vision training where reading your eye chart is one of the only practices you need to do. This is because while you are reading your chart you are applying all the principles from all the vision practices. Vision building is the amalgamation of everything in this book into one streamlined practice. It is the pinnacle of vision training and it ought to be done either every day or every other day. Leave your eye chart hung up in a well-trafficked area so that you have ample opportunities to glance at it and play with it on a regular basis. Even once you get your distance vision back to normal, keep reading fine print far away every day in a relaxed way to keep your distance vision superb.

Keep in mind that vision building is not confined to only reading the eye charts in this book. Take the vision building techniques out into the world with you. Read road signs, storefronts, menus at restaurants, subtitles on television or movies. Go beyond just reading flat two-dimensional surfaces too. Use the distance techniques to gaze at natural beauty far away on three-dimensional objects like trees, clouds, birds, buildings, mountains, or the ocean. Teach your eyes to see all things clearly at all distances.

Hypermetropia & Presbyopia

Hypermetropia is 'farsightedness' and presbyopia is 'middle age' or 'old-age sight.' Both are often brought about by a strain or an effort to see something up close. The strain associated with trying to force focus up close causes a malfunction in the four recti muscles that keep the eye 'stuck' in the short position for focusing at the far point. Farsighted eyes are therefore too short. The lenses inside farsighted eyes tend to lack the flexibility to get thicker in order to focus light reflecting off up-close objects, making them appear blurry.

Even when looking near, the eyes remain focused far away and blur is experienced up close because the light reflecting off near objects focuses behind the retina. When reading glasses are worn, the light reflecting off near objects gets brought forward to focus on the retina, which clears the near point but ignores the chronic tension in the four recti muscles around each eye. The plan for reversing hyperopia/presbyopia is to utilize the clear vision you already have by focusing on clear objects at farther distances and to gradually stretch the vision, imagination, visualization, attention, and focus closer and closer in over time.

If you are farsighted, imagine that a bubble surrounds you. Everything beyond the bubble is clear. Everything within the bubble is blurry. Improving your vision is shrinking your bubble so that you are able to focus closer and closer. Maybe eventually your bubble will get so small that you can see clearly at six inches or closer without any strain or effort. Remember that the harder you try to see clear up close, the blurrier it becomes. The less you try to see clear up close, the clearer it becomes.

On an emotional level, farsightedness is often caused by anger or frustration. Anger as a reaction to a traumatic experience or a significant life transition is usually what prompts us create those bubbles of rejection as we push the clarity farther away and pay more attention to others and the outside world rather than ourselves and the inside world. Farsighted people tend to have more extroverted personalities. In order to shrink your bubble and see up close clearly again, you must overcome old and new angers or frustrations that are keeping your vision in a constricted and limited state.

By releasing angers and frustrations, your eye muscles will become more relaxed. The eye muscles to pay particular attention to are the four recti muscles that attach on the top, bottom, left, and right of each eye. Once they stop chronically straining, your other two oblique eye muscles will be more adept at lengthening your eye to focus better up close.

Morning Relaxation: (Chapter 3) Think about tapping and massaging acupressure points as efficient ways to release the recti muscles. When tensing and releasing, try to feel your recti muscles squeezing your eye on all the four cardinal directions and then totally letting go when you exhale. Nose draw on a piece of paper five to ten inches from your nose to stretch your imagination and visualization in closer by creating clear mental pictures near.

Sunning: (Chapter 3) Think about the warm bright light loosening your tight recti eye muscles and melting away your mental stresses and frustrations.

Palming and Visualizing: (Chapter 3) Palming ought to be practiced for several minutes every day. For best results, palm for a few minutes every hour. Let the warm darkness soothe your tight recti muscles and remind them that they do not need to squeeze your eyes when you palm. While palming, stretch your imagination in and visualize things up close perfectly clearly, even if they are blurry with eyes open. For example, imagine the letters in a book up close, or the details of a beautiful flower as you lean in to smell it.

Swinging: (Chapter 4) Break the bad staring habit with long swings, medium swings, and short swings. Try noticing oppositional movement on up close objects when you do small head swings or optical swings. Blink as you read each sentence.

Centralization: (Chapter 5) Practice centralization far away where you can already tell a significant difference between your central and peripheral vision. The better you get a centralizing far away, the better you will get at centralizing up close where you might not notice as much of a difference between central and peripheral yet if they both look blurry. Look for little details on things up close. Keep your point of focus small and keep your eyes moving from one part of a near object to another.

Gateposts: (Chapter 6) When reading books with both eyes open (without an eye patch) hold up one finger, pen, pencil, or pointer vertically in front of your nose. When you look at the book in your hand, the near object will split into two and you can read the words in between the two 'gateposts.'

Near to Far Shifting: (Chapter 6) Imagine your near thumb and your far thumb perfectly clearly when you repeat this practice mentally with your eyes closed, even if they are blurry with your eyes open. Apply the 5-10-15 rule to all near work like reading books and working on computers.

Rope Fusion: (Chapter 6) Use a 1 to 3 foot long rope to track up and down with to help stretch your focus in. Even if the rope gets blurry up close, you can still see the V, X, and A shapes the rope makes.

Lens Flexor: (Chapter 6) Start far away and move your flexing object (thumb, pen, alphabet card, etc.) slowly closer toward your nose until you reach the edge of your bubble. Come a little closer than the edge so that it becomes a little blurry, and then send it back outside your bubble so it becomes clear again. Over time your bubble will get smaller so you can flex farther closer in.

Convergence Games: (Chapter 6) Farsighted eyes tend to have trouble converging. Since the comfort zone is in the distance, most farsighted eyes are more comfortable diverging. Use your two thumbs, two pencils, or the fusion cards to train your eyes to both turn in and aim at the same point up close at the same time for fusion and focus. Anything to practice crossing your eyes will help increase accommodation up close. If you have a convergence insufficiency, hold the tip of a pen halfway in between the fusion card in your hand and your nose. Focus on the tip of the pen and try to notice the illusion of a third object appearing in the background, until you can actually lower the pen and focus on that third object without uncrossing your eyes.

Vision Building Near: (Chapter 7) Reading fine print up close is by far one of the most important practices for helping with farsightedness. Relaxed reading is where near vision is built, strengthened, and maintained. Hold your practice reading material just inside your 'edge,' right where the letters switch from clear to blurry. Do plenty of reading warm ups like sunning, palming, swinging, and space riding to prevent straining while reading. Pay more attention to the white space of the page than the black letters on the page. Each time you do your reading practice, move your material one or two inches closer until you can read it three inches from your nose. The vision building phase is when you will experience and observe most of your clear flashes, since the reading card acts as an objective measurement tool of your visual acuity. In a matter of time you will be able to read the next smaller line down on the card when you used to not be able to. Keep clearing the card until you can read all the way down to the very bottom line. Why stop there?

As you learned in Chapter 6, all of the vision building techniques can be applied both to distant eye charts and to reading cards up close. Always read your reading cards or microprint with each eye separately and then both eyes together. It is best to wear an eye patch so that your head is free to access easy and fluid movement. Even once you have improved your near vision, you need to continue to read fine print up close every day to keep your near vision superb.

As described at the end of the myopia section, do not confine your near vision improvement to only reading flat two-dimensional surfaces. Gaze at other beautiful three-dimensional things with fine details up close, like the palm of your hand, a painting, a leaf, a flower, or a crystal. Teach your eyes to see all things clearly up close.

Astigmatism

Astigmatism can accompany nearsightedness, farsightedness, or both. In astigmatism, the curvature of the eyeball in one principal meridian is greater than in the one at right angles to it, which makes the eyeball lopsided and the curvature of the cornea uneven. The transparent surface of the eye, the cornea, is supposed to be perfectly round in shape. When there is uneven strain or tension from one or more of the extraocular muscles, it makes the cornea misshapen. The light entering the eye fails to focus into one small point, and certain light rays shoot off into different directions landing on the wrong parts of the retina. All forms of astigmatism - nearsighted, farsighted and mixed - change the direction of the light entering the eye, which leads to doubling, tripling, or quadrupling of images.

Many people with astigmatism see these as shadows, ghost images, or overlapping images. Dr. Bates called these illusions 'astigmatic images.' Once again, the astigmatism is rooted in strain; so all the relaxation practices will help since they all replace strain with relaxation.

If you're not sure whether you have astigmatism or not, look at the *Astigmatism Chart on Page 303.* Do all the lines look equally black? If so, you probably don't have astigmatism. If any of the horizontal, vertical, or diagonal lines appear less black, more blurry, distorted, or wavy in any way, that may be an indication of astigmatism. The number at the end of the line that looks different gives an approximate reading of your axis, or angle of astigmatism.

Astigmatism is often caused by imbalanced eye movements in relation to head movements. Dr. Elliott Forrest put forth a functional explanation of astigmatism that blames incorrect ergonomics and poor vision habits for the development of astigmatism. He calls our attention to the difference between eye scans and head scans. Eye scanning is when we keep our head still and just move our eyes, like how most people normally read. Head scanning is when we move our head and our eyes follow, like looking up from reading a book when someone calls your name. Forrest found that if people have incongruous eye scanning and head scanning while performing daily tasks, an astigmatism usually appeared at an angle that corresponds with that imbalanced use.

For example, if you only move your eyes horizontally when you read a book, but never move your eyes vertically because you do a head movement to look up instead, then you are likely to develop a horizontal astigmatism (180 axis) because the left and right rectus muscles are getting more toned than the top and bottom rectus muscles. If you constantly move your eyes vertically from your computer screen to your keyboard, but never move your eyes horizontally because you do a horizontal head movement to look side to side instead, you will likely to develop a vertical astigmatism (90 axis) because the top and bottom rectus muscles are getting more toned than the left and right rectus muscles.

Pay attention to how you use and move your eyes and head throughout your daily tasks. Do you tend tilt your head to one side or the other? Do you rest your chin on your fist while sitting at a computer desk? What is your workstation setup like at school or work? Do you read books or look at smartphones in bed while lying on your side? Once you become aware of your imbalances, you can begin to correct them and either move your eyes horizontally and vertically equally or move your head horizontally and vertically equally. An important caveat is that it is not always simply the imbalanced use of the eyes and head that manifests the astigmatism; it is actually more to do with the rigidity or relaxation associated with that usage. The more you learn how to relax your eyes in general, the imbalanced usage won't even matter as much. However, if you already have an astigmatism, figure out which tasks or activities are contributing to the imbalanced use and see if you can bring more balance and harmony into your eyes, head, and body.

The long swing (Chapter 4) is very beneficial for helping with astigmatism, since it greatly loosens and equalizes the muscles around the eyes. The yogic eye movements (Chapter 8) can also be very beneficial for reducing muscular imbalance. The ring of life mental focus practice (Chapter 8) is especially good for astigmatism.

There are also some additional physical techniques to address astigmatism.

The first is called: 'up and in.' Close your eyes, look up and in toward the center of your forehead, and hold for a few seconds. Breathe deeply as you look up and in and make a big sigh noise when you release. The astigmatic images will disappear after looking up and in a few times in a row. It is likely that you will feel a sensation of soreness when looking up and in. This is because you have found an area of strain and tension that is starting to release. Depending on your astigmatism, it may work better to cross your eyes down and in instead.

A second technique is called: 'sweep the ceiling.' With your eyes open, pretend that you have a long broomstick extending from your nose and sweep the ceiling with it. Come back down to your eye chart or book and see how this technique decreases astigmatic images. Even if you do not have astigmatism, sweeping the ceiling is an excellent habit to form while doing up close work, like reading this book, because it prevents your eyelids from drooping too far down and putting too much pressure on your eyes.

A third technique is called: 'fusion fix.' If you experience astigmatic images, gently bring your focus closer in by slightly crossing your eyes. This will make whatever object you are looking at split into two slightly. Uncross your eyes and send your focus back out to the object and watch it fuse back into one object. Repeat several times. Each time you fuse the object back into one there will be less shadows and doubling.

A fourth technique is called: 'oscillating.' When looking at a distant object or chart, relax your right ear toward your right shoulder and then relax your left ear toward your left shoulder. This oscillation of your head will make the astigmatic images appear to rotate around the real image. This technique helps loosen the two oblique muscles specifically and will help you differentiate between the real image and the astigmatic images.

More powerful than the physical techniques for astigmatism are the mental techniques.

Dr. Bates taught people with astigmatism to banish all astigmatic thoughts and illusions. It is natural to want to look at and analyze the astigmatic aberrations that appear, but you must begin ignoring them. Take for example feeding a stray cat. If you feed a stray cat once, it will return tomorrow and keep coming back. If you ignore the stray cat, it will not return; therefore, you need to stop 'feeding' the ghost images. When they appear, try not to pay much attention to them, and instead try to remain focused on the real single image.

If, when you look at your eye chart you see shadows or doubling, close your eyes and imagine the letters and lines perfectly clear and singular. If they still appear as doubled in your mind, imagine the two images slowly coming closer together, merging together, and becoming one. Open your eyes back up. If they are still doubled, you can try merging them as described above with your eyes open. As you look, breathe, blink, centralize, and keep reminding yourself that there is only one image or one letter. You know for a fact that the shadowing, doubling, or tripling is not real. They are only illusions; you know that there is only one. That is what Bates meant by banishing astigmatic thoughts. Do not let the illusions fool you. Keep reminding yourself of what you know the image truly is until you start to see it how it really is. Determine which one is the real letter and which one is the fake astigmatic letter.

On an emotional level, astigmatism is often a side effect from self-doubt or indecisiveness. When you never commit to one path or are never sure of yourself, you are constantly juggling different options or outcomes, which contributes to the illusion of seeing multiple images. A psychological way to decrease astigmatism is to practice being more decisive and more confident in your decisions. Try to go with your gut instead of second guessing yourself all the time. Do not be afraid to make mistakes or make guesses.

Astigmatism correction ought to be left out of your weaker prescription training glasses if your cylinder is -1.50 or lower. If your cylinder is higher than -1.50, it may be better to gradually decrease the cylinder in increments. In that case, you would keep the axis the same. The axis is just the angle of the cylinder, so you would drop the cylinder by half or whole diopter drops while keeping the axis the same each time. However, as long as there is astigmatism correction in the lens in front of your eye, the astigmatism will remain stuck in your eye. Only once the astigmatism correction is removed from the lens can the astigmatism begin to fully unwind from the eye.

Strabismus, Amblyopia & Diplopia

Strabismus, or squint, is known as 'turned eye.' In strabismus one or both eyes may turn up, down, left, right, or in any diagonal direction. The issue is a muscular imbalance in the eye muscles, with strain or tension causing one of the muscles to pull too much. If both eyes do not aim at the same point at the same time, there is no fusion. This often leads to diplopia, or double vision. Oftentimes instead of trying to interpret two different images that do not match up, the brain will 'shut off' one eye and only use the image from the straight eye. The orthodox fix for strabismus is to surgically cut or tuck the imbalanced muscle to point the eye forward. This is purely cosmetic though and does not address any vision issues associated with it like a lack of fusion or lack of depth perception. There are much more natural ways to both straighten out the eyes and remove any underlying vision issues associated with the turned eye.

Amblyopia is known as 'lazy eye.' In amblyopia the brain still shuts down one eye and only uses the other, but one or both eyes are not always turned like in strabismus. The issue can either be because of blindness on certain parts of the retina or because of a disconnection between the eyes and the visual cortex in the brain. Based off the recent successes of neuroplasticity research, it has been proven that new neural pathways can be carved at any age and the amblyopic eye can reconnect with the visual cortex through vision training.

The term 'lazy eye' is a misnomer because it makes one think that the reason their eye is misaligned or not seeing correctly must be because it is lazy or weak, and therefore must be strengthened. The opposite is the case. The 'lazy' eye is actually more strained than the normal eye, and it needs more relaxation and rest.

Strabismus, amblyopia and diplopia are all caused by mental strain. More often than not, an operation to 'fix' these issues creates more strain and can make the vision worse. On the contrary, anything that relieves strain and tension will benefit all three of these issues.

Movement is very important for loosening up and equalizing the muscles around the eyes, so the long, medium, and short swings (Chapter 4), the picket fence shifter (Chapter 4) and the yogic eye movements (Chapter 8) will help a lot. Sunning (Chapter 3) will be very important as well. Your eyes are naturally drawn toward the light of the sun so you can modify your sun drills to encourage the light to pull your eye toward the direction you want it to go. Palming (Chapter 3) will help increase relaxation levels and encourage the eye muscles to straighten out. In general, you want to begin to 'favor your phoria.' Esophoria is when an eye turns in toward the nose. Exophoria is when an eye turns out toward the temple.

If your left eye is esophoric, or turns to the right in toward your nose, you can favor your phoria by finding more opportunities to for your left eye to turn out to the left more. For example, when you go to the movies, sit on the right side of the theater so your left eye looks out toward the left. When doing the lens flexor (Chapter 6) with your right eye patched and your left eye open, instead of going straight out in front of your nose, stretch your flexing object out to the left a little bit to encourage your left eye to point left of the midline. The opposite would be the case if you had an exophoria in your left eye. In that case, your left eye would point out to the left away from your nose, and you would need to favor the phoria by finding ways to encourage your left eye to turn in to the right more. So you would stretch your flexing object out to the right a little bit to encourage your left eye to point right of the midline.

In addition to using an eye patch during a vision training practice as described above, you may also wear an eye patch while doing everyday activities. Patching your dominant eye give your 'lazy eye' a chance to work correctly independently without being ignored by the brain. Patching your 'lazy eye' will give it a little rest while your dominant eye does the seeing.

An additional practice to help with strabismus is called: 'canthus' writing. The canthus is the place where your upper and lower eyelids meet, so you have an inner canthus on the nasal side of each eye and an outer canthus on the temporal side of each eye. To perform canthus writing, place the back of your thumb on the bridge of your nose near your inner canthus if your eye turns out, or on your temple near your outer canthus if your eye turns in. Pretend like you are writing the alphabet one letter at a time on the pad of your thumb with the tip of your index finger. This helps coax your eye in or out by enticing it to look toward the little imaginary letters you draw on your thumb with your index finger.

By far, the most important practices for both amblyopia and strabismus are the fusion practices (Chapter 6). In most cases of amblyopia and strabismus, fusion is not present. So the main goal is to achieve fusion first and then work on vision improvement. Spend lots of time practicing the gateposts and rope fusion. Wear an eye patch on your stronger eye when doing your vision practices or when relaxing at home to help your weak or blind eye improve.

Computer Vision Syndrome (CVS)

A more recent addition to the arena of vision problems is computer vision syndrome. Many people rely heavily on technology and incorporate frequent use of screened instruments such as cell phones, tablets, laptops, desktop computers, and televisions into their daily lives. The short and long-term effects of these new instruments on the eyes are now beginning to become apparent. Extended and repeated use produces different types of strain in different users, but some symptoms of CVS include eyestrain, dry eyes, fatigue, eye pain, headaches, light sensitivity, blurred vision, and double vision. Studies have found that screens lead to both a lower blink rate and a higher number of incomplete blinks as compared to printed material.[10] When the eyes are left wide open for long periods of time, more evaporation of the tears occurs, which leads to dry eyes.

Your eyes really dislike being held at one focal distance for long periods of time. You may have experienced that after a long amount of time spent staring at a screen your eyes take longer to readjust and focus upon looking away from the screen. As screens become smaller and more portable, the ergonomics of technological interaction becomes compromised. Even when working at a desk, most people do not utilize the most ideal setup for screen viewing.

It is my suspicion that it is not necessarily the screens themselves that are harmful to our eyes, but rather how we use the screens is harmful to our eyes. CVS can be both prevented and reversed if the eyes are used properly while looking at screens. If good vision habits are learned and applied, one can use computers and read for long periods of time without experiencing the symptoms of CVS.

The best habit to utilize for long stints of computer use is the 5-10-15 rule. Every 5 minutes, take at least a 10 second break to look at something at least 15 feet away. During your mini-break, make sure to yawn (Chapter 3) several times and butterfly blink (Chapter 4) to refresh your eyes. To enhance this habit even more, stand up and stretch during your mini-break or do your favorite relaxation or vision practice like the long swing (Chapter 4), palming (Chapter 3), or body looseners (Chapter 8). This simple habit not only keeps your eyes healthy and strain-free for longer periods of time at the computer, but it can also increase your levels of mental focus and productivity because you are resting your eyes and your mind before they feel fatigued.

It is also smart to arrange the most ergonomic working layout by setting the correct viewing distances and angles. Try to keep your computer display slightly below eye level and avoid slouching. It is best to prevent glare on your screen and to work in an adequately illuminated environment. Working in the dark is not recommended because you cannot use the 5-10-15 rule in that scenario. Adjusting the brightness and contrast levels of your monitor according to the changing light levels throughout the day and night can be of real benefit as well. The simplest remedy is reducing your computer use time.

More research continues to surface that blames the high intensity, short wavelength blue light for the negative side effects of screens. Environmental blue light is not normally as much of a problem, because when you are outdoors the brightness of the sun constricts your pupils and decreases the amount of blue light that enters the eyes. It is the artificial blue light from screens that poses more of a risk, because when you are indoors it is never as bright as the sun so your pupils dilate wider, allowing more of this blue light to enter the eye. There are a handful of ways to remedy this issue. The best way is to use blue blocking software on your computers and devices. Most smartphones and tablets have a 'night shift' mode that decreases blue light. You can download Iris or Flux onto your laptop or desktop to automatically or manually decrease the blue light coming from your screens. You can also consider using a removable blue blocking filter that fits over your laptop screen or desktop monitor or using prescription or non-prescription blue blocking glasses that also filter blue light out. It is also advisable to consume dark leafy greens or supplements that contain lutein and zeaxanthin, which can help absorb blue light inside the eye.

Dry Eye Syndrome

Dry eye is a disorder where there is an insufficient tear film on the surface of the eye, particularly on the cornea. The cornea is the most sensitive area of the human body, as it has more nerve endings per square millimeter than any other part of the body. Therefore, when the cornea dries out it can create all kinds of discomforts, irritations, and feelings of dryness, itchiness, grittiness, burning, and redness. Dry eye has many potential causes including not blinking enough, tear film evaporation, not enough tear production, contact usage, hormonal changes or menopause, environmental conditions, smoking, drinking alcohol or caffeine, and over-the-counter or prescription medications.

It is important to understand that tears are not simply salt water. Tears contain a cocktail of ingredients including electrolytes, oils, proteins, antibodies, nutrients, and vitamins. There are also three different types of tears: emotional tears, reflex tears, and basal tears. Emotional tears are produced when humans experience extreme emotions like sadness, grief, anger, fear, or joy. Reflex tears are produced when an irritant is introduced to the surface of the eye to try and wash it off. Basal tears are produced to lubricate the eyes. Dry eye syndrome is most often associated with an issue concerning the basal tears.

The job of the tears is not only to provide the surface of the eye with the nutrients and oxygen it needs as well as an extra layer of protection, but a healthy tear film is also a factor in accommodation or focus. The tear film is the first part of the eye that light strikes, so if the first step of the focusing process is compromised then all the following steps will be lacking.

The two most simple and natural remedies for dry eyes are yawning (Chapter 3) and blinking (Chapter 4). Each big yawn stimulates the lacrimal glands to produce tears, and each blink releases small amounts of oil from the tarsal glands near the eyelashes. If you have dry eyes, chances are you do not blink enough. The average blink rate is between 15 and 30 blinks per minute, or once every 2 to 4 seconds, which can add up to 1,200 blinks an hour or 28,800 blinks a day. Reading books and looking at screens both tend to decrease blink rates, so make a conscious effort to blink more all day long. When your eyes feel dry, take several big yawns to stimulate some natural tear production. Vitamin A and Vitamin C are both essential for healthy tear films, as is enough hydration. Most over-the-counter eye drops contain preservatives and other unwanted ingredients. Look for more natural or homeopathic eye drops like Boiron Opthique 1s or Similasan brand, which contain homeopathic ingredients that nourish the eye tissues. High quality castor oil eye drops may also be of benefit. Giving yourself an eye bath using an eye cup filled with saline or with Dr. Christopher's Eyebright Solution diluted in distilled water may help. Surprisingly, neti pots can also increase tear production (Chapter 8).

Eye Floaters

Floaters are particles that get suspended in the fluid inside the eye and cast shadows upon your retina. They often look like transparent squiggly clusters or worm-like objects that move around whenever you move your eyes or head. They are often most visible when looking at a plain background or a bright blue sky.

Floaters are fairly common and usually harmless. If you notice a large number of floaters appearing suddenly, or the appearance of flashing lights, it could be a sign of something more serious like a retinal detachment, in which case you need to see an eye doctor right away. More often than not though, they are just a byproduct of aging and you may experience just a few of them that are sometimes noticeable and sometimes not.

The fluid inside your eye is called the vitreous humor. The vitreous is a clear gel-like substance that fills the space between the lens in the front of your eye and the retina in the back of your eye. The vitreous is responsible for maintaining the round shape of your eye. It is like the scaffolding supporting the retina, and if the vitreous becomes compromised in any way, the retina loses its support and can 'detach.' The retina is not actually attached, but rather suspended by the vitreous.

The vitreous consists of about 99% water and 1% other elements, including a network of hyaluronic acid and collagen. Hyaluronic acid retains water molecules, but over time the network breaks down as a result of the hyaluronic acid releasing its trapped water molecules, forming a watery center inside the vitreous body. As you age, pieces of the gel-like hyaluronic acid collagen network break off and float around within the watery center of the vitreous. When light enters the eye, the floaters get in the way and cast shadows on the retina, which is what you're actually seeing when you see the floaters. You cannot see the floaters themselves because they exist within the eye. When you move the floaters move, and when you stop moving the floaters stop moving as well.

Diet, nutrition, and supplementation are important in preventing and working with floaters. Sometimes the floaters can be a sign of a nutrient or mineral deficiency. Some people benefit from taking Silica, which is good for the skin, hair, nails, and eyes because it increases collagen production. Floaters may also indicate heavy metal toxicity, so any form of detox can also help the eye health as well. Drinking plenty of water, whether detoxing or not, is crucial for the vitreous health since it consists of 99% water.

The Bates Method can be a good way to work with the floaters naturally. Palming and sunning (Chapter 3) opens up all the channels of the eyes to allow more blood flow and lymph flow, as well as more intraocular drainage. Swinging (Chapter 4) stimulates movement of the fluid inside the eye, which could potentially flush the floaters out over time. The lymph system is the 'cleanup crew' of the body, so anything you can do to increase lymph flow like various forms of physical movement or exercise, can potentially decrease floaters. Your eyes are nourished by the lymph system, so increasing the lymph flow to the eyes can help purify the eyes in general. If the floaters were stationary, your brain would actually tune them out, just like it tunes out the presence of blood vessels that line the inside of the eye. The reason you do not perceive the blood vessels is because they are stationary relative to the movement of your eye. The only reason you see the floaters is because they move around.

So aside from the physical ways to deal with floaters, also utilize the power of your mind to actually tune them out or 'see through' them. When your vision is blurry, you pay more attention to the floaters. When your vision clears through the steps described in this book, you will not notice the floaters as much because you will be more focused on the clearer world all around you instead of the microscopic contents within your eyeballs.

Cataracts

Cataracts are opacities of the lens inside the eye. The lens is a flexible, biconvex structure made up of extremely thin layers. When focusing 15 feet or farther, the lens thins and the layers come closer together. When focusing 15 feet or closer, the lens thickens and the layers spread apart. The flexing of the lens is an automatic and involuntary process that is meant to last for life. If the eyes aren't used properly or glasses are worn, the lens loses its own flexibility and becomes more rigid. This loss of flexibility is accompanied by the accumulation of particles, debris and waste material depositing in between the layers of the lens, which blocks the light rays that enter the eyes. This cloudiness, or opacity, is called a cataract.

Many of the practices in this book can benefit cataracts. Ideally, they are to be used to prevent cataracts from forming in the future by keeping the lens young and flexible. However, if cataracts are caught early enough in their formation process, the relaxation practices can help break up the cataracts and clear up the lens. Even cataracts are fluid, and it is important to understand that relaxation can clear one layer of the lens, but tension can cloud it up again.

The most basic explanation of cataracts is that they are caused by a lack of circulation to the eye. Since the lens is transparent, no blood vessels run through it to supply it with oxygen, nutrients, etc. The way the lens gets what it needs is by getting 'bathed' by the fluids in the aqueous and vitreous chambers in front of and behind the lens. If there is constriction due to tension, the eye lacks circulation and the lens does not get 'bathed' enough, leading to the formation of cataracts. Therefore, one of the number one priorities for people with cataracts is to open up all the channels of the eyes through relaxation, to purify the bloodstream, to increase circulation, and increase the movement of the eyes. Some of the best practices in this book for addressing cataracts are palming and sunning (Chapter 3), swinging and picket fence shifter (Chapter 4), near to far shifting, lens flexor, and rope fusion (Chapter 6), as well as peripheral expansion (Chapter 5). The lens flexor tends to be the most important for cataracts and needs to be practiced every day to start to flex and clear the lens.

There is also a strong nutritional component to cataract development. A diet high in sugar and starches and low in proteins and amino acids often leads to cataracts. Vitamins A, B complex, C, D, E and K, as well as the minerals zinc and selenium have been found to be important for healthy lenses. Many people with cataracts have a deficiency of one of the above vitamins or minerals. The homeopathic herbs in Dr. Christopher's Eyebright solution *(Page 263)* are designed to help address cataracts by using the eyewash externally and taking the capsules or tea internally. Some people use high quality castor oil eye drops or Can-C eye drops that contain the N-Acetylcarnosine compound.

The conventional solution to cataracts is a cataract surgery, where your lens is completely removed and replaced with a synthetic lens. In order to accomplish this, the ciliary muscles that surround the lens must be severed, and therefore lose their ability to flex the lens. The synthetic lens can either be made to help you see near, requiring glasses to see in the distance, or to help you see far, requiring glasses to see up close. Some eye doctors put a near lens in one eye and a distance lens in the other eye, so you have to switch back and forth from one eye to the other depending on where you are looking. This surgery is only done when the cataract is considered 'ripe' or at a full stage of development. If you have cataracts that are 'ripe', there may not be as much potential to reverse them. However, if you have caught your cataracts early on in their development, there is more hope.

A cataract is only a cataract when it interferes with your vision. If the cataract is not interfering with your peripheral or central vision, you may be able to reverse it gradually over time. If it is severely affecting your vision, the surgery might be the more realistic option, in which case the practices in this book will help you to prepare for and recover from the surgery.

Glaucoma

Glaucoma is characterized by a hardness of the eyeball due to a rise in intraocular pressure. The eyes are filled with a fluid called aqueous humor. This fluid is replenished and secreted constantly and is meant to drain out through the Canal of Schlemm in between the iris and the cornea. If the iris adheres to the cornea or if debris builds up, the drainage canal can become obscured, which can create a blockage that leads to ocular hypertension. Excess strain or tension in the ocular muscles around the eye may also increase the pressure inside the eye.

Most eye doctors treat glaucoma with certain types of medicinal eye drops that constrict the pupil and lower the pressure of the eyes. If the pressure cannot be controlled with drops, there are several surgical options that create channels to drain the fluids and relieve the pressure of the eyes. However, the eye drops cause dependency and the operations often make the vision worse since nothing is done to address the underlying root cause of the glaucoma, which is strain. If you are using prescription drops, it is better to wean off them than to stop taking them immediately. Practice the relaxation and vision training while taking the drops. As the tension naturally decreases your eye doctor may inform you that fewer drops are needed.

As opposed to cataracts, which are essentially caused by a lack of circulation to the eye, the most basic way to understand glaucoma is that it is caused by a lack of circulation or drainage away from the eye. Once again, the primary goal is to open up all the channels of the eye through relaxation, to increase circulation, and to increase the movement of the eyes.

The Bates Method offers more natural ways to help decrease and eliminate glaucoma through relaxation. Therefore, anything that helps relax the muscles of the eyes and increase the flow of the fluids inside the eye will help. The best way to accomplish both of those is through gentle movement practices like swinging (Chapter 4), sunning and palming (Chapter 3) as well as the acupressure points (Chapter 3), centralization (Chapter 5) and all the relaxation and mental focus practices.

Macular Degeneration

Macular degeneration is a neurodegenerative disease that affects the retina. The retina is the most active part of the human body and receives the most blood flow 'per capita' of any other organ, including the brain and heart. The most active part of the retina is the macula in the center. Due to its high activity levels, the macula creates a lot of 'debris' as a waste byproduct of its work. This waste called: 'drusen' includes the discs of the photoreceptors, which are shed and replenished every day. Each photoreceptor contains hundreds of discs at their base designed to detect light photons. Once light strikes the rod or cone, discs are shed and it is the job of the retinal pigment epithelium to clean them up by absorbing and ingesting thousands of these discs. If the cleanup crew gets overloaded or falls behind it can lead to a buildup of drusen, which can lead to oxidative damage, inflammation, blurred vision, loss of vision, and macular degeneration.

There are two main types of macular degeneration: dry and wet. The majority of people with macular degeneration have the dry kind, while some others develop the wet kind, which is essentially the dry kind with even more retinal complications and abnormal blood vessel growth. Lutein and zeaxanthin are important because they help filter and absorb the harmful short-wave blue light that can be one of the contributing factors to macular degeneration and other retinal issues. Leafy greens and other vegetables tend to have the highest concentration of these two powerful carotenoids. In addition, the lutein, zeaxanthin, Vitamin A, vitamin C, vitamin E, and zinc, there are five specific compounds that can target drusen: phytic acid, carnitine, coenzyme Q10, chromium, and methionine. The saffron herb has also shown promising results for macular degeneration, and there are supplements that contain saffron powder or saffron extract.

Other forms of alternative treatments for macular degeneration include acupuncture, micro current stimulation therapy, chelation therapy, and stem cell therapy.

Mental Focus #1: Positive Affirmations

Positive affirmations can be used to retrain your subconscious mind and help establish new beliefs about your ability to see clearly. Repeating these mantras helps switch your outlook from, "I'll believe it when I see it," to, "I'll see it when I believe it." Do not deny any feelings that arise as a result of vision training. Learn to let yourself feel whatever feelings emerge, without necessarily acting upon them, but just feeling and expressing them as clearly as possible. The primary repressed emotion for nearsightedness is fear and the primary repressed emotion for farsightedness is anger.

- *It is possible for me to see clearly again without glasses.*
- *I am willing to see clearly again without glasses.*
- *I deserve to see clearly again without glasses.*
- *Clear vision is my birthright.*
- *I see more clearly every day.*
- *I see more clearly today than I did yesterday.*
- *My vision gets clearer as I get older and wiser.*
- *I can see so much without my glasses on.*
- *My depth perception is better without my glasses on.*
- *My color vision is more vivid without my glasses on.*
- *I am more connected to the environment and other people without my glasses.*
- *My intuition is stronger without my glasses on.*
- *I am totally relaxed and my eyes love it.*
- *My mind is free of strain, stress and worry.*
- *My memory is stronger now and I recall things easily.*
- *My imagination is fuller, brighter and more fun than it has ever been.*
- *My visualization is effortless and vivid.*
- *My attention is sharp and my mental focus is strong.*
- *It is such a clear day today.*

- *I believe in my innate ability to heal and see clearly without effort.*
- *Clear vision is only possible by letting go.*
- *I embody clarity on all levels of my life.*
- *I see equally clear near and far.*
- *My eyes are free.*
- *My eyes feel soft.*
- *My eyes feel amazing.*
- *I love myself.*
- *Every day is a new opportunity to improve my own eyesight and insight.*
- *I can do anything that I truly put my mind to.*
- *I am focused.*
- *I am determined.*
- *I am confident.*
- *All my senses are heightened and I am more sensitive to external stimuli.*
- *I embrace my true vision.*
- *There is no rush.*
- *Don't worry, be happy.*
- *I am strong and capable of accomplishing goals that I have set for myself.*
- *Clear thoughts and clear vision happen automatically and effortlessly.*
- *I give myself permission to relax and heal.*
- *Good vision habits all day long.*
- *Centralize, centralize, centralize.*
- *Relax, relax, relax.*
- *Let go.*
- *Thank you for my vision.*
- *I am seeing clearly and I love it!*

Vision Work #1

- ✓ Copy or print your eye charts and vision tools.
- ✓ Create your starting point by recording the results of your near and far vision.
- ✓ Begin breaking your addiction to prescription glasses. Quit contacts, if possible.
- ✓ Begin using weaker prescription 'training glasses' when possible.
- ✓ Read, write, say, and think lots of positive affirmations.
- ✓ Fill out your daily practice checklist and vision journal.

Daily Practice Checklist Week 1

M Tu W Th F S Su			
☐☐☐☐☐☐☐		Take Off Your Glasses	5-60 minutes
☐☐☐☐☐☐☐		Mental Focus Practice	1-5 minutes

◩ = *done once per day*
☒ = *done twice per day*

Vision Journal: ____

____

____

____

____

____

"I also like to take my glasses off and look at people. The faces around me, all of them, seem kind and pretty and smiling. What's more, when my glasses are off, I don't ever think about arguing with anyone at all, nor do I feel the need to make snide remarks."

-Osamu Dazai

Chapter 2

Phase 0.3:
Pre-Practice Groundwork
Addressing Your Root Causes

"The eyes represent the capacity to see. When there are problems with the eyes, it usually means there is something we do not want to see, either about ourselves or about life: past, present, or future. Whenever I see small children wearing glasses, I know there is stuff going on in their household they do not want to look at. If they can't change the experience, they will diffuse the sight so they don't have to see it so clearly. Many people have had dramatic healing experiences when they have been willing to go back into the past and clean up what it was they did not want to look at a year or two before they began wearing glasses. Are you negating what's happening right now? What don't you want to face? Are you afraid to see the present or the future? If you could see clearly, what would you see that you don't see now? Can you see what you are doing to yourself?"

-Louise Hay

Vision Beyond Eyesight

Before even beginning any physical eyesight enhancing practices, you must first identify and address your own unique underlying root causes of your vision problems. As you just learned in the introduction, vision is only one tenth physical and nine tenths mental. To only focus on your eyesight would be a mistake that would prevent you from healing your vision to the fullest extent. To improve your vision completely and holistically you must also focus on your insight. At first glance, one might think that improving vision depends on strengthening the eye muscles through repetition of physical eye exercises, but this turns out not to be the best way. I wish to emphasize the importance of exploring all the non-physical realms of your vision, and I encourage you to expand your definition of vision to encompass more than just eyesight.

This much larger non-physical realm of your vision includes things like insight, inner vision, intuition, memory, imagination, visualization, creativity, hindsight, foresight, desires, dreams, goals, aspirations, self-image, identity, personality, worldview, beliefs, perceptions, knowledge, thoughts, ideas, emotions, and the subconscious. When you experience blurry eyesight on the physical level it is usually just an indication of a deeper imbalance on a mental or emotional level. So now is the time to dive a little deeper and explore some of the subtler realms of vision to initiate the healing process. You will begin by examining your past vision and analyzing your own vision story, which will lead you up to your present vision, and then forward to look ahead to your future vision.

"If we deny our good in any way, it is an act of not loving ourselves. I remember a client I worked with who wore glasses. One day we released an old fear from childhood. The next day she awakened to find her contact lenses were bothering her too much to wear. She looked around and found her eyesight was perfectly clear. Yet she spent the whole day saying, 'I don't believe it, I don't believe it.' The next day she was back to wearing contacts. Our sub-conscious mind has no sense of humor. She couldn't believe she had created perfect eyesight."

-Louise Hay

Clearing Your Past

How do you feel about your past? What parts of your past do you love and enjoy looking back on? What parts of your past make you feel uncomfortable or make you want to ignore or forget? It's usually the things that make you feel uneasy to reflect upon that were, and still are, connected with your current vision problem. Dr. Bates pointed out that physical eyestrain is merely a product of mental strains. Therefore, vision problems are often rooted in psychological stress, worry, anxiety, fear, or trauma. It was, and may continue to still be, the mental and emotional strains that caused your eye muscles to misbehave and malfunction. If you want to heal your present vision you must address the contributing factors and underlying root causes from your past. These deeper individual influences are what caused your vision problems to develop in the first place. If these remain unaddressed, no amount of vision practices in the present will help you obtain perfect vision. Do not get stuck simply blaming your age or your genes for your vision problems, try digging deeper to discover more. Start by asking yourself the following questions:

- *What has led you up to this point?*
- *What was going on in your life around the time you developed a vision problem?*
- *How old were you?*
- *What stage of life were you in?*
- *Where did you live? What was your house like?*
- *How was your relationship with your mother?*
- *How was your relationship with your father?*
- *Do you have any siblings? What was your relationship like with them?*
- *Were you a student in school? What grade were you in? Who were your teachers? Who were your classmates?*
- *Were you bullied or made fun of growing up?*
- *Were you an employee at a company? Where did you work? Who was your boss? Who were your coworkers?*
- *What was going on at home, at school, or at work?*
- *Was there something stressful?*
- *Were you going through some sort of physical, mental, or emotional transition or transformation?*
- *Did you witness or experience a physical, mental, or emotional trauma?*
- *What were you afraid of?*
- *What were you not willing to look at?*

- *What are you still not willing to look at?*
- *What lies were you telling others?*
- *What lies were you telling yourself?*
- *Have you made any enemies in the past?*
- *Are you holding onto grudges from the past?*
- *What was going on in the world, locally or globally, around the time you developed a vision problem?*

These are the kinds of questions that conventional eye doctors rarely pose. Yet these are your own unique and individual root causes to your vision problems and when they are not acknowledged or dealt with, the problem will never be solved. Instead of asking you these deeply provocative life questions, which could have potentially brought back the clarity and averted the need for glasses in the first place, your eye doctor swiftly prescribed you a pair of distance or reading glasses to help you ignore these inner imbalances and get back to your life. But they are still there, burrowing even deeper and may continue to negatively affect your body, mind, and vision until they are looked at and dealt with. When I say, "dealt with", I don't necessarily mean that you must relive traumatic experiences from your past, but rather commend yourself that you have made a valuable discovery about one of your own individual root causes and acknowledge that it is connected to your current vision and life. The first step in overcoming them is letting them be known. Write your discoveries down. Say them out loud to yourself or to someone you trust. Let it out.

Some people realize these contributing causes right away, whereas other people require more time and introspection. Sometimes it is apparent and it stares you right in the face immediately upon opening the door up to your past. Other times it is subtler or buried deeper. If nothing arises at first, do not give up. If your vision problem developed at a very young age or a very long time ago, try jogging your memory by visualizing photographs of yourself at that time or remembering home movies taken of you back then. Sometimes it is a big event like the death of a loved one, the divorce of your parents, a traumatic car accident, losing your job, moving to a new city, or some sort of public humiliation. Other times it is a small event like watching a scary or gory movie, being picked on or embarrassed, hiding or denying certain aspects of yourself, trying to fit in or conform, transitioning from elementary school to middle school, from middle school to high school, from high school to college, or from college to a job, or even telling a lie. Rarely is it just one thing, but rather an amalgamation of many factors.

When exploring your underlying root causes, try to boil them all down to the base emotion of fear. What fears or angers were instilled into your mind by experiencing those things in your past? Have those patterns of fear or anger remained to this day?

The main emotion associated with nearsightedness is fear, and more specifically the suppression of fear. The main emotion associated with farsightedness is anger, or more specifically the suppression of anger. When it comes down to it though, anger is just a form of fear. Not only do you need to identify what you were afraid of, but also more specifically, which fears did you bottle up and keep inside? Sometimes it can be a physical fear like fear of the dark, fear of scary movies, fear of a bully, fear of a teacher, parent, or boss, while other times it can be mental or emotional fear, like fear of rejection, fear of failure, fear of embarrassment, fear of the future, or fear of the unknown. It's usually not the fear itself, but rather the lack of expression of the fear.

For example, when I was in elementary school my parents signed my sister and I up for dance classes after school. I was put in a jazz dance class with three other boys around my age. I didn't mind taking the dance classes, but I soon became self-conscious about it. I didn't think that jazz dance was the most masculine activity and was therefore embarrassed about it. In an attempt to protect myself, I decided to keep it a secret. I didn't tell a single one of my friends I was a jazz dancer. No one at school knew. I was terribly afraid of what people would think of me if they found out. I feared I would become the laughing stock of the entire school. I was afraid people would think I was girly, that I was not cool, that I wouldn't fit in. So essentially my solution was to omit the truth; to lie. Whenever we tell a lie, it automatically creates an accompanying fear of being found out. I was not being honest with the people around me and therefore I was not being honest with myself. I was literally covering up or blurring over a part of my life so people couldn't see who I was or what I was doing. I was in this class for over a year, and the fear and anxiety built up more and more. Interestingly enough, this was right around the time I began wearing glasses. It wasn't the dance class itself, but rather the suppression of my own fears about what would happen if people found out about the dance class that manifested physical blur in my eyesight. Over a decade later when I learned about holistic eye care, I realized that I still had not told anyone about this and therefore was still holding onto certain fears and embarrassments. My vision teacher helped me identify this as one of many of my own personal contributing factors. Once I understood the connection, I was able to share this story, express my feelings, and finally release this decade-old issue.

So, you can see that the blur can initially form as a type of defense mechanism, an attempt to protect ourselves from the scary things around us or within us. This can certainly be a helpful evolutionary tool in the moment, but the problem arises when we get stuck in this fear-based state and never let our guards down even when we are safe again. Once you put on a pair of prescription glasses, it fixes your vision in that state and lodges that emotion or fear in your system. That's why sometimes these suppressed emotions resurface upon removing your lenses.

I encourage you to become an emotional archaeologist, to dig deeper into your mind, and shine your inner light on some of the darker or partially forgotten areas and unresolved issues that you have been putting off looking at. Get clear about your past, present, and future fears. Each time you investigate a possible contributing factor, ask yourself, "What am I afraid of?"

Since the problem stems from suppressing emotions, the best way to fix the problem is by releasing and expressing emotions. Use this formula to frame your emotional clearings: "I am afraid of ____________ because if ________ then _________." You can fill in the blanks with any of your own personalized emotions, fears, or mental blocks. Either write them down, state them out loud, or share them with your trusted friends or family. Own your feelings and let them out for others to see. Stop hiding them or blurring them from view.

If you have discovered some unresolved emotions or untold lies, it may feel really good to either come clean and tell the truth or fully feel that emotion now that you are older and more equipped to handle it.

This may result in what I consider to be one of the most powerful and overlooked eye exercises: crying. Your eyes are not only for receiving light and seeing. They are also for releasing emotions through your tears. Letting emotions pass through you and granting yourself permission to cry can result in a big release of pent up emotions, stresses, worries, anxieties, fears, and strains.

Your past vision story and your current present vision is totally unique from every other human on the planet. I want you to rewrite your vision story and reconnect with your true vision. Not the artificial vision that was prescribed to you by an eye doctor, but the true vision you were given when you were born. That's what you do when you take off your glasses, is reconnect with your true vision. Once you get clearer about your past vision, you can then begin to bring your attention to your eyesight and insight in the present moment.

Clearing Your Present

Taking a look back at your vision story ought to give you a deeper perspective into how you have gotten to this point with your vision. Now, what is the current state of your vision? Not just your eyesight, but also your insight. How do you feel about your life in the present? Is it what you thought it would be? What about your life differs from your previous vision of your life. What unexpected twists and turns have come up that you didn't foresee? What parts of your present life are you content with, that you enjoy seeing? What parts of your present life are you not content with, that you'd rather not see? It could be where you live, where you work, who you spend your time with, how you feel physically, mentally, emotionally, or spiritually, what you're doing, or if you feel aligned with your life purpose or calling. Are you satisfied with the state of things? If not, why not? What can you do to make a change and get more in alignment with your ideal life?

Another factor in your present vision is your personality type. What kind of person are you? Nearsighted people tend to be more introverted and remain in their small, safe bubble without venturing out beyond their comfort zone. They may be less outgoing and spend more time doing up close work and reading. They may have certain fears of the distance or fears of the future. Farsighted people tend to be more extroverted and do not spend enough time with themselves, always caring for others. They may avoid up close or introspective activities and may have certain resistances to their past or present. Astigmatic people tend to be more indecisive, never certain which decision to make or direction to go. They may lack confidence or commitment. By identifying your tendencies and understanding the connections between the way you live your life and the way you see your life you may start to balance these out to compensate. If you know you are shy or introverted, try putting yourself out there more. If you know you are extraverted, try looking within more and taking care of yourself instead of always seeking external validation. If you know you are indecisive, try being more confident in your decisions, listening to your intuition, and going with your gut feelings without second guessing yourself so much.

Another avenue to explore is your identity. How do you define yourself as a person? Do you identify with your vision problem? Do you describe yourself as a nearsighted person or a farsighted person? Are your glasses or contacts a part of who you are as a person? Do your friends and family associate you with your glasses? If you have worn glasses for a long time it will take an adjustment for you and the people around you to get used to your new glasses-free look. This process is not just about improving your eyesight. It is about going through a personal transformation, nourishing a new identity, one free of visual ailments.

Maybe you will be reminded of the person you used to be before you wore glasses. Maybe you will create a new identity altogether.

To make these positive changes permanent you need to observe your self-talk. What do you tell yourself or others about your eyes and vision? Have you ever said something like, "I'm blind as a bat," or "I can't see anything without my glasses," or "My vision is terrible," or "I hate my eyes, I hate my vision!" or something along those lines? Your eyes are quite close to your mouth and they can hear what you say about them. Even if you just think these things to yourself mentally, your eyes will know you're talking behind their back. Your vision is 90% mental so choose your thoughts and words wisely. That type of negative self-talk only reinforces the vision problem and solidifies the state of blur. To reverse this, try some positive self-talk, or the positive affirmations at the end of Chapter 1. When you get a flash of clarity in your eyesight, confirm it by stating, "I am seeing clearly!" These types of inner shifts are what I refer to when I say, "Take off your mental glasses." It's one thing to remove your physical glasses from your face, but you also need to remove your mental glasses from your mind. Removing the barriers and obstacles that have been built up by yourself or others.

A powerful exercise is to look at your reflection in a mirror. Look yourself directly in the eye and tell yourself that you love and accept yourself no matter what. Tell yourself you are beautiful. Try several different positive affirmations while facing your reflection and see what surfaces. Study your eyes. Look at your left eye. Look at your right eye. Watch what happens when you blink your eyes. Observe the minute changes of your iris and pupil. Close your eyes for a few seconds to allow your pupils to dilate. Watch as your pupils constrict upon opening your eyes. See if you can notice the little tiny movements of your eyes as you shift from one eye to the other. See yourself in the now, in the present moment.

One final attribute of your present vision is paying attention to the present moment. Perfect vision is only possible in the present moment. When your mind leaves the present moment and wanders into the past or the future, it disconnects from your eyes. Your eyes look at one thing but your mind thinks of another thing. There is a difference between looking and seeing. True vision takes place only when your mind sees what your eyes are looking at. A scattered mind that is constantly thinking about the next task or replaying previous events is a stressed mind. Therefore, when exploring your past and future vision, or when daydreaming in general, close or palm your eyes to prevent staring. Creating and maintaining a daily holistic vision routine and repeating your vision practices every day is by far the best way to bring your present vision back into balance.

Clearing Your Future

How do you feel about your future? What do you envision happening in the future? Where do you picture yourself one year from today? Where do you picture yourself in two years, five years, or ten years? What are your short-term and long-term goals and aspirations that you hope to accomplish? What do you hope to look like or feel like? Who do you want to be with? Where do you want to live? Where do you want to work? What do you want to learn? What parts of your future are you excited about and anticipate? What parts of your future are you putting off or dreading? If you are not clear about your future path, you may feel lost, like you lack direction, or like you are walking blindly.

Sometimes your bigger vision refers to your life purpose. Do you know what your purpose is? If so, what are you doing to get closer to making it your reality? If not, contemplate what you are passionate about. Oftentimes the things you care most deeply about act as clues pointing you toward your purpose. If you already are clear about your purpose but don't feel like you are aligned with it, or you feel unable to pursue your purpose, that may be contributing to a feeling of strain or imbalance on a deep level. Ask yourself, does your school or work nourish your soul or drain your soul? Is what you spend your time doing every day bringing you closer to fulfilling your purpose or does it feel like a distraction that is taking you farther away from it? Keep in mind that life purposes and callings do not necessarily have to be limited to just one, and they can also change over time. It is a good idea to periodically check in with yourself to see how you are growing and evolving over time and make adjustments as is necessary. It is never too late to make a change in your life. People go back to school. People change careers. People move to new cities. You are the director of your own life. You can take action to make what you see with your eyes align with what you see in your mind and feel in your heart.

Do you have trouble setting goals and following through to completion? It may not be enough to just set a goal in your mind. Writing your goals down could increase the probability of you sticking to it. Sharing your goals with a friend or colleague and asking them to hold you accountable for it will increase the probability of you completing it even more. With that added accountability you will be more likely to hold true to your aim. When it comes to your vision goals, that is where a vision teacher comes in. Just reading this book or doing your vision practice on your own may not take you all the way to completion. When you have a vision coach holding you accountable, your success will be more ensured. Write down some of your vision-related and non-vision-related goals:

This year I will:

Next year I will:

Mental Focus #2: Past Self, Present Self, Future Self

Sit in a comfortable position or lie down on your back and close your eyes gently.

First, picture the past version of yourself around the time you first developed a vision problem. If you are nearsighted that may be sometime early in life between the ages of 5 and 10. If you are farsighted that may be later in life between the ages of 40 and 60. What did this younger version of you look like? Where were you then? Were you in school? Were you at a job? Picture your younger self in the house where you lived, the school you went to, or the job you held. Imagine walking up to your younger self and looking him or her in the eyes. Listen to what your younger self has to say to you. Once you have heard the message from him or her, communicate something back. What do you want to tell your younger self? What did he or she need to hear or know at that time? Reconnect with your inner child or younger self and see what insights arise.

Next, picture the present version of yourself in this very moment. Imagine looking back at yourself from across the room sitting there with your eyes closed. Experiment with different perspectives. What do you look like from straight ahead, from the left side, from the right side, from behind, from above? Now bring your attention inward, tuning into how your body feels. What parts of your body are comfortable? What parts of your body are uncomfortable? Scan your body from your toes, to your feet, ankles, shins, calves, knees, thighs, hips, genitals, abdomen, organs, ribs, lungs, heart, shoulders, arms, elbows, wrists, fingers, neck, throat, chin, jaw, tongue, teeth, cheeks, nose, ears, eyes, eyebrows, forehead, scalp, and brain. Pay special attention to your breath and your heartbeat. Feel your lungs expanding and contracting with your breath. See if you can feel or hear your heart beating.

Finally, picture the future version of yourself once you have successfully accomplished your goals. What do you look like without glasses? Imagine yourself doing everyday tasks without glasses and seeing everything clearly and easily, like driving, walking, reading, writing, talking, working, typing, playing sports, traveling, swimming, and spending time with friends and family. How will your life be different with independently clear vision? What new activities or tasks will you be able to take on? What other goals do you have beyond your vision improvement? Think about those and picture yourself having already accomplished or achieved them. What does that look like for you? What does that feel like to you? The more you play out these scenarios mentally, the higher the chances are of seeing and experiencing them physically.

Vision Work #2

- ✓ Identify and process some of your underlying root causes from your past.
- ✓ Take stock of your present.
- ✓ Envision your future.

Daily Practice Checklist Week 2

M Tu W Th F S Su			
☐☐☐☐☐☐☐		Take Off Your Glasses	5-60 minutes
☐☐☐☐☐☐☐		Mental Focus Practice	1-5 minutes

Vision Journal: ____

____

____

____

____

____

____

____

____

"The eyes are not viewers. They are also projectors that are running a second story over the picture that we see in front of us all the time."
-Jim Carrey

A FRIENDLY REMINDER

. . . .

Before you begin your first set of physical vision practices throughout the next six chapters...

Remember that it is mainly mental!

Your vision is happening in the back of your brain, not just in your eyes.

This is both a form of brain training and eye training.

You are learning a brand new way to see the world in a relaxed and receptive way.

You are not just trying to learn a series of physical eye exercises.

The practices you are about to learn are simply meant to help you achieve the sensation of relaxation.

Your approach to the practice matters and dictates the results you get.

If you're not in the mood to do the practices, or you feel like you're forcing yourself to do a chore or exercise, you might as well not do the practices.

If you are in the mood to do the practices and you're doing them because you want to be doing them, and treat it more like a game than an exercise, you'll get much better results.

Vision cannot be forced. It can only be coaxed.

So have fun and keep a smile on your face as you practice.

Chapter 3

Phase 1.1:

Relaxation Foundations

Your Daily Vision Routine

"All methods of curing errors of refraction are simply different ways of obtaining rest. Patients who do not succeed with any particular method of obtaining rest for their eyes should abandon it and try something else. The cause of the failure is strain, and it does no good to go on straining." *-Dr. William H. Bates*

"According to Dr. S. Weir Mitchell, there is but one disease, congestion; there is but one cure, circulation... Authorities agree that relaxation improves any bodily condition or any function because relaxation is the natural state of the normal body."

-Margaret D. Corbett

"The evidence is conclusive... errors of refraction [vision problems], are purely functional troubles; and since they are always relieved by the relief of the strain with which they are associated, it follows that any of the methods which promote relaxation... may be employed for their cure." *-Dr. William H. Bates*

Morning Relaxation Routine

Now that you have thoroughly explored the non-physical aspects of your past, present, and future vision, you are now ready to begin exploring the physical and mental practices taught by the Bates-Corbett Method, starting with passive and dynamic relaxation.

To get your vision routine established, perform this chapter's practices first thing in the morning upon waking up. You can even do the first five practices in bed before you even get up and start your day. Once you do a few or all of the first five practices lying or sitting up in bed, you can get up and complete your morning vision routine with a short sunning and palming session. If the sun is shining, you can step outside or take the sun through a window. If the sun has not come up yet, you can use your indoor sun lamp to wake your eyes up with some bright, warm light. Right after sunning your eyes, palm your eyes and visualize. Once you memorize the practices, your morning vision routine ought to only take between 2 and 10 minutes, which even the busiest person can fit into their schedule. It may require setting your alarm earlier to carve out some extra time to set your eyes up for success for the whole rest of your day. Something very powerful begins to happen when you start every single day with a handful of simple and relaxing vision practices.

For best results, repeat any or all of these practices again in the afternoon, evening, and night, or whenever needed. Only doing these practices once a day in the morning will not be enough. Some of these practices, like the eyebrow raises and nose drawing, can be repeated multiple times a day without anyone even noticing that you are doing vision practices, if you learn how to perform them in a conspicuous way. You may prefer to perform others, like sunning and palming, in private at first. Keep in mind that the more you repeat the practices, the more results you get in a shorter period of time... except for sunning; that is one practice where less is more.

In addition to learning and repeating the physical practices, you can also begin to replace bad vision habits with good vision habits during all waking hours. The more you repeat your physical relaxation techniques, the more you will understand what it means to keep your eyes dynamically relaxed while using them. You will also become more aware of when your eyes are not relaxed, or when they are straining. Check in with your eyes and mind multiple times a day. Ask yourself, "Am I straining?" or "Am I relaxing?" If you are straining, consciously let go of the strain, and replace it with relaxation.

Stretch & Yawn

Purpose:

- Wake up the physical body and loosen muscles after lying still all night.
- Oxygenate the eyes and brain.
- Activate the lacrimal glands, which produce tears to lubricate eyes.
- Release tension in the jaw.

Directions:

1) Inhale deeply through the nose to initiate the yawn.
2) Open your mouth and take in even more air as you yawn.
3) Stretch your limbs out in all directions, spreading your fingers and toes.
4) Move the eyes in all directions, with lids open or closed to stretch all eye muscles.
5) Pay special attention to loosening the neck because a tight neck leads to tight eyes.
6) Take 3 to 6 big yawns in a row and blink to spread the new tears.

Time: 1 to 2 minutes *(longer if you have your own stretching/yoga morning routine).*

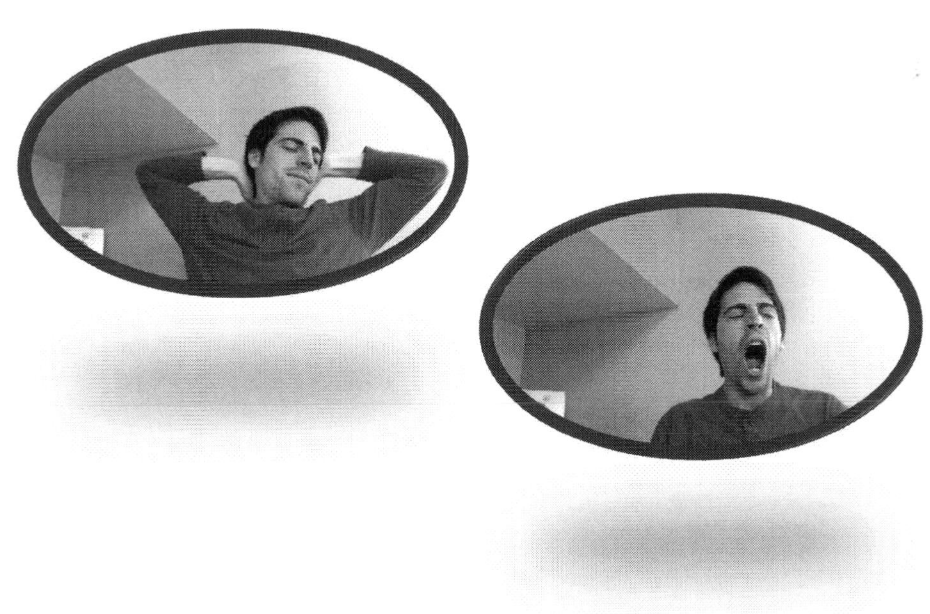

Description:

If you have ever owned a cat or dog you will know that this is the first thing they do upon waking up before anything else. Not just once either... they stretch their limbs and yawn several times to start each day and continue to yawn throughout the day and night.

Take note from other animals and make sure you don't skip over this primal necessity. There is a good chance that your day will be more stressful if you forget to stretch and yawn in the morning. Bring awareness, movement, and energy into every joint in your body. Begin by wiggling your fingers and toes. Then roll your wrists and ankles. Bend your elbows and knees. Circle your hips in all directions. Fold your whole body forward and bend your whole body backward gently. Hug your knees into your chest and get as small as you can, then stretch your limbs out and get as large as you can.

Yawning is one of the best things you can do for your eyes and is a great natural remedy for dry eyes. Each time you yawn you take in a healthy amount of fresh oxygen, which the eyes need to function properly. Each yawn also stimulates your lacrimal glands on the upper outer corner of each eye, which are about the size and shape of an almond. These glands produce tears, which not only cleanse and lubricate your eyes but also improve the quality of vision.

Eyes are never meant to be dry. The eyes are filled with liquid internally and are meant to maintain a fine layer of liquid externally on the surface. People with dry, red or itchy eyes have low functioning lacrimal glands. Regular yawning can help eliminate the need for eye drops because you will begin producing your own tears instead of relying on artificial tears.

Unfortunately, yawning is sometimes stigmatized with either being tired or bored. I encourage you to leave behind this stigma and yawn dozens of times a day in order to keep your eyes healthy, your brain oxygenated, and your eyesight sharp. Demonstrate that you see so much more clearly with moist eyes than dry eyes.

Tapping

Purpose:

- Increase circulation and lymph flow to the face and eyes.
- Stimulate the nerves in the face connected to the eyes.

Directions:

1) Extend your index and middle fingers of both hands.
2) Begin gently tapping on your chin.
3) Continue tapping and slowly make your way up your jaw line, over your temples, over your eyebrows, and meeting at the center of your forehead.
4) Keep tapping and make your way back over your eyebrows, over your temples, over your ears, behind your ears, to your visual cortex in the back of your head.
5) From chin to cortex counts as one trip.
6) Take 5 to 10 trips.

Time: 1 to 2 minutes.

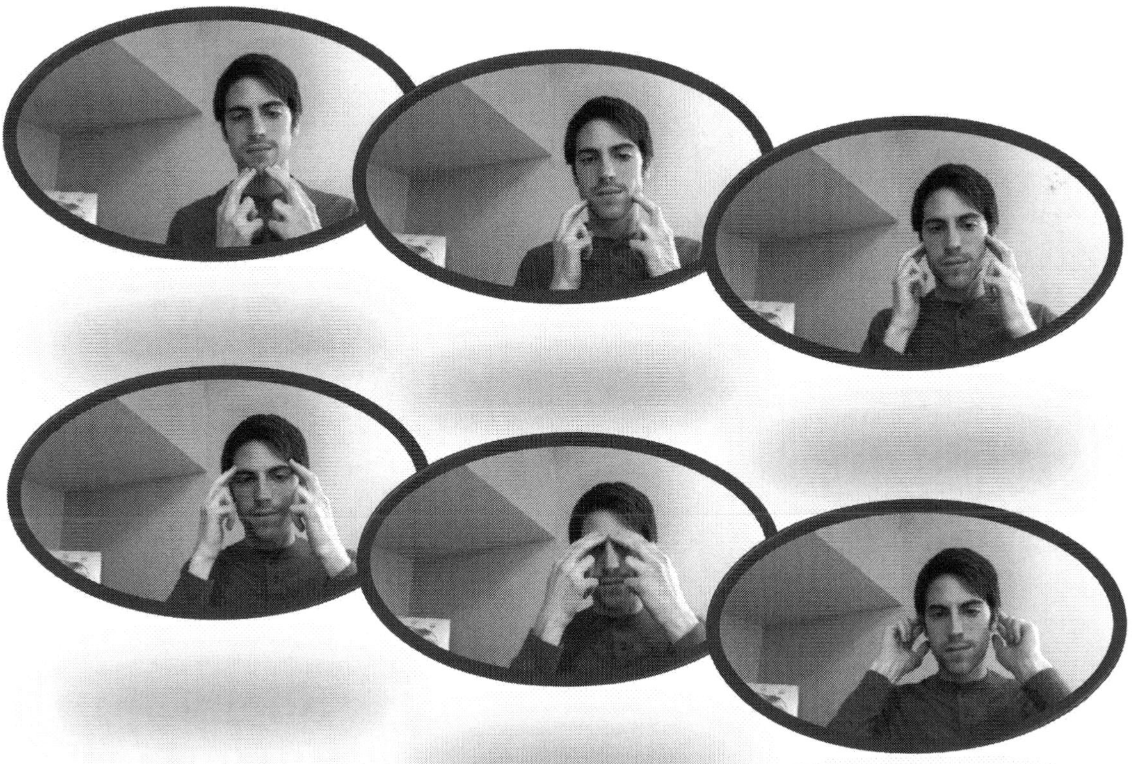

Description:

Gently tap your face in a heart-shaped path from your chin to your forehead with the fingertips of your index and middle fingers, as shown in the pictures. Tapping has been known as an effective method for thousands of years with roots in Classical Chinese Medicine, which mapped out the entire human body with meridian lines and acupressure points.

In regards to the vision, there are several sympathetic nerves in the face that connect with the eyes and the visual system. By gently tapping these nerves you stimulate and activate them to 'switch on' for the day after being dormant overnight. You may feel as you travel along the heart-shaped path that different areas feel more sensitive than others. These are the different acupressure points that may have more or less tension or strain stored in them.

The gentle tapping also encourages more blood and lymph flow up and around the face and eye orbits. Tapping the upper temporal side of each eye may stimulate your lacrimal glands so watering and tearing of the eyes is normal and beneficial. Tapping can also be very energizing and a great way to start your day. You may tap in the morning to help you wake up or anytime throughout the day when you feel tired or fatigued. Taking about 10 tapping trips takes about 1 to 2 minutes.

You may also try tapping all around your eye orbits, above your eyebrows, on your cheekbones, or on your temples, as well as on the crown of your head, on your upper and lower lips, below your collar bones, and on your ribcage. Do not tap directly on your eyeballs.

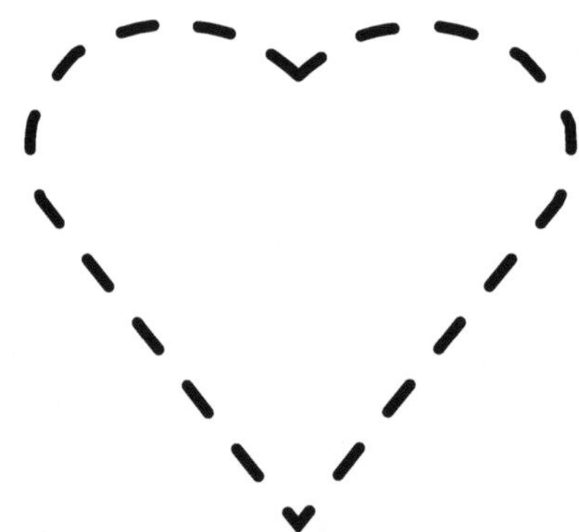

Acupressure Points

Purpose:

- Increase circulation to the face and eyes.
- Ease tension in nerves around eyes.
- Cultivate and increase energy flow.

Directions:

1) Begin by using your right thumb and index finger to squeeze the space between your left and right thumb and index finger. Repeat on the other hand and press until the spot feels less tender.

2) Move up to your face and begin gently pressing, pulsing or wiggling your fingers on each of the acupressure points around each eye orbit for 5 to 10 seconds each.

3) Finish with one more acupressure point on the cheekbones.

Time: 1 to 2 minutes.

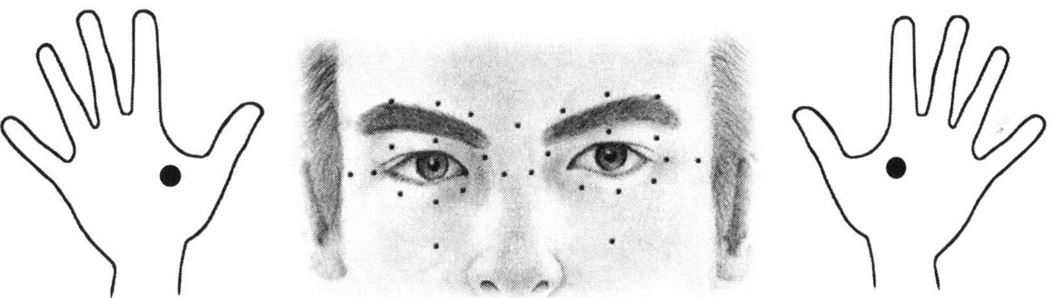

Description:

The acupressure points begin with one point on each hand and all the rest around each eye orbit.

The first point is located in between the thumb and index finger. This spot is called the 'Hoku' point and is known as a 'headache melter' because it is connected with the entire body but specifically the head, face, and eyes. The point is fairly central, but you can explore the whole fleshy area in between your thumb and forefinger in search of tension. After you press there on each hand, you can move up to the remaining points around each eye.

The eye orbits are the bony cavities in which the eyes sit. These orbits, in addition to the cushiony layers of fat surrounding each eye, help protect your precious eye organs. All around each eye on the edges of each eye orbit are tiny grooves. These grooves allow nerves, veins, and capillaries to pass through them. According to many traditions, these are also the locations of important acupressure points. In acupuncture these are the points that thin needles can be inserted into for highly concentrated energy attraction or dispersion. However, these points can be just as easily accessed with your fingers to achieve similar results. When you use needles, it is acupuncture. When you use fingers, it is acupressure.

There are three points on the upper eye orbit, three points on the lower eye orbit, three points above each eyebrow, points on the temples and bridge of the nose, one point on the third eye in between the two eyebrows on the forehead, and one point on each cheekbone about an inch below each eye. Explore your own orbits to find these little grooves since they may be slightly different for everyone. Make sure you are right on the edge of your eye orbits and not actually touching your eyeballs at all. You can hold your fingers on the spots, gently pulse them in and out, or gently wiggle them side-to-side. No matter which way you choose to do it, you want to give attention to each point for 5 to 10 seconds. Some points may be more sensitive than others. Only apply a little bit of pressure. Since the acupressure points are dealing with subtle energies it is less of a massage and more of a gentle cultivation of energy and awareness.

Eyebrow Raises / Tense & Release

Purpose:

- Let go of unconscious tension through progressive muscle relaxation.
- Relaxing muscles in eyes, face, scalp and head.

Directions:

1) Precede tense and release with a few eyebrow raises.
2) Inhale, squeeze all the muscles in your face toward the tip of your nose.
3) Exhale, release all the muscles in your face opening your eyes wide.
4) Repeat 10 times.

Time: 1 to 2 minutes.

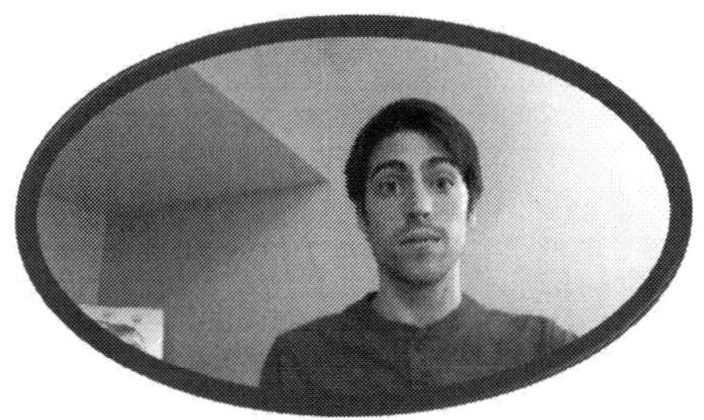

Eyebrow Raise

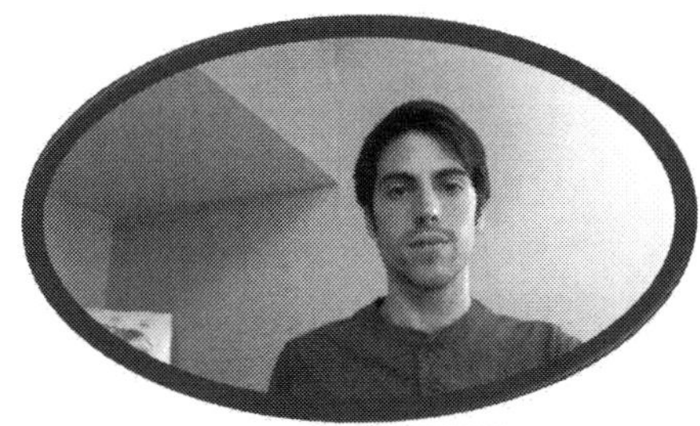

Relaxed

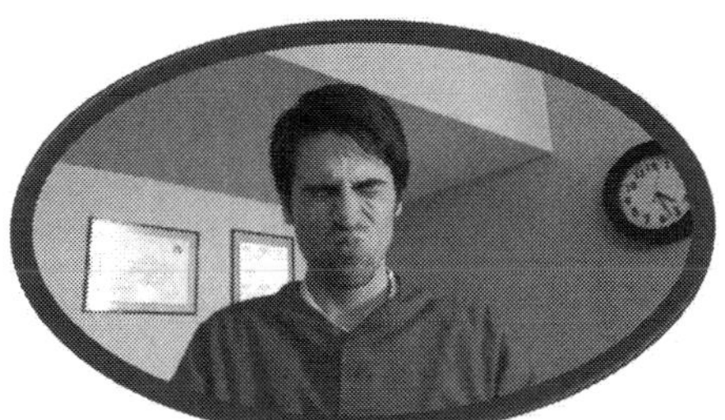

Inhale, Tense

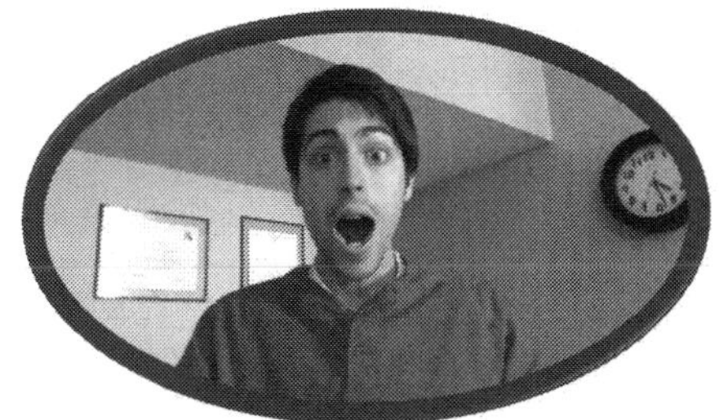

Exhale, Release

Description:

Eyebrow raises are performed by raising both eyebrows at once and then relaxing them back down. Your eyes can be open or closed, but make sure you isolate your brow muscles from your eye muscles. Do not look up when you raise your eyebrows. Keep your eyes relaxed and pointing forward. Not only do eyebrow raises release tension in your brow and forehead but the relaxation even spreads over your entire scalp all the way to the back of your head and to the base of your skull. Eyebrow raises are especially important for people who have a tendency to scrunch their brow when reading or concentrating. When you catch yourself scrunching your brow, do five to ten eyebrow raises to relax your forehead, keep your eyebrows relaxed, and your eyes open comfortably.

Tensing and releasing is based on a technique called 'progressive muscle relaxation,' which was developed by the American physician, Edmund Jacobson, in the early 1920s. The concept is that the body's muscles can hold both conscious tension and unconscious tension. Conscious tension is more often found in voluntary muscle groups while unconscious tension is more often found in involuntary muscle groups. Most of the tension in the eyes is unconscious since most of the eye muscles are involuntary muscles. Stress can be a significant factor in unconscious tension. If you have a particularly stressful day or week then your involuntary systems like breathing, heart rate, blood pressure, or digestion may be under more unconscious tension and function less than optimally. So how can you let go of unconscious tension? Jacobson's studies found that nearly all of the test subjects recorded lower levels of stress and tension in a particular muscle group after consciously tensing it more and then releasing it. For example, let's say that tension is measured on a scale of 1 to 10 and you begin with a tension level of 6 in your right arm. By consciously raising that tension to 10 by squeezing all the muscles in your right arm, holding for a few seconds and then totally relaxing all the muscles in your right arm, your tension level will always measure lower than 6 afterward.

This is what you are doing with your eyes. In order to release the unconscious strain in both the outer and inner eye muscles, tense and release all the muscles in your face, including your eyes. As you inhale deeply squeeze all the muscles in your face toward the tip of your nose, like a prune face, and hold for 2 to 4 seconds. As you exhale release all the muscles in your face and gently stretch them away from the tip of your nose, opening your jaw and eyes wide and lifting your eyebrows, like a surprised face. Repeat between 2 and 4 times. Tensing and releasing is very potent so you don't need to do it very many times to absorb the benefits.

Nose Drawing

Purpose:

- Improve imagination, visualization and memory.
- Stretch the imagination further in and/or out.
- Calm the limbic system through oscillations in the cervical spine.

Directions:

1) With eyes closed, pretend that you have a black magic marker attached to the tip of your nose. If you are nearsighted the magic marker is between 3 and 15 feet long. If you are farsighted the magic marker is between 3 and 15 inches long.
2) Imagine there is a bright white piece of paper, a blank canvas, or a large billboard, either up close or far away for you to draw on.
3) Move your head to move your nose marker, as you draw one of the shapes below, seeing the lines appear as you drag your nose marker along the imaginary surface.
4) Once you complete your first nose drawing, write your signature and today's date in the bottom corner, and take a moment to gaze at your beautifully clear creation.
5) Your magic nose marker turns in to a magic nose eraser for you to erase your drawing with, going back to a blank surface for your next nose drawing.
6) Repeat a few more of the suggested drawings below, or make up your own.

Time: 1 to 2 minutes.

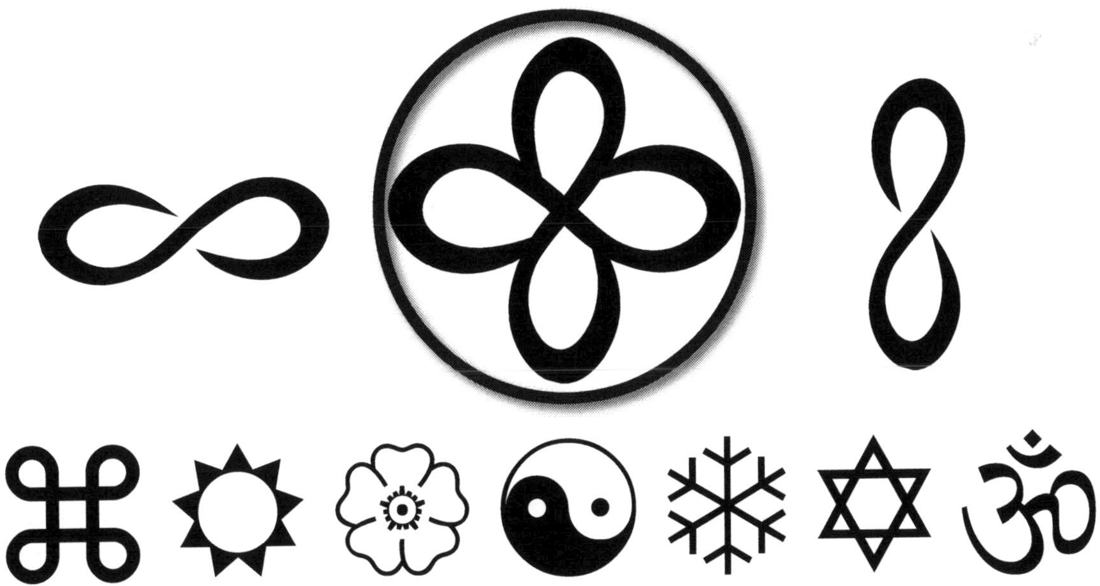

Description:

This practice not only helps improve your imagination, visualization and memory, but it's fun too! It will really begin to help you stretch your vision either further in or further out depending on where you are experiencing blur. If you are farsighted and experience blur up close, you will be nose drawing on an imaginary piece of paper very close to your face and picturing your drawings perfectly clear near. If you are nearsighted and experience blur in the distance, you will be nose drawing on an imaginary piece of paper or billboard very far from your face and picturing your drawings perfectly clear far away. Once again, you cannot begin to improve your external vision until you can imagine clarity with your internal vision, or imagination. Since you may be uncomfortable in your area of blur, the imaginary paper may move further away or closer in as you draw, so take notice if this happens and readjust it accordingly in your imagination. You can't nose draw on a paper at arm's length with a 6 inch nose marker or a 10 foot nose marker. Try to keep your imaginary drawing surface at the same distance.

With your eyes closed, draw an infinity sign on your imaginary paper near or far with your magic nose marker. Through the center of the infinity sign draw a vertical figure eight. Encompass your four-leaf clover in a circle outlining it clockwise and counterclockwise a few times in each direction. Always sign and date each drawing you make. Take a moment to gaze at your creation. Your black magic marker turns into a magic eraser and erase your drawing so your paper returns to a blank slate. Next pick another drawing, whether one of the other suggestions on the previous page or make up your own. Sign and date and admire your drawing, seeing it with perfect clarity in your mind. Erase your drawing to start again. Whatever you draw, make sure the lines appear perfectly crisp, clear, and black against a bright white background. Maybe you want to try other colors, or draw things floating in midair instead. Make sure you are still drawing either close up if farsighted and far away if nearsighted. Sign and date your nose drawing. Admire and erase. Repeat.

Another beneficial aspect of nose drawing is that the subtle movements you make with your head help to stimulate and relax your first two vertebrae in your cervical spine, the axis and the atlas. This is the place where your spinal cord connects to your brain stem, which is associated with your limbic system. The limbic system plays a large part in how the auntonomic nervous system responds to stress and anxiety, with one of the reactions being the sympathetic 'fight or flight' response. Nose drawing helps trigger the parasympathetic 'rest and relaxation' response instead, which will help your eyes and mind calm down to allow for easier and clearer vision.

Light Therapy

Once you complete your first five relaxation practices in bed, you can get out of bed and feed your eyes their breakfast: sunlight. Before learning and trying the sunning practice though, make sure you read this to learn how light affects sight and begin overcoming any mental resistance or fear of light.

Your eyes are the only organs in the body constituted to receive light. Receiving light is the primary purpose of your eyes, and if there is any resistance, fear, or discomfort in the process of receiving light, that is an indication that there is something fundamentally out of balance with the visual system. Before improving any other visual issue, you must overcome light sensitivity. The best way to overcome light sensitivity is by repeating the next practice called sunning, where you gradually begin exposing your closed eyes to bright light in tiny doses in a safe, gentle, and comfortable way. The better your eyes get at handling bright light in a relaxed way, the better they will do at all their other functions, including seeing.

It is true that excessive exposure to sunlight can be harmful. Anyone who has stayed out in the sun too long without protection knows from experience that the sun can burn the skin, and prolonged exposure over many years can increase the chances of developing certain types of skin cancers. Likewise, overexposure to sunlight through the eyes can burn the retinas and increase the chances of developing cataracts or other vision problems. The takeaway is this though: just because something in excess is harmful does not mean it needs to be avoided altogether. Not getting enough sunlight is just as bad as getting too much sunlight.

> *"It is not light but darkness that is dangerous to the eye. Prolonged exclusion from the light always lowers the vision and may produce serious inflammatory conditions."*
>
> *-Dr. William H. Bates*

The retina, which is the inside 2/3 of the back of your eyeball, is lined with millions of photoreceptor cells, or light sensitive nerves. These rods and cones require stimulation by light and begin to perish if they do not receive the type of light they need. Full-spectrum sunlight is the highest quality of light. Artificial light from electric bulbs and screens is a lower quality light because it is only a limited sliver of the visible light spectrum. The eyes need a balance of the entire visible light spectrum, plus a trace amount of the invisible light spectrum that is unperceivable to the human eye, including ultraviolet and infrared. The key is balance; you do not want to get too much, and you do not want to get not enough.

While sunglasses can act as helpful tools to protect your eyes from overexposure to light, when they are worn too much they actually lead to light sensitivity, weaken the eyes, and begin the eyes down the road toward poorer vision by decreasing their ability to perform their number one function: receiving light. The more you wear sunglasses, the less you can handle bright light, and soon you will not be able to leave the house without them. Some people even need to wear sunglasses on cloudy or overcast days, or at night in artificial light. Often times light sensitivity is actually caused by the fear of light rather than by the light itself. If this is the case, by changing your mind and understanding of how crucial light is for sight, you can begin improving your relationship with the life-providing sun. You may use sunglasses when driving or when you need protection for long hours outdoors but try to use lightly tinted or yellow tinted ones rather than darkly tinted ones.

Sunlight is like food for your eyes. Sunlight stimulates the optic nerves, which are some of the largest nerves in the entire body. Sunlight revitalizes the retinal nerves, the rods and cones. Sunlight regulates your lacrimal glands for healthy and natural tear production, preventing dryness, redness, and itchiness. Sunlight speeds up the reproduction of visual purple, which is a visual pigment in the retinas that aids night vision. Sunlight speeds up the transition from light to dark by activating the involuntary muscles of the iris to constrict and dilate the pupil appropriately. Sunlight relaxes all the muscles, tendons, and nerves of the entire body. Sunlight opens up all the channels of your eyes to improve blood flow, lymph flow, and energy flow. Most importantly, sunlight soothes tense minds. If you are feeling stressed or anxious, your mental state can be immediately improved by letting the warm rejuvenating sunlight shine upon your face. The sun can be the best medicine for the eyes, if used responsibly.

When you starve your eyes and cut them off from their essential environmental nutrient, light sensitivity is not the only negative side effect. Eyes that do not get enough light are dim of vision, with sluggish optic nerves, and slow replacement of visual purple. The shock associated with brightness to a light-sensitive eye tightens all the muscles of the eyes and constricts circulation, which may even produce pain or discomfort, which wrongly perpetuates the mistaken belief that light ought to be avoided. In short, lack of light can lead to a condition known as 'mal-illumination'.

Mal-illumination

n. an environmental condition characterized by a lack of full-spectrum light.

Dr. John Ott, the father of photobiology, inventor of the full-spectrum light bulb, and pioneer of time-lapse photography, coined the term 'mal-illumination' to explain the negative mental and physical health implications that come from a lack of exposure to sunlight. Like the similar word malnutrition, which refers to the negative physical and mental health implications that come from a lack of proper diet and nutrition, mal-illumination can have some significant and serious effects on the human body and mind.

Through his years of scientific experiments with vegetation, flowers, and lab mice, Dr. Ott proved that a trace amount of full-spectrum ultraviolet light from its source, the sun, is essential not only for optimal health but also for the regulation of the involuntary functions and rhythms of the entire organism. Flowers that were secluded from the sun and exposed to only artificial light fell out synch with their natural bloom cycles or failed to bloom at all. Mice that were secluded from the sun and exposed to only specific wavelengths of artificial light became lethargic and developed tumors. Dr. Ott did not limit these findings to plants and animals; he claimed that humans were affected in similar ways.

The amount of light and darkness you experience throughout the day influences the release of hormones that induce sleep, initiate waking, and set your circadian rhythms. Sunlight is food for your eyes. They need a minimum daily dose of sunlight to be optimally healthy. If your daily does falls below the minimum, not only will your vision begin to diminish, but your mental health may plummet as well. Depression, obesity, and disease can all be rooted in a basic lack of sunlight. Some people who live far from the equator and go many months in a row with little to no sunlight experience Seasonal Affect Disorder, or SAD, which is often treated by using one of Dr. Ott's full-spectrum 'sunlamps.'

Human eyes have evolved over millennia under the full-spectrum ultraviolet light from the sun. Only in recent times have we waged war against the life-providing orb in the sky after being told by medical professionals to avoid it at all cost. As you will see, however, light is necessary for sight.

Eliminating any type of light sensitivity or fear of light is essential for regaining normal eyesight. Do not starve your eyes of what they need to see - vitamin D. The Institute of Ophthalmology at University College London published research in the journal *Neurobiology of Aging* in 2012 that "...found vitamin D reduces the effects of aging in mouse eyes and improves vision of older mice significantly." Further research suggests that getting 14 hours of sunshine a week can help prevent myopia development in children. Keep in mind though that adults need the sun just as much as children do. How many hours a day do you spend outdoors? If it is less than two, make a conscious effort to increase it. If you go to a playground you will see little kids happily playing in bright sunlight and almost all the adults wearing sunglasses. UVB light, or ultraviolet B rays, play a role in the cellular production of vitamin D, which helps the eyes focus light on the retina. Many people are vitamin D deficient. It can be taken in the form of Vitamin D3 supplements or in its natural form from direct sunlight shining on the skin or indirectly entering through the eyes.

Biomimicry is a term for mimicking nature and working with, instead of against fundamental laws of nature. When you look to nature for guidance on this topic, almost every living thing on Earth thrives on sunlight. Plants and flowers face toward the sun. Reptiles, birds, and mammals all depend on sunlight. Animals that live underground and fish that dwell in the ocean depths where light does not penetrate are blind. Donkeys that were used to work in coalmines lost their vision after working in the dark caves, but then regained it once they emerged and were returned to live in sunny fields once more. Most animals with eyes need the sun to see and function. We human animals are no exception.

There are simple ways to take in this daily dose of sunshine safely and efficiently. The simplest and most direct way is by 'sunning' your eyes as described in the next practice. If you do have any type of light sensitivity or aversion toward the sun just take it slow. If direct sunlight is too bright at first, try standing in the shade of a tree and the light will get filtered through the leaves and branches. If that is still too bright, try sunning indoors facing a window. If that is still too bright, you will be better off starting with a sunlamp instead, to give you more control over the intensity of the light. Incandescent or full-spectrum lights are the only types of light bulbs you want to use for indoor sunning. You can start with a dim incandescent light bulb, and gradually work your way all the way up to 75, 100, or 150 watts. My favorite sunlamp is a 150-watt incandescent flood light that screws into a porcelain clamp. Incandescent is the best because it not only provides a nice warm colored light, but it also produces heat, which emulates the sun. Sun your eyes gently and frequently in small short doses. Follow the rules of sunning: a little bit often, palm twice as long, and always let comfort be your guide. It is not advised to look directly at the sun with your eyes open. Do not confuse the Bates Method sunning with sun gazing, which is the practice of gazing directly at the sun for long periods of time. Getting the light indirectly by sunning with your eyes closed the whole time is just as efficient and is safer.

"Be gentle about it; do not rush out and attempt to stare into the heavens. You should never stare, least of all at the sun. Instead, lessen the shock of contrast by accustoming the eyes to light in easy stages."

-Margaret Corbett

In addition to repeating your specific sunning practice once or twice a day, try gradually spending more time outdoors in general without wearing sunglasses, prescription glasses, or contact lenses. Wear a wide-brimmed hat instead, which will provide shade and protection from direct light, but will still allow the absorption of indirect light reflecting off of objects around you. If you are driving or plan on spending many hours outdoors, it is okay to use sunglasses for protection to avoid overexposure. However, for short periods of time outside, start to try walking around without them and also without squinting. The end goal is to be able to be outdoors on a brilliant sunny day and keep your eyes totally relaxed.

If you have any type of aversion toward the sun or fear of the sun harming you, trace back to the root of that feeling. Sometimes the fear of the sun comes from a bad childhood experience of sunburn or sun poisoning. Perhaps the fear is fueled by misinformation from the optical and sunscreen industries. It is true that overexposure to the sun can damage the skin and the eyes. However, just because something is harmful in excess does not mean it must be avoided altogether. This idea applies to many things in our world. An excess of anything can be harmful. Drinking too much water can be fatal, but that doesn't mean to stop drinking water. Dehydration is fatal too. Moderation is key here, and finding a balance between too much light and not enough light is up to you based on your own experience and comfort level. Sunning helps you redefine your relationship with the sun and changes your perception of the sun from a harmful enemy to a vision-sustaining friend. Sunshine instills deep relaxation into the muscles, tendons, and nerves surrounding the eyes very efficiently, so it doesn't take much at all. A little bit of sunshine goes a long way. Start small and gradually increase the length of your sunning sessions, without ever going overboard.

You can even sun your eyes on a cloudy day. This is called 'clouding'. The healing light from the sun that filters through the clouds is still more beneficial on an overcast day than what you get from using an artificial sunlamp indoors. Artificial lights may be used in replacement of the sun if you are light sensitive or if environmental conditions make it difficult to get enough sunlight. Starting every single day with a short sunning session is a perfect way to wake your eyes up, get them ready for a full day of vision, and to lighten your mind for a positive and bright day ahead.

Sunning

Purpose:

- Reduce photophobia (fear of light) and photosensitivity (sensitivity to light).
- Stimulate and revitalize the rods and cones on the retina.
- Retrain the ciliary muscles and iris to constrict and dilate the pupil properly.
- Relax nerves, tendons, muscles and mind.
- Activate the visual system.
- Remedy for red, dry, or itchy eyes.
- Reduce inflammation, swelling, or pressure in and around the eyes.
- Increase circulation to shoulders, neck, head, face, and eyes.
- Open tear ducts and regulate tear glands.
- Brighten the eyes.

Directions: *(<u>always follow the rules for sunning and times for sunning on next page</u>)*

1) Face the sun, clouds, or sunlamp with closed eyes.
2) Slowly pivot your head side to side, keeping your eyes and face totally relaxed.
3) Turn left enough to shade left eye and turn right enough to shade right eye.
4) Continue for as long as is comfortable.
5) Palm for the same amount of time you sunned for.
6) Sun your closed eyes a little more after palming to readjust to the light.

Time: 30 seconds to 10 minutes, 1 or 2 times a day.

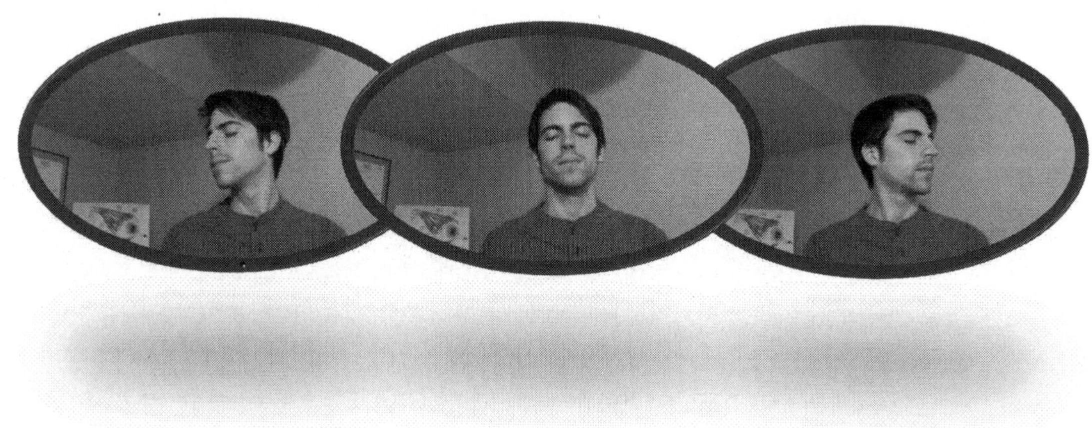

There are additional advanced sun drills that are not included in this book because they must be taught directly by a certified Bates Method teacher. Feel free to contact me to schedule an online or in-person vision training lesson to learn the advanced sun drills.

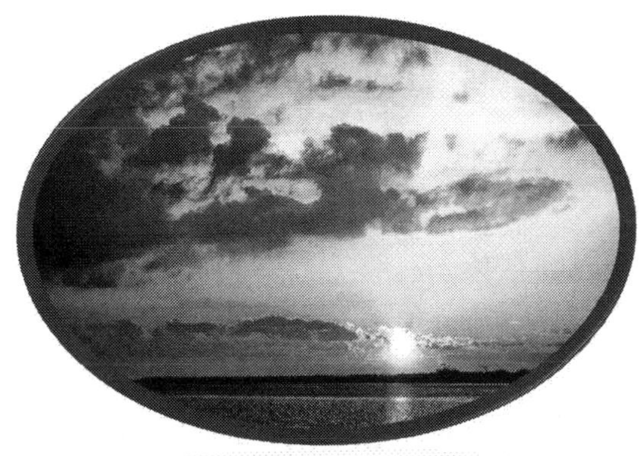

Rules for Sunning

1. **Always let comfort be your guide** – listen to your own body, don't sun too much.
2. **A little bit often** – take the sun in tiny doses rather than a lot all at once.
3. **Always palm your eyes** for as long or twice as long as you sun.
4. **Never stare directly at the sun** with your eyes open.

Times for Sunning

Depending on where you live, sunning between 6:00 to 9:00 am in the morning, or 4:00 to 7:00 pm in the evening is ideal. The closer the sun is to the horizon the better. Morning and evening are the best times for sunning because the sun is less intense with a lower UV index, plus you won't have to tilt your head as far back when the sun is lower in the sky. Aim as close to sunrise or sunset if possible. If you can only sun mid-day, don't do it for as long since the sun is brighter, hotter, and has a higher UV index.

"We are all light deficient and this deficiency may be the source of our physical and emotional problems."

-Dr. John Ott

Description:

Sunning is the most basic way to gently teach you how to accept and receive bright light safely and easily. Sunning is like feeding your eyes their primary food source: light. Simply face toward the sun with your eyes closed and pivot your head side-to-side. Keep your chin lifted as you breathe deeply and rhythmically. Coordinate your breath and movement. Optionally, you can lift your eyebrows without opening your eyes, which thins your eyelids and allows even more light to pass through them. Since your eyes are closed, you are not allowing any light directly into your eyes. Even though the light that penetrates through your eyelids is indirect light, it still stimulates and activates the photoreceptor cells in your retina that feed off of light: rods and cones.

Do not squint your eyes or furrow your brow. Lift your eyebrows while you keep your eyes closed. Do not resist the light. Receive the light into your body through your closed eyes. Make sure you pivot your head far enough in each direction to shade whichever eye is facing away from the sun and stretch your neck muscles. With repetition this will retrain the involuntary muscle components of the iris to respond correctly to varying light levels. Your pupils will be constricting and dilating in response to your head movements. Increasing the flexibility and response of your iris will allow your eyes to remain relaxed in all light levels and can also contribute to your eyes' ability to focus better. The ultimate goal is to be able to be outside on a bright sunny day without sunglasses, without feeling the urge to squint or strain.

Another dynamic of this practice is to incorporate *oppositional movement*. As you slowly swing your head left to right begin to notice that the sun appears to move in the opposite direction your head moves. It will be fairly simple to imagine the oppositional movement of the sun while your eyes are closed due to the change in brightness as you pivot your head.

You can sun your eyes standing or sitting for anywhere between 30 seconds and 10 minutes close to sunrise and sunset. Not only will sunning benefit your eyes, but it will also give you your daily dose of Vitamin D, the sunshine vitamin. Oil glands in the skin all over your body secrete *ergosteral*, which reacts with sunshine to produce Vitamin D naturally. Deficiency in Vitamin D is very common so make sure to sun your eyes regularly to help get your levels up while recharging and refreshing your eyes and mind. Sunning at sunrise and sunset helps set your internal clocks and circadian rhythms. It helps keep your body and mind balanced and in tune with nature. Sunning can be a very peaceful and centering practice, and happens to be my personal favorite vision practice.

Palming

Purpose:

- Rest and relax the eyes and mind.
- Soothe the optic nerves.
- Improve imagination, visualization, and memory.
- Improve mental focus and attention.
- Increase circulation to the eyes.

Directions:

1) Rub your hands together briskly to warm up your palms.
2) Rest your elbows on a soft and stable surface, keeping spine erect.
3) Cross the fingers of one hand over the fingers of the other hand on your forehead.
4) Place your palms over your eyes without touching them or applying any pressure.
5) Adjust your hands as necessary to block out all the light.
6) Breathe deeply and begin any one of your favorite mental focusing practices.
7) Do not stare while you palm. Let your eyes move freely in response to the movement of your thoughts.

Time: 30 seconds to 30+ minutes, 3 to 10 times a day.

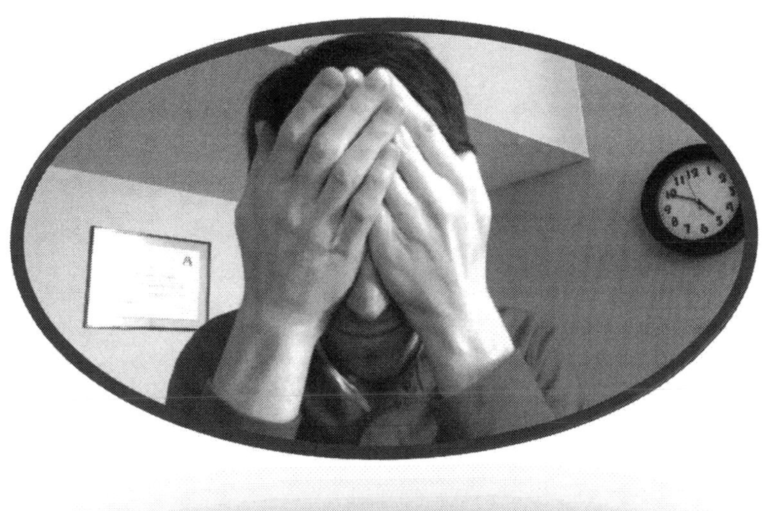

You probably overwork your eyes. If your feet get tired you search for a seat to rest them. But when your eyes get tired you watch television, play on your phone, or read a book. Modern lifestyles may even demand overuse of the eyes. However, a little rest often goes a long way and prevents exhaustion and fatigue.

Palming is one of the most important and beneficial forms of relaxation in the Bates Method. The warmth of your hands relaxes the six muscles around each eye and attracts more energy and blood flow. The darkness relaxes the ciliary muscles, retina, and optic nerves. The palms contain dozens of nerves, which can create an electromagnetic connection with your optic nerve bundles when you place your palms directly over your eyes. Your eyes work by contrast between light and dark. Palming helps balance out the amount of light and darkness you get. While in the darkness your eyes are reconstituting a visual pigment called *rhodopsin* or visual purple, which is produced in the dark and helps your night vision.

Palming can greatly enhance your performance as well. If you sprinkle mini palming breaks into your daily tasks, you will tire less easily and maintain steady energy levels. After each chapter you read, palm your eyes and mentally go over what you just learned. At work, palm every hour for a few minutes and watch your productivity soar.

It is very important to find a comfortable and sustainable position to palm in. Your back ought to remain supported and maintain its natural curvature. You don't want your head to thrust forward or back, but to be lined up with your backbone. You don't want to be tight or uncomfortable anywhere because that will constrict your blood flow. Do not let the weight of your head press into your hands. No pressure ought to be applied to the eyes. If lying down you can place a large blanket or pillow under your arms to support them. If seated in a chair you can hinge at your hips and rest your elbows on your knees, a desk or a table with blankets or pillows under them for comfort and finding the perfect height. Experiment with finding your favorite position to palm in so you can maintain comfort and focus for several minutes at a time.

The best position of the hands for palming is to lay the four fingers of one hand over the four fingers of your other hand on your forehead at an angle that allows for easy breathing through your nose. The heels of your hands ought to be gently touching your cheekbones. Make any adjustments to allow your cupped palms to rest completely over your eye orbits and block out 100% of the light. It is quite remarkable how perfectly your palms can fit over your eye orbits, like they were made for this application. Take time to find your perfect fit. No pressure ought to be put on your eyes so they remain free to be open or closed, to blink, and move around in all directions. Applying too much pressure will constrict blood flow, so you want to very gently rest your hands on your face. Look around inside your palming caves to see if there are any light leaks and adjust your hands accordingly without constricting your breath. Once there is no light coming through any cracks you can close your eyes and begin a mental focusing practice of your choosing.

Palming itself is one of the most physically relaxing practices, but it is even more important to be focusing and relaxing your mind while palming your eyes. Palming loses its beneficial affects if the mind is not relaxed or focused. Palming your eyes is useless if your mind runs wild or stresses out. Learning how to harness your mind and get better at playing mental pictures in your head while you palm is one of the most important skills you will learn from this book and will lead to the biggest improvements in your vision. I want to reemphasize the importance of the mental side of this practice. Each time you palm is a new opportunity for you to access the mental side of seeing, activate your insight, replay a pleasant happy memory, go to your happy place, or imagine clear things near, far, and everywhere. In order to see clearly on the outside, you must learn to see clearly on the inside.

Since palming is such an important practice, it is recommended that you do it several times a day, especially when first starting your vision practice. Anytime throughout the day when you get a chance you can easily palm your eyes to rest them. There is no maximum time limit for palming. I encourage everyone improving their own eyesight to try palming for 30 to 60 minutes while listening to music or an audio book to experience maximum benefits. It takes between 2 and 5 minutes for your optic nerve to fully relax so if you are only palming for 1 or 2 minutes you may not achieve the full results. However, even palming for 30 seconds can be enough to reset your visual system and help you tune in with the sensation of relaxation. Make it a fun challenge to see how long you can palm.

"Palm, if your eyes are tired. Palm, if your eyes hurt. Palm, if a headache threatens. Just as strained eyes sap the vitality and drain the nervous system, so relaxing the eyes sends ease and relaxation throughout the entire body, resuscitating and rejuvenating tense nerves and tired muscles."

-Margaret D. Corbett

Mental Focus #3: Picturing Black

The previous section describes how to get into a physical palming posture. This is only the first step. The second step is mental palming. Physical palming can be beneficial on its own, but if your mind is wandering freely, going through to-do lists, wondering what's for dinner, or stressing about anything at all it defeats the purpose of palming. Remember that your vision is 90% mental and 10% physical. So how can you achieve the greatest relaxation and benefit from palming? By giving your mind something to focus on. There are several different mental focusing practices you may use to help keep your mind focused while palming. Each chapter of this book will provide you with a new mental focus practice.

While palming after sunning, it helps to visualize the color black in order to balance out taking in the bright light. The color black is soothing to your optic nerves and mind. The retinas need a balance between light and dark. Darkness prompts the production of *rhodopsion* or *visual purple*, a visual pigment that allows for night vision. While sunning in the bright light your cones are activated and allow for aspects of vision like fine details, central vision, and colors. When you palm and picture the color black your rods are activated and visual purple is produced. It can take several minutes for your optic nerve to relax. If you do not see blackness at first, it is because your optic nerves are still active. Keep palming until a deeper shade of black can be imagined. The level of blackness can be an indicator of your relaxation level. Pure black represents mental relaxation and focus, while lack of total blackness indicates mental strain or lack of mental focus. Picturing black can be both a means to relaxation and a result of relaxation.

Start by simply thinking of the color black spreading across your entire visual field. Since you are literally blocking out all external light, any remaining colors, shades, shapes, or images are simply products of your mind. They are being produced from the inside, not from the outside. Since your mind is projecting your inner vision, by focusing your mind on the color black you will be able to 'see' the color black more and more. If just picturing the color black is difficult try to picture familiar objects that are black like a black dog, black cat, black hat, black pants, black car, black umbrella, black jacket, etc. The object you choose to picture does not matter as much as your ability to imagine it the darkest black you possibly can. Some people succeed by thinking about touching black silk or satin, while other people succeed by imagining spilling black ink or black paint spreading out in all directions.

Dr. Bates wrote extensively on picturing a tiny black dot. To experiment with that while palming, begin by picturing a tiny vertical black line, only a few centimeters tall. Shift your mental attention from the top of the vertical line to the bottom of the vertical line. Even though your eyes are palmed and closed, you ought to still feel them moving in response to the movement of your thoughts. Shift up and down rapidly without any effort. It takes effort to consciously move your eyes, but no effort to move your mind or attention. Next, picture a horizontal line a few centimeters long going through the center of the vertical line, creating a plus sign. Shift your mind back and forth from the left side to the right side of the horizontal line quickly. Next, rotate the plus sign on its side so it creates an X. Rapidly shift your mind diagonally up and diagonally down in both directions. Next, draw a circle encompassing the X and trace the outline of the circle clockwise and counterclockwise. Finally, close the circle in so all that remains is a tiny black dot. Do not stare at the black dot. Continue to shift mentally up and down, side to side, diagonally, or circularly. Imagine taking that tiny black dot with you everywhere you go. Wherever you look, you can remember or imagine shifting on a tiny black dot upon the surface of the object you gaze at.

Vision Work #3

Repeat your morning relaxation routine of stretching and yawning, tapping, acupressure points, eyebrow raises/tense and release, and nose drawing before you even get out of bed. Right after you get out of bed, either step outside to sun your eyes, sun your eyes through an open or closed window, or use your indoor sun lamp to do a short light therapy session. Follow your sunning practice with an equal amount of time palming your eyes practicing a mental focus technique to develop your memory, imagination, and visualization skills. Within 5 or 10 minutes you have already completed your first vision routine of the day. Repeat any of these relaxation techniques whenever you need to later in your morning, afternoon, evening, or night. Feed your eyes some sort of light every day, whether outside in the sun, inside through a window, or inside with a light bulb.

Remember that a little bit goes a long way so don't overdo it. Start small and slowly work your way up. The first week only sun for one minute, the second week sun for two minutes, the third week for three minutes, etc. Always palm after you sun and always let comfort be your guide.

Daily Vision Practice Checklist Week 3

M Tu W Th F S Su			
☐☐☐☐☐☐☐		Morning Relaxation Routine	3-6 minutes
☐☐☐☐☐☐☐		Sunning	1-3 minutes
☐☐☐☐☐☐☐		Palming & Mental Focus	2-6 minutes
		Daily Target:	***5-15 mins***

Vision Journal: ____

____

____

____

____

____

"Remember that you don't have to do every single practice every single day. Success is more about the good vision habits you learn from the practices, and learning how to maintain them in between your practices."

-Nathan T. Oxenfeld

"There are as many hours in the day to use the eyes well as to use the eyes badly."

-Dr. William H. Bates

Chapter 4

Phase 1.2:

Relaxation Foundations

Movement – Blinking, Shifting, Swinging

"The world moves. Let it move. All objects move if you let them. Do not interfere with this movement, or try to stop it. This cannot be done without an effort which impairs the efficiency of the eye and mind."

-Dr. William H. Bates

In **Chapter 3** you began establishing your daily vision routine with a handful of basic relaxation practices to begin replacing eyestrain with relaxation. Once your tight eye muscles begin to relax in response to your overall physical and mental relaxation, the next step is to get them to start moving more. Most people with blurry vision or vision problems have tight, tense eyes that lack movement and have the tendency to stare or freeze.

Staring is one of the worst vision habits and goes directly against the nature of the eye. Unlike other parts of the body that rest when you stop moving them, the eyes are actually most rested and relaxed when in a state of movement. The lack of movement, or staring, leads to strain and tension and lowers the eyesight. The way the eyes stay focused is by constantly adjusting and moving from one point to another. So that will be your next objective in this process, to get your eyes to start moving more freely, effortlessly, and automatically through the practices of blinking, swinging, and shifting.

There are two types of staring: unconscious and conscious. Unconscious staring is when you park your eyes on an object and let your mind wander, or daydream. Your mind travels back into the past or forward into the future, and they are totally disconnected from what your eyes are looking at. You are spacing out or zoning out and your eyes freeze. Conscious staring is when you hold your eyes at the same focal distance for too long, but your mind remains actively focused on what you are looking at. Examples of conscious staring include near work like reading a book, writing a letter, working on a computer, or staring at any other type of screen like a smartphone, tablet, laptop, or television. Eyes crave movement and adjustment and become very unhappy and uncomfortable if you force them to stay stuck at the same distance for too long. Make sure that you give your eyes what they crave: regular and frequent blinking, movement, shifting, and adjusting to various different distances from near, to middle, to far.

When I learned how important motion, movement, and shifting were to obtaining healthier eyes, it actually stressed me out at first. I wondered, "How am I going to get anything done if I have to spend all day constantly moving my eyes around?" That was before I learned that the shifting is supposed to be involuntary, not a conscious effort. So, do not think that you have to be consciously moving your eyes around 24/7. Know that the more you relax your eyes using the practices from the previous chapter, and the more you repeat the practices contained in this chapter, your eyes will reawaken to their natural state of easy movement and they will begin moving a lot more on their own without you controlling them.

Butterfly Blinking

Purpose:

- Encourage more frequent and proper blinking habits.
- Cleanse the cornea and surface of the eye.
- Instill deep and rhythmic abdominal breathing to oxygenate the eyes.

Directions:

1) Take deep belly breaths with eyes closed *(instructions on Page 245).*
2) On your long slow inhale, blink blink blink softly and rapidly.
3) Close your eyes after your inhale, pivot head side to side as you exhale.
4) Repeat 10 times.

Time: 1 to 2 minutes.

"When an effort is made to stop blinking, whether successful or not, the vision is always lowered. When the eyes are permitted to blink regularly, easily, continuously, the vision is usually benefited."

–Dr. William H. Bates

Are you still following the 13 Rules of Relaxed Reading from Page 12-13?

How is your posture? How are the muscles in your face, eyes, and brow? How is your breathing? How is your blinking? Are you stopping at the end of every few sentences to close your eyes and picture the last word you read clearly? Are you looking off into the distance every so often? Can you see an imaginary bright white line underlining the sentences as you read? Can you imagine a bright white line underlining these words with your eyes closed?

Description:

Blinking, although simple, is crucial for healthy eyes. The average blink rate is between 15 and 30 blinks per minute, or once every 2 to 4 seconds, which can add up to 1,200 blinks an hour or 28,800 blinks a day. Where do you stack up against the average? Do you blink more or less? Are you even aware of how little or how often you blink? Start to pay more attention to it, and consciously start blinking more. Did you know it is possible to blink a right way and a wrong way? The wrong way is labored, heavy, and effortful where you squeeze the eye shut tight and involve other facial muscles. The right way is soft, easy, and effortless where your vision is barely interrupted and your eyelid muscle works independently. This blinking practice is called butterfly blinking because I want you to think about your upper eyelid moving as soft and fluttery as a butterfly's wing when it flies. Think about your upper eyelid lowering down to give your lower eyelid a tiny little kiss, and then lifting back up immediately.

Breathing in and out through the nose allows your belly to contract on the exhale and expand on the inhale. Feel free to rest one or both hands on your belly to feel the movement more. Now as you inhale through your nose and expand your abdomen, gently lift and lower your upper eyelids in quick, fluttery motions. Try blinking 3 to 6 times per second throughout your entire inhale. At the top of your inhale close your eyes. Keep your eyes closed as you exhale out of your mouth making an exaggerated 'sigh' noise, pivoting your head gently side to side. Repeat this 5 to 10 times: inhale and blink, blink, blink, close your eyes, exhale and pivot your head left to right.

This practice will encourage you to breathe from your belly more throughout the rest of the day and it will greatly increase your oxygen intake. The eyes need sufficient oxygen to function properly and this is a great way to ensure they do. Most of the action of a blink is in the upper eyelid. This drill helps bring more awareness to the eyelids and blinking movements. Most people do not blink enough which leads to staring, dried out, and tired eyes. Each blink is a tiny resting period for the eyes and also breaks the stare by shifting your visual attention. Blinking helps clean the surface of the eyes and corneas, wiping away any debris from the environment like dust, dirt, or other foreign objects.

Remember how yawning several times made your eyes feel nice and lubricated? Well this gentle blinking drill helps spread all that fresh fluid around the surface of the eyes and keep your eyes nice and refreshed. The more lubricated your eyes are with a complete tear film, the better they will see.

Eyerise & Eyeset

Purpose:

- Relax the blinking muscles in your eyelids.
- Relax your eyes and your mind.
- Coordinate your eyes and your breath.
- Connect your eyes and your mind.

Directions:

1) Close your eyes and begin belly breathing *(instructions on Page 245).*
2) Very slowly lift your eyelids up as you inhale until your eyes are open.
3) Very slowly lower your eyelids down as you exhale until your eyes are closed.
4) Keep coordinating your breath and eyelids, going as slow as you can.

Time: 1 to 2 minutes.

Description:

The muscle that elevates your upper eyelid is called the *levator palpebrae superioris* muscle. You may associate blinking with the act of closing your eyes, but this muscle is actually responsible for opening your eyes. When you blink, this muscle temporarily inactivates as the upper eyelid meets the lower eyelid, and then reactivates to lift the upper eyelid back up. Just like breathing, blinking can be both involuntary and voluntary. By consciously controlling the blink with a few blinking practices, you can influence a more rhythmic and regular blinking pattern to maintain itself without you thinking about it.

This eyerise and eyeset practice is designed to help teach you how to blink properly and gently. Normally your blinks are extremely rapid. By slowing down the blink and coordinating it with belly breathing, you can retrain your blinking muscles to act without strain or effort. Even when you speed your blinks back up to the normal rate, remember the fluidity and softness you felt during the eyerise and eyeset. An average healthy blink rate is once every 3 to 5 seconds, or 12 to 20 times a minute. If you realize you're blinking less than that, try resetting your blinking pattern by blinking once every 5 seconds a few times, then every 4 seconds a few times, then every 3 seconds, every 2 seconds, every second, and every half second. Try to maintain the rhythm that feels best for your eyes.

Picket Fence Shifter

Purpose:

- Loosen tight extrinsic eye muscles.
- Loosen tight head, neck, and shoulder muscles.
- Invite the eyes to shift more rapidly and subtly.
- Increase saccadic eye movements.
- Break the habit of staring.

Directions:

1) Move your shifter left to right, pivot your head oppositely.
2) Repeat 10 times eyes open and 10 times eyes closed.
3) Move your shifter up and down, pivot your head oppositely.
4) Repeat 10 times eyes open and 10 times eyes closed.
5) Move your shifter diagonally one way, pivot your head oppositely.
6) Repeat 10 times eyes open and 10 times eyes closed.
7) Move your shifter diagonally the other way, pivot oppositely.
8) Repeat 10 times eyes open and 10 times eyes closed.

Time: 1 to 4 minutes.

Picket fence shifter as one sheet.

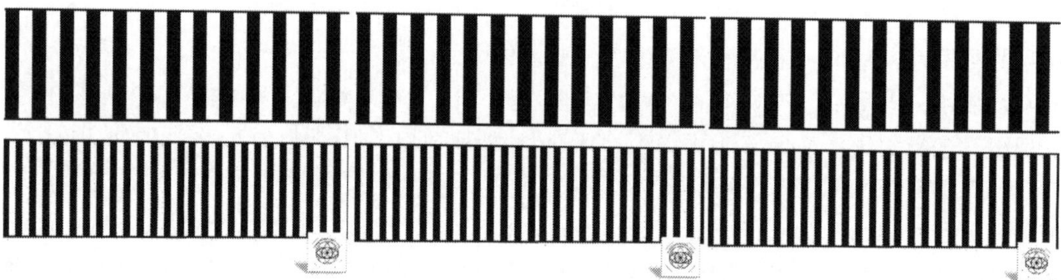

Multiple picket fence shifters taped together.

Description:

You can use your picket fence shifter *(Page 307)* as one page, but the longer your picket fence shifter the more your eyes will shift. Mount two or three copies of the picket fence onto a poster board or cardboard to make it sturdier. Regardless of length, it is very effective in getting your eyes to shift more. The micro movements of your eyes are called 'saccades', and you are using the pickets to increase the rate of saccadic eye movements. Don't try to focus on the picket fence shifter - just let it slide by effortlessly in the opposite direction that your head is pivoting. The pickets should not all just blur into one gray blob passing by though, so experiment to find the best distance to hold the picket fence shifter from your face and the perfect speed to move the pickets in order to feel the most saccades.

When you move the shifter horizontally, pivot your head right to left in the opposite direction. When you pivot the shifter vertically, pivot your head up and down oppositely. When you pivot the shifter diagonally, pivot your head diagonally in the opposite direction. The more you practice the more you will be able to feel the subtle sensation of your eyes shifting rapidly. It's almost like they're making little jumps or jerks. Normal eyes can vibrate up to 50-100 times per second, and the picket fence shifter is the best way to encourage these micro-movements and vibrations. Closing your eyes and remembering the pickets passing by in your mind helps strengthen your memory and visualization. You may even be able to feel the saccadic eye movements happening beneath your closed eyelids. The gentle pivoting of your head in the opposite direction of the picket fence helps loosen up tight neck muscles and increase circulation to your face, head, neck, shoulders, and eyes.

- Pivoting horizontally loosens the two recti muscles on the left and right of each eye.
- Pivoting vertically loosens the two recti muscles on the top and bottom of each eye.
- Pivoting diagonally in each direction loosens the two oblique muscles that wrap around the middle of each eye.

Unlike conscious eye movements, the picket fence shifter promotes unconscious, involuntary eye movements. This helps relax and retrain the involuntary muscles in and around the eyes. Increased movement of the head and eyes also stimulates the movement and replenishment of the fluids inside the eyes. The main goals of the picket fence shifter are to get your eyes shifting more, to loosen tight eye muscles, to experience oppositional movement, and to relax your eyes and mind. Always palm your eyes after using your picket fence shifter. You can also look for real picket fences, railings, blinds, or other actual objects to access the saccadic eye shifting throughout your day if you don't have your shifter.

The Long Swing / Body Swing

Purpose:

- Create a sense of motion and become aware of *oppositional movement.*
- Increase circulation and lymph flow to the entire body and eyes.
- Increase movement and shifting of the eyes.
- Break the habit of staring.
- Loosen tight eye muscles.
- Relax voluntary and involuntary muscle systems.
- Loosen all vertebrae, relax inner organs.
- Bring ease to entire nervous system.
- Activate the *fovea centralis*, encourage flashes of clear vision.
- Improve memory, imagination, visualization, and balance.

Directions:

1. Stand comfortably with feet a little wider than hip's width apart.
2. Have your eye level slightly below the horizon, notice stationary objects.
3. Turn upper body 90° to the right while lifting the left heel off the ground.
4. Turn upper body 90° to the left while lifting the right heel off the ground.
5. Swing back and forth from right to left letting your eyes remain soft.
6. Repeat 10 swings with eyes open noticing the *oppositional movement.*
7. Repeat 10 swings with one arm lifted relaxing your gaze on your thumb.
8. Repeat 10 swings with eyes closed continuing to visualize *oppositional movement.*
9. Repeat steps 6-8 for 4 to 6 minutes.

Time: 1 to 6 minutes, 1 to 3 times a day.

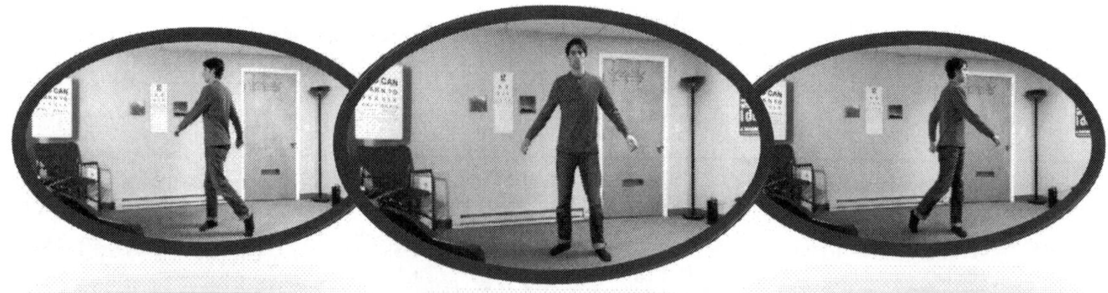

Description:

Do you remember how much fun you had playing on swing sets as a child? Think about how relaxing it is swing gently in a hammock or to sway back and forth in a rocking chair. These activities are not only fun and relaxing, but they can benefit your eyes as well.

At first the long swing may seem like a simple and repetitive movement, but there is a lot happening. The long swing increases circulation of the blood throughout the entire body, which nourishes the eye muscles, choroid, and retina. In addition to blood flow, the long swing also increases lymph flow. The lymphatic system is like the 'cleanup crew' of the body; it helps to eliminate toxins and other unwanted waste products. Did you know the human body has twice as much lymphatic fluid than blood? Whereas the circulatory system has a heart to push blood throughout the body, the lymphatic system has no such organ. Instead, lymph fluid circulates through the body via movement and gravity. Since your eyes are nourished by and contain lymphatic fluid it makes sense that if there is a lack of movement then lymphatic fluid can stagnate within the body and the eyes, which can slow down the visual process. Swinging 180 degrees not only stirs up lymph fluid, but it also encourages more subtle movements of the eyes. Normal eyes vibrate at least 3 times per second, if not many more. Vision declines when we slow down or stop that natural movement by staring. Swinging breaks the deeply ingrained habit of staring by helping to loosen up any tight muscles in and around the eyes.

The long swing is one way to turn on your 'auto-focus' because it activates your central vision. The *fovea centralis*, or central pit in the back of the retina, is your center of sight that allows you to see fine details and colors. The *fovea centralis* is filled with cones, which are stimulated and activated by movement. When you stare your center of sight does not get stimulated and you may experience blur. You can demonstrate this to yourself simply by staring at this page. If you stare at anything for too long without shifting or blinking you will begin to witness your visual field shrinking or disappearing. On the contrary, movement is the key to clarity. Flashes of clarity only come while in motion.

Like many of the Bates Method practices, the long swing is performed with eyes open and with eyes closed. The purpose of repeating the practice with the eyes closed is because vision is so much more mental than physical. Closed-eye swinging allows you to begin strengthening your memory, imagination, visualization, and even balance. In order to stay present with the practice and to avoid any dizziness while swinging with eyes closed, try to remember and visualize what you saw while swinging with your eyes open. Notice that everything appears to move in the opposite direction that your body moves. This *oppositional movement* can be noticed virtually anytime you are moving in any direction. You can experience *oppositional movement* by noticing that when you walk forward in one direction the ground appears to be moving backwards in the opposite direction. This is even more exaggerated when riding as a passenger in a car or train.

If you are nearsighted and objects appear blurry with eyes open then imagine them perfectly clear with eyes closed. There is no limit to what you can imagine. In order to see clearly with your eyes open, you must first be able to see clearly with your eyes closed by using your imagination, memory, and visualization. Do not twist or turn your head or neck while swinging. Simply rotate your shoulders, torso, and hips and allow your head and eyes go along for the ride. Do not try and focus on any one object in particular along your path. Instead, keep your eyes moving and jumping from point to point along the 180 degree path. The more you swing, the more your eyes will loosen and the more rapidly they will shift.

Continue cycling through the three steps of the long swing for four to six minutes or longer; rotating back and forth between ten swings with eyes open and arms down, ten swings with eyes open looking at your thumb, and ten swings with eyes closed and arms down. Six is the magic number because after swinging for six minutes all the muscles in the body relax, several cycles of blood circulation occur, and the entire nervous system relaxes by switching from the sympathetic nervous system, which is geared for the fight or flight stress response, to the parasympathetic nervous system, which is geared for rest and relaxation response. To finish the long swing, close your eyes and begin slowing down, making your swings shorter and shorter until you return to stillness in your own center.

If you experience any motion sickness or dizziness, try the swing seated, or modify the swing to make it more comfortable for you. Remember to take deep breaths as you swing. Oftentimes dizziness comes from trying to resist or stop the motion. Instead, accept the motion and allow everything to slide by easily. When you swing with your eyes closed it is very important to stay present and remember the sense of motion and your surroundings. This will not only prevent dizziness but it will actually improve your balance and memory. If you still experience dizziness, modify the swing further by performing it sitting down in a chair and making the movements smaller. You can also modify the swing or even make up your own type of long swing. Since movement is key, it does not matter what type of movement you do. Swings can range from a gentle sway to a square dance. Have fun with it and reconnect with the constant motion of this world.

The Medium Swing / Head Swing

Purpose:

- Loosen tight muscles in the eyes, neck and shoulders.
- Increase circulation and lymph flow to the head, neck and eyes.
- Increase the movement and shifting of the eyes.
- Strengthen memory and visualization.
- Practice observing oppositional movement.

Directions:

1) Hold your index finger 3 to 6 inches from your nose.
2) Eyes closed, pivot head left to right 5 to 10 times, imagine *oppositional movement.*
3) Eyes open, pivot your head left to right 5 to 10 times, see *oppositional movement.*
4) Repeat alternating between eyes closed and open for between 50 and 100 swings.

Time: 1 to 2 minutes.

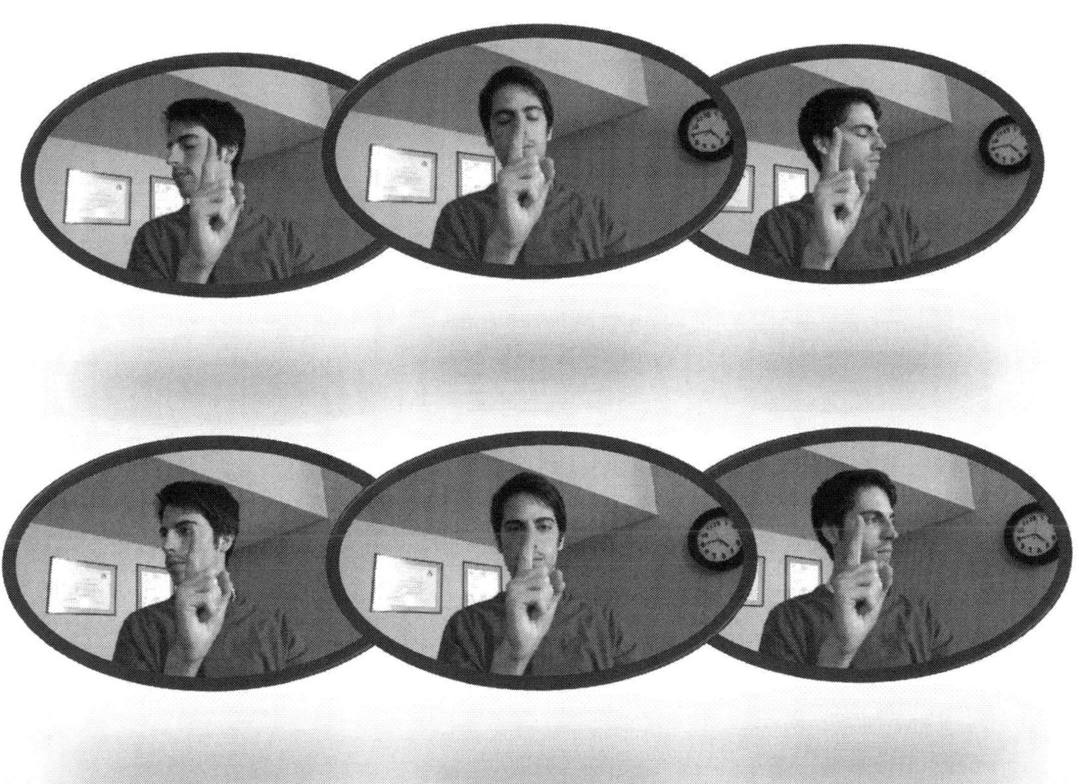

Description:

If you ever wake up with a stiff neck you will likely have stiff eyes as well. The head swing not only loosens tight neck muscles but it also loosens tight eye muscles. After practicing for a couple of minutes you will get increased circulation to your upper body, neck, head, and eyes as well as increased lymph flow. Begin with your eyes closed. Let your head sway gently side to side, pointing your nose over your left shoulder then over your right shoulder at a comfortable pace. Make sure you maintain the deep, rhythmic breathing while you swing your head left to right.

This is another experience observing what Dr. Bates called *oppositional movement,* which is the illusion that stationary objects appear to be moving in the opposite direction your head is moving. It is the same oppositional movement that you saw when doing the Long Swing, but maybe a little less pronounced since only your head is moving instead of your entire body. However, you need to still be able to perceive the illusion on a smaller scale.

When doing the head swing with your eyes closed, you can start to visualize and feel your index finger seeming to travel from cheek to cheek or ear to ear in the opposite direction that your head is moving. Holding your index finger close to your nose makes it easier to sense the *oppositional movement.*

After swinging 5 to 10 times with your eyes closed, open your eyes and swing 10 more times, looking past your finger into the distance. Notice that when you look to the left your finger is by your right cheek or ear. When you look to the right your finger is by your left cheek or ear. The next time you close your eyes it will be easier for you to remember and visualize your finger because you just witnessed it happening in front of you. Repeat the cycle of 10 times eyes closed 10 times eyes open for 1 to 2 minutes or longer if you enjoy it.

The head swing can be used anytime throughout the day, with or without holding up your finger in front of your nose, whenever your eyes feel tired or if your neck and shoulders feel tight. Let your eyes remain soft as you pivot your head and they will begin shifting more freely and rapidly, pronouncing the illusion of oppositional movement even more. Do not try to focus on anything, just practice relaxing your eyes and watching objects swing in the opposite direction of your head.

The Short Swing / Optical Swing

Purpose:

- Encourage more natural and effortless use of the eyes.
- Increase the movement and shifting of the eyes.
- Strengthen memory and visualization.
- Practice observing oppositional movement.

Directions:

1) Keep your head and body still, facing a near or far object.

2) With eyes closed think about the left side of the object, then the right side of the object. Keep wondering what the left side looks like and what the right side looks like.

3) As your attention moves from the left side to the right side, notice how your eyes automatically shift from left to right. As your attention moves from the right side to the left side, notice how that makes your eyes automatically shift from right to left.

4) As you shift from left to right, imagine the object jumping to the left slightly. As you shift from right to left, imagine the object jumping to the right slightly.

5) With eyes open look from the left side to the right side of your object and observe it appearing to jump to the left slightly. Look from the right side to the left side of your object and observe it appearing to jump to the right slightly.

6) Close your eyes and think about the top of the object, then think about the bottom of the object. Keep wondering what the top looks like and what the bottom looks like.

7) As your attention moves from the top to the bottom, notice how that makes your eyes automatically shift from up to down. As your attention moves from the bottom to the top, notice how that makes your eyes automatically shift from down to up.

8) As you shift from top to bottom, imagine the object jumping up slightly. As you shift from bottom to top, imagine the object jumping down slightly.

9) With eyes open look from the top to the bottom of your object and observe it appearing to jump up slightly. Look from the bottom to the top of your object and observe it appearing to jump down slightly.

10) Repeat going between eyes closed and open until you are able to physically see the subtle oppositional movement as well as you can imagine it mentally.

Time: 1 to 3 minutes.

Description:

The optical swing or short swing is like your eyeballs doing the long swing inside your eye sockets. Your body and head remain still, and just your eyes swing gently. If you control your eyes consciously too much, the shifting will be labored and full of effort and strain. Instead, try moving your mind first and letting your eyes follow.

"The eyes attend the thoughts." –Dr. Jerriann Taber

Utilize your own curiosity to initiate automatic, effortless eye movements. Gaze at a near or far object with your eyes open for a moment, and then close your eyes and remember it. Ask yourself, "I wonder what the left side of that object looks like?" The thought alone will make your eyes instantly point to the left without any conscious control. Let them move on their own. After looking at the left side for a few seconds, ask yourself, "I wonder what the right side of that object looks like?" The new thought impulse will make your eyes instantly point to the right without any conscious control. Even without being able to physically see the object, you can feel how your mind controls your eyes beneath your closed eyelids.

Try the same thing with your eyes open, now being able to physically see the near or far object. Are you able to allow your eyes to attend your thoughts? Move your mind, attention, and curiosity first, your eyes will follow like excited little hunters. Let your head follow the movement of your eyes if it wants to. Feel the difference between moving your mind first and letting your eyes follow versus moving your eyes first and making your mind follow.

Once you can tune into the automatic and effortless tiny short swings and shifts, see if you can begin to notice the oppositional movement on a very subtle scale. You get the most apparent oppositional movement when doing the long swing, and maybe a little less apparent oppositional movement when doing the medium swing. The oppositional movement when doing the short swing is extremely subtle. As opposed to your body moving 180 degrees, or your head moving 90 degrees, your eyes will just be shifting a few inches, centimeters, or millimeters. Therefore, the object you are short swinging on will only shift oppositely a few inches, centimeters, or millimeters. Being able to see the tiny little oppositional shifts of the objects you're shifting on is an enormously important and relaxing visual skill to develop. Don't get frustrated if you cannot see it right away. Just notice that when you centralize on the left side of the object the majority of the object is in your right peripheral field, and when you centralize on the right side of the object the majority of the object is in your left peripheral field. As you shift back and forth from the left side to the right side, the object seems to jump from your right periphery to your left periphery. That is the tiny horizontal oppositional movement.

What about vertical? Close your eyes and ask yourself, "I wonder what the top of that object looks like?" and feel your eyes automatically shift up. Then ask yourself, "I wonder what the bottom of that object looks like?" and feel your eyes automatically shift down. Some people find it easier to imagine the tiny oppositional movement mentally first, before they can see it more physically with their eyes open.

Dr. Bates said that the shorter the swing, the greater the relaxation. At first, the long swing might feel the most relaxing, and the short swing may not work as well. That is because your eye muscles might still be quite tight, and they do better at big long shifts versus these tiny micro movements. The more you practice your long swing and medium swing, the better you will get at your short swing.

Constant shifting is necessary to maintain centralization. These short shifts are refreshing to your retinas and allow you to maintain clear central vision in the fovea. The moment you lose the shifting and begin to stare at one point for too long, your retina loses its sensitivity and your central focus begins to diffuse out to your peripheral field, which leads to blurry vision.

Just remember that everything is moving all the time. On a macro scale, we exist on a constantly spinning and rotating globe hurtling through space. On a micro scale, the protons, neutrons, and electrons contained in the atoms that make up all material things are constantly shifting and vibrating. Even though it's too small to see, if you think about those microscopic movements happening within even the most stationary and solid objects, it will initiate more microscopic movements happening within your eyes and mind. Movement is necessary for sight. The more you move, the more you see. The less you move the less you see. Remember though, that these movements are beyond your conscious control. Your eyes have the ability to shift more than three times per second, adding up to over 170,000 shifts per day. It is not up to you to shift your eyes 170,000 times per day though. Your eyes already want to do that by themselves, and they do a much better job when you keep them soft and relaxed. The more relaxed you keep them, the faster they shift. If your eyes feel like they are not shifting enough, then the next practice will shake them loose and teach them how to shift much more with the help of a new vision tool.

Mental Focus #4: Pleasant Happy Memory

One of the simplest methods for keeping your mind focused is recalling something of interest. It is much easier to focus on something you enjoy than to try and force focus on something you don't. It's sort of like getting lost in a great book. At first you are still tuned into your surroundings. Once you get into a flow after a few chapters you get so focused on the story that you don't even hear people calling your name.

So while palming, recall or relive a pleasant happy memory, whether it is a vacation you took, your favorite game as a child, experiences with friends or family, or even dreaming of places you'd like to go in the future. What you imagine is not as important as how you imagine it. There is no limit to what you can imagine, so make your visualization as finely detailed as possible.

This is also another chance to continue stretching your imagination, or insight, further in or further out into the blur. So, if you are nearsighted, imagine looking off into the distance and seeing objects perfectly clear. If you are farsighted, imagine holding small objects in your hands very close to your face and examining all the fine details perfectly clear. The first step to clearing up vision with your eyes open is to imagine what that looks like with your eyes closed.

During this pleasant happy memory picture practice 'seeing' with your eyes closed and also practice recalling your other specialized sensations of smelling, tasting, touching, and hearing from your memory. Incorporate all five senses into your visualization. Accompany your mental pictures with sounds, smells, tastes and feelings from the scene you choose to imagine. Make sure there is plenty of movement involved in your memory and visualization to avoid mental staring. Do not stare when you are palming. Allow your eyes to be free to gaze around in the darkness as they 'look' for what you are picturing mentally.

Dr. Bates taught that the mind cannot do two things at once. The mind cannot simultaneously strain and relax at the same time. Therefore, as long as you are focused on your pleasant happy memory, you are not straining or stressing. Enjoy that mental relief.

Get into a comfortable position for palming and go to your happy place that makes you feel warm and fuzzy inside. See the next page for some examples.

Example 1:

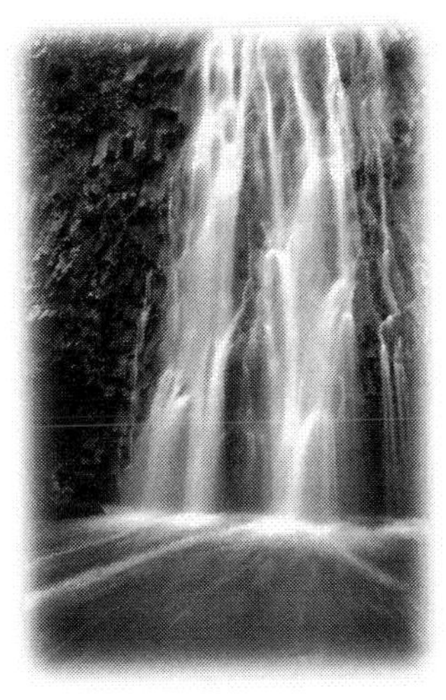

Imagine that you are walking barefoot on a path through a field. The sun is shining and you can feel its warmth on your skin and face. The earth is soft and cool beneath your feet. A warm breeze blows the scents of flowers into your nose from the field. You bend over and get very close to one flower. Take a big inhale and smell it. Examine every fine detail of the flower up close. What type of flower is it? What color are its petals? How many petals does it have? See this flower perfectly clearly. Then stand up and look up into the distance. Off to the left there is a majestic mountain range. Scan your eyes over each snowy peak and see the mountains perfectly clearly. Straight ahead, the path you are on enters an inviting forest. Meander on the path and enter the trees. The air feels different and there is a different scent in the air. Look around at all the trees. Approach a tree and touch its bark. Is it soft or rough? You can hear the sound of rushing water a little further along, so you continue walking on the path. You reach a clearing where you see a tall but gentle waterfall plunging into a clear pool. Dip your hands into the cool water and splash your face. How does the water feel? Go ahead and take a dip in this safe and serene pool. Let the water hold you up and relax all your limbs. Float weightlessly and bring your visualization to a close.

Example 2:

Imagine you are walking barefoot on a sandy path on a warm summer day. You see a sign that reads: Welcome to the Beach. *You crest over a sand dune and your gaze scans the horizon of the flat ocean. Continue down onto the beach and feel the soft sand sift between your toes with each step. Breathe in and smell the salt in the air. Listen to the waves crash and watch the ocean spray disappear into the air. Approach where the water meets the land. Look down and spot a seashell. Pick it up and examine it closely. What type of seashell is in your hand? What does it feel like? See all the fine details of your beautiful seashell closely easily. Lovingly toss your gorgeous seashell out into the ocean and watch it make a splash. Dip your feet in the water and let your eyes look up. Off in the distance you can easily see a black number 4 on the bright white triangular sail of a tiny sailboat moving swiftly across the ocean. Turn around and walk back up toward the flora. You see a little wooden stand near some palm trees. Approach the smiling man behind the counter and request a fresh fruit smoothie. Pay him and then take a big sip of your refreshing drink.*

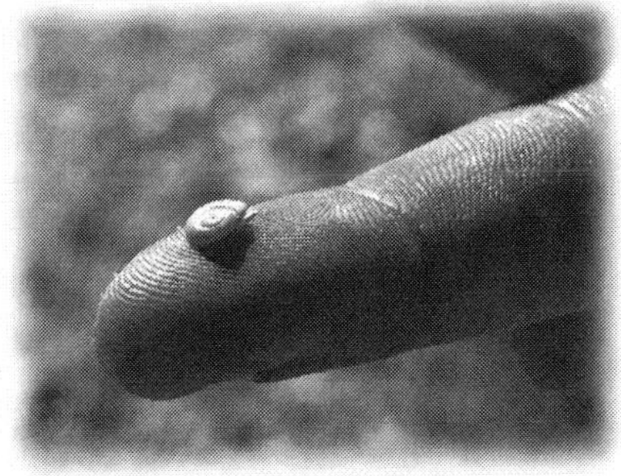

Vision Work #4

Add breathing, blinking, shifting, and swinging to your daily relaxation routine of relaxing, sunning, palming and visualizing. Increase your saccadic eye movements using the picket fence shifter and encourage more saccadic eye movements while swinging or moving in general. Allow your eyes to shift more automatically and effortlessly all day.

Daily Practice Checklist Week 4

M	Tu	W	Th	F	S	Su			
☐	☐	☐	☐	☐	☐	☐	♥	Morning Relaxation Routine	3-6 minutes
☐	☐	☐	☐	☐	☐	☐	◀◀ ▶▶	Swinging	2-6 minutes
☐	☐	☐	☐	☐	☐	☐	☼	Sunning	1-4 minutes
☐	☐	☐	☐	☐	☐	☐	💭	Palming & Mental Drill	2-8 minutes
☐	☐	☐	☐	☐	☐	☐	|||||	Picket Fence Shifter	1-4 minutes
								Daily Target:	***9-18 mins***

Vision Journal: ____

____

____

____

____

____

"The eyes do not see. They merely record sense impressions, which are then used by the mind to see with."

-Aldous Huxley

Chapter 5

Phase 1.3:

Relaxation Foundations

Centralization of the Eyes and of the Mind

"Dr. Bates coined the term 'Central Fixation' and defined it to mean 'seeing best where you are looking,' at the point of greatest mental and visual focus. This centralization accurately describes the phenomena of seeing with perfect vision, that is, the bringing into play of the retinal nerves which are equipped to do our keenest seeing. The fovea, which is the most sensitive part of the center of sight, or macula, has been called the light-finder, the child of impulse. It unfolds to do its duty only when the physical eye and the mind are relaxed, that is, relieved from the compulsion originated by the mind. Any compulsion from mind or eye muscles closes the cone-shaped nerves of the fovea tight like a sensitive plant, then only general or blurry vision takes place since the other nerves of the retina are not equipped to do the keenest seeing. When the sensitive light-finding nerves of the fovea become active, every portion of an object regarded stands out in extreme vividness while the cones are vibrating over it with such speed that the entire object seems to be seen all at once. For this reason, if you determine to see one thing best or one part of a thing best, you are attempting to do the impossible, trying to command an impulse. If, however, you will relax the eyes and mind, release them from compulsion and just let vision take place – that is, give way to impulse – the eyes will assume their normal shape and the light-seeking cones will be vibrated by the light reflected onto them from every portion of the surface of the object regarded. In this way, the object is clearly outlined as a shadow. Thus, for the fraction of a second it takes the fovea to be stimulated by the light from each part of the object, you see that part more clearly than any other. The mind, being relaxed, interprets accurately for size, shape, depth and distance, and clear vision has taken place."

-Margaret D. Corbett

Centralization of the Eyes – A New Way to See

Integral Eyesight Improvement teaches two different categories of vision practices: practices and habits. Most of the practices that have been covered so far in this book have been physical in nature, which require you to set aside time and energy to consciously perform them. Habits, on the other hand, are performed unconsciously all day long. Centralization is an example of a vision habit. There are some practices that can help you demonstrate and strengthen centralization that you will learn in this chapter, but centralization itself is not a physical practice. It is more of a mental vision habit that you can become aware of 24/7. It is a new way to see and a new way to think.

This is good news because it has the potential to drastically expand your vision practice to include many of your preexisting activities, since you will start centralizing while walking, talking, reading, writing, working, driving, exercising, and more. Every second of the day becomes an opportunity to centralize your eyes and mind, whether you have glasses on or not. It is the anatomically correct way to use your eyes and is a totally new way of seeing the world around you. Once you learn about centralization there is no reason for you to go back to how you previously used your eyes. So, what is centralization?

Dr. Bates considered centralization (or central fixation) as the fundamental principle of his method and defined it as 'seeing best where you are looking'. It is the key to seeing clearly without glasses. The opposite of centralization is diffusion (or eccentric fixation). Diffusion results from the bad habit of staring and glasses usage. If you lack central fixation, you lack focus. Your visual field is made up of your central vision and your peripheral vision. Your central vision is whatever you look directly at, while your peripheral vision is whatever you don't look directly at. Therefore, Dr. Bates' definition of 'seeing best where you are looking' means that objects you look directly at using your central vision ought to look better than objects you don't look directly at using your peripheral vision. At first glance this may seem quite obvious, but upon further investigation it becomes more complex. To understand centralization, it helps to revisit the anatomy of your eyes.

Light enters the eye by passing through the cornea, the aqueous humor, the pupil, the lens, and the vitreous humor, to land on the retina, which is covered in photoreceptor cells called rods and cones. In the very center of the retina is the *macula lutea* and in the center of the macula is the *fovea centralis*. This tiny center of sight only covers a 1.5 mm area of the retina, yet it is the only part of the retina where 20/20 vision is achievable because it is filled with cones. Your approximately 7 million cones provide your central vision and are equipped to see fine details. There are red, green, and blue cones, so they are also responsible for your color vision. Cones are more active in bright light and give you your daytime vision. No rods are found within the *fovea*. The rods are dispersed throughout the whole rest of the retina. Your approximately 120 million rods provide your peripheral vision, but are not equipped to see fine details or colors. Instead, they detect motion and contrast. Rods are more sensitive to dim light and more active in the darkness, giving you night vision.

So, based on the anatomy of your eyes, it makes sense that a very tiny central point that you are looking directly at will be more distinct and more colorful than everything else in your peripheral field that you are not looking directly at. Compare this to how your vision looks through glasses or contacts, which make nearly everything in your visual field seem equally crisp and clear. Artificial lenses decrease the difference between central and peripheral vision. In other words, lenses decentralize your vision. Natural vision is more like a spherical spectrum, where the center is the highest definition and the image loses definition as it moves concentrically outward toward the edges. It is anatomically impossible to see centrally and peripherally equally clear at the same time. Vision works by contrast. In order for your brain to see one part of your visual field clearly, it has to blur the other parts of your visual field that you are not looking directly at, whether that means two objects side by side on the same plane or two objects at different distances in the foreground and background. To focus the foreground the background must blur, and to focus the background the foreground must blur.

So, if you can only see one tiny point clearly, how are you supposed to see big objects? You move your central vision! The reason I usually call it centralization instead of central fixation is because the word 'fixation' makes me think of staring. You cannot see a whole house all at once by staring at it. You can only see one part at a time, one doorknob, one windowpane, or one shingle. You cannot see a whole tree all at once. You can only see one leaf at a time. Therefore, centralization relies on movement. This is where all that shifting you have been practicing pays off. Dr. Bates said that, "constant shifting is necessary to maintain central fixation." Your eyes shift so subtly and rapidly that they automatically drag your tiny central point all around objects and your brain pieces together thousands of tiny points into one continuous image. Think of a connect-the-dots drawing. You can't tell what the image is until you connect the dots with lines. Shifting is like connecting the dots. Avoid 'blotter vision' where you try to take in too much through your eyes all at once. Only take in one part of the picture at a time.

Make sure not to confuse centralization with staring. The longer you stare, the less you centralize. In order to maintain centralization, your eyes have to shift continuously to observe different portions of objects with your fovea. At first it sounds like a lot of work to keep the eyes constantly shifting, but remember that the goal is to make this an unconscious and involuntary process. It will be conscious at the beginning while you are reading about it, thinking about it, and practicing centralization. With repetition though, it will simply become the new way you use your eyes all the time, of looking at individual parts of objects rather than the object as a whole. Do not try too hard to see one point more clearly than another point. You will end up straining. Instead, just allow your eyes to centralize automatically on their own as you keep reminding yourself that one tiny point is seen clearer than the rest. There is nothing you have to do to make it clearer, except to stay relaxed while moving. Margaret Corbett poetically reminds us that the cones are like sensitive plants that constrict in the presence of strain and open up in the presence of relaxation. This is further proof of why relaxation is the key to clear vision, because your cones only function optimally when relaxed. Since your retinas are extensions of your brain and your rods and cones are specialized neurons made up of brain tissue, mental relaxation is your best bet.

At first, you may not be able to demonstrate to yourself that you see best where you are looking, especially if you currently experience blur near or far. In this case it may help to define centralization oppositely; as 'seeing worse where you are not looking'. As you look at this book, realize that peripheral objects in the background behind the book appear less distinct than the page. Now look up at one of those objects and realize that the page in the foreground is now less distinct than the object you are looking at. To develop centralization in your blurrier zones, keep practicing it and noticing it in your clearer zones. The more you demonstrate the truth of this visual and mental phenomenon in areas where you can easily see the distinction between your central and peripheral fields, the more you will begin to see it at more challenging distances. If this is still difficult to demonstrate, try using lights. Find a place where there are two lights a few feet apart from each other. Look at the left light and see it as brighter than the right light. Look at the right light and see it as brighter as the left light.

If you experience blurry vision near or far, it may be because you are using the wrong part of your retina to see with. Dr. Bates could tell if one of his patients lacked centralization when they were able to see peripheral objects as clearly or clearer than central objects. He called this phenomenon "eccentric fixation" or diffusion. When you diffuse your focus to too large of an area and try to force your rods to do the job of your cones it can add significant stress to your visual system. Instead of trying to focus on everything in your entire visual field at once, hone your physical and mental attention down to a much smaller area. It ought to be a big relief to learn that clear 20/20 vision can only be found within the center 1% of your visual field without having to worry too much about the other 99% that lies off center. Even though the fovea takes up less than 1% of the retina, it takes up 50% of the visual cortex in the brain, so centralization is as much a mental habit as it is a physical strategy. Practicing centralization reeducates your retina to properly use the cones in the fovea to see clear details instead of using the rods in the periphery.

Centralization is arguably the most important concept to understand and practice on both the physical and mental levels if you hope to improve your eyesight. Clear vision is a result of proper centralization. Although centralization is more of an idea or a habit, there are still a handful of practices designed to help you get better at centralizing all the time.

"The macula lutea is thus one of the most extraordinarily interesting features of the human eye, yet, although it is described in every ophthalmic textbook, most are vague about its purpose and take little interest in it unless it happens to become diseased. Dr. Bates, however, took a great deal of interest in it and discovered that the function of the fovea in relation to the rest of the retina was crucial to all the operations of vision. The point of fixation is the point to which attention is directed at any given moment. Central fixation, then, means that the point of immediate attention is always regarded directly by the fovea centralis. This does not imply that the eye should be fixed in the ordinary sense: on the contrary, in order for central fixation to be maintained, the eye must be constantly moving. Dr. Bates found that the tiny eye movements he had observed in normal vision were essential to stimulate the fovea properly - according to his reasoning, if the eye stares fixedly, the fovea becomes no more sensitive that the surrounding retina. If this happens all kinds of aberrations of vision follow, simply because the eye literally loses its sense of direction."

-Peter Mansfield

One Thing Best / Other Thing Worse

Purpose:

- To demonstrate and develop centralization.
- To distinguish between central and peripheral vision.
- To make the area you see best smaller and smaller.

Directions:

1) Hold 2 thumbs (or any 2 things) up in front of you two feet apart from each other.
2) Centralize on your left thumb and realize your right thumb is less distinct.
3) Centralize on your right thumb and realize your left thumb is less distinct.
4) Repeat a few times eyes open and then a few times eyes closed repeating mentally.
5) Move your thumbs closer together, one foot apart and repeat steps 2-4.
6) Move your thumbs closer together, to six inches apart and repeat steps 2-4.
7) Move your thumbs, closer so that they are touching and repeat steps 2-4.
8) Hold one thumb up in front of your nose.
9) Centralize on the left side of your thumbnail and see it better than the right side.
10) Centralize on the right side of your thumbnail and see it better than the left side.
11) Repeat a few times with eyes open a few times with eyes closed repeating mentally.

Time: 2 to 4 minutes.

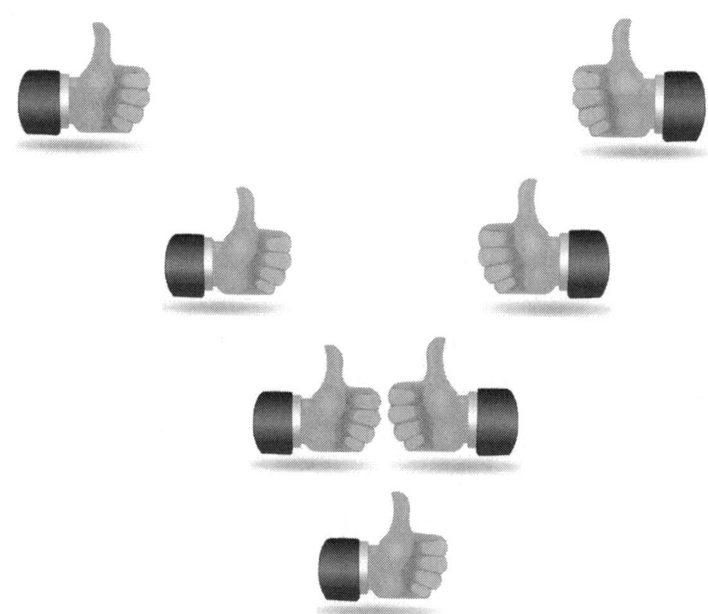

Description:

To truly grasp the concept of centralization you must practice seeing best where you are looking even when two different points are very close to each other. An ongoing goal is to hone your central vision down to a smaller and smaller area. Dr. Bates taught that the central vision needs to be infinitesimally small; almost so small that it has no surface area. The one thing best practice helps shrink your point of central focus down and distinguish the subtle difference between central and peripheral vision.

This is accomplished by beginning with your thumbs two feet apart from each other and bringing them closer together in intervals until they are touching. It is simple to demonstrate to yourself that you see one thumb better than the other when they are two feet apart because the thumb you're not looking at is in your far peripheral field, but it may become more challenging as you bring them closer together so that the thumb you're not looking at moves into your mid peripheral field and your near peripheral field.

Point your nose at the thumb you are centralizing on as you shift back and forth and either say out loud or think to yourself, "one thumb best, other thumb worse." After shifting from thumb to thumb a few times with your eyes open repeat with your eyes closed. Using your memory and imagination, keep imagining one thumb clearer at a time in your mind. Before opening your eyes back up, bring your thumbs a little closer together and open your eyes on an exhale to continue shifting from one thumb to the other, pointing with your nose.

When your two thumbs are touching each other, continue shifting from one to the other saying, "One thumb best, other thumb worse." Keep reminding yourself mentally that the thumb you are not looking at is less distinct than the thumb you are centralizing on, even if they look somewhat similar. The more you picture the difference in your mind with your eyes closed, the more apparent the difference will become with your eyes open.

Once you are able to demonstrate centralization with your thumbs touching, then you can try practicing with just one thumb by shifting from the left side of your thumbnail to the right side and seeing one side better than the other. Experiment to see how small you can get your central field to become. Try substituting other objects for your thumbs, like toothpicks, pens, pencils, or eye charts.

The above description helps you practice centralizing on two objects within arm's length on the same plane by shifting left and right. To practice centralizing on two objects at different distances, hold one thumb near your nose and your other thumb out at arm's length. When you centralize on your near thumb in the foreground, the background becomes less distinct and doubles. When you centralize on your far thumb in the background, the foreground becomes less distinct and doubles. This version is still within arm's length though, so make sure to practice centralizing side to side and near to far on objects at farther distances as well.

If you are nearsighted, centralization will be easier up close and harder far away because everything in the distance may appear equally blurry. If you are farsighted, centralization will be easier far away and harder up close because everything up close may appear equally blurry. However, even if you don't necessarily 'see best where you are looking' near or far, you can still demonstrate to yourself that the objects in your peripheral field that you're not looking directly at appear relatively blurrier than the objects in your central field that you are looking directly at. In that case, using the opposite definition of 'seeing worse where you are not looking' may be easier.

This is one tangible way for you to 'work with the blur'. By allowing your peripheral vision to have some blur in it, you are allowing your central vision to heighten its clarity. If you cannot let go of the desire for clarity in the periphery, your central vision will never see as clear as it could. It is paradoxical because only when you let go of trying to see clearly in the periphery does your central vision sharpen, which can then spread out and clear the periphery a little bit. Are you willing to invite some blur into your peripheral vision in order to achieve clear central vision? If so, start asking or telling peripheral objects that you are not looking at presently to "blur off". When you want to see a blurry peripheral object clearly, all you need to do is shift your attention and central vision over to it and let go of the last object you were just centralizing on. You cannot centralize on two things at once.

You cannot force centralization to happen. The cones in your *fovea centralis* will only cooperate when your eyes and mind are relaxed, so don't strain to see one thing best. Just keep shifting from one point to another and observe centralization happening.

Reverse Blinking (The Fundamental Principle)

Purpose:

- To practice centralization.
- To distinguish between central and peripheral vision.
- To make the area you see best smaller and smaller.
- To cultivate and experience clear flashes.

Directions:

1) Look at the letter B in the word **B L I N K**.
2) Notice if the B looks better, the same, or worse than the letters L I N K.
3) Close your eyes for 10 seconds and remember any color to rest your mind and eyes.
4) When your eyes feel rested, open your eyes on the letter B for 1 second, then close.
5) Think about what you saw; did the B look better, the same, or worse than the others?
6) If you relax and centralize, you'll have a flash of improved clarity and see the B best.
7) Keep repeating steps 3-5 until you get a clear flash, then try a longer reverse blink.
8) Keep your eyes closed for 10 seconds, thinking about your color until they feel rested.
9) When your eyes feel rested, open your eyes on the letter B for 2 seconds, then close.
10) Think about what you saw; did the B look better, the same, or worse than the others?
11) Keep repeating steps 8-10 until you can hold a clear flash, then try a second longer.
12) With your eyes closed again, think about your color until your eyes feel rested.
13) When your eyes feel rested, open them on the letter B for 3 seconds, then close.
14) Think about what you saw; did the B look better, the same, or worse than the others?
15) Repeat steps 1-14 on the K and practice seeing the last letter of the word best.
16) Repeat steps 1-14 on a distant letter or object to cultivate clear flashes far away.

Time: 2 to 4 minutes.

Description:

"Do you read imperfectly? Can you observe then that when you look at the first word, or the first letter, of a sentence you do not see best where you are looking; that you see other words, or other letters, just as well as or better than the one you are looking at? Do you observe also that the harder you try to see the worse you see?

Now close your eyes and rest them, remembering some color, like black or white that you can remember perfectly. Keep them closed until they feel rested, or until the feeling of strain has been completely relieved. Now open them and look at the first word or letter of a sentence for a fraction of a second. If you have been able to relax, partially or completely, you will have a flash of improved or clear vision, and the area seen best will be smaller.

After opening the eyes for this fraction of a second, close them again quickly, still remembering the color, and keep them closed until they again feel rested. Then again open them for a fraction of a second. Continue this alternate resting of the eyes and flashing of the letters for a time, and you may soon find that you can keep your eyes open longer than a fraction of a second without losing the improved vision.

If your trouble is with distant instead of near vision, use the same method with distant letters. In this way you can demonstrate for yourself the fundamental principle of the cure of imperfect sight by treatment without glasses.

If you fail, ask someone with perfect sight to help you."

-Dr. William H. Bates

(See page 309 for a Fundamental Principle reading card.)

Nose Drawing, Counting, Colors, and Shapes

Purpose:

- To practice centralization.
- To prevent staring.
- To distinguish between central and peripheral vision.
- To pique curiosity, interest, and attention.
- Define edges and get rid of hazy lines or shadows around objects.

Directions:

Nose Drawing

1) Pretend you have a magic marker extending straight out from the tip of your nose.
2) Look at an object, outline its perimeter with your nose marker by moving your head.
3) Go around the object in both directions and trace over some details within the object.
4) Your mind, eyes, and nose all travel together.
5) Close your eyes and repeat mentally, visualizing drawing the world around you.

Counting

1) Look for repetitive patterns around you (lights, cars, windows, bricks, outlets, etc.).
2) Nose draw each one as you count them out loud or mentally.

Colors

1) Assign the 7 colors of the rainbow to the 7 days of the week.
2) Search for as many objects that are the color of the day.

Shapes

1) Start categorizing objects into four basic shapes: squares, rectangles, triangles, circles.
2) As you nose draw objects, determine which of the four basic shapes it resembles most.
3) It may be obvious or abstract.

Time: All day long.

Red	**Monday**
Orange	**Tuesday**
Yellow	**Wednesday**
Green	**Thursday**
Blue	**Friday**
Indigo/Violet	**Saturday/Sunday**

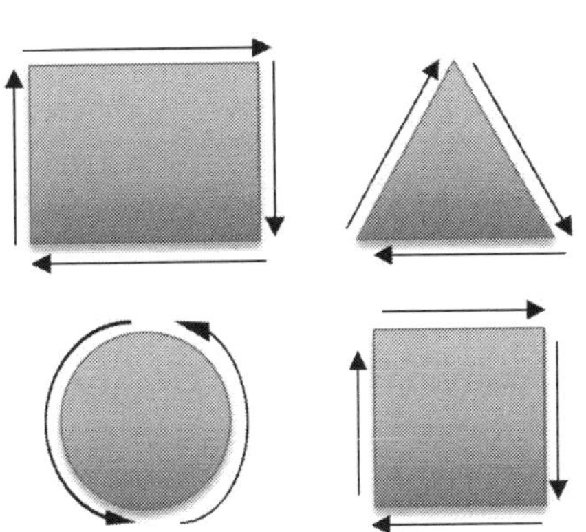

Description:

Nose drawing and counting objects promotes physical centralization and prevents your eyes from staring. Searching for different colors and shapes promotes mental centralization and prevents your mind from staring. Nose drawing turns you into the artist creating the world you see. Pretend that your nose has a magic marker, pen, pencil, laser, or pointer attached to it that you can use to trace around the perimeter of objects by moving your head. You can outline anything, anytime, anywhere... doors, windows, houses, cars, people, clouds, poles, signs, letters, etc. Anything with edges can be outlined.

As your nose and eyes travel around the edges of objects, realize that you see the part that you are nose drawing better than the parts that you aren't nose drawing. Do not force it; allow it. Do not try to see one part best. Allow your eyes to see one part best. Soon nose drawing will become subconscious and your eyes will habitually perform this automatically without you moving your head so much.

Counting objects expands curiosity, which is an important factor in vision. You become more aware of your surroundings. Just like nose drawing, you can count anything, anytime, anywhere. Search for repetitive patterns like the number of lights in the room, the number of paintings on the wall, the number of cars passing by, the number of people in a room, the number of items on your desk, etc. Point your nose toward each object as you count it.

Taking counting a step further, you can also incorporate colors. Assign the seven colors of the rainbow to the seven days of the week and become hypersensitive to the color of the day. Count the number of red objects you see on Mondays and the number of blue objects you see on Fridays. This practice contributes to improving centralization because on Thursdays you see green more distinctly than the rest of the colors and on the weekends you see purple more distinctly than the rest of the colors. The color of the day compares to your central vision and the other six colors compare to your peripheral vision - less distinct than the color of the day because you are not paying as much attention to them.

Do you remember playing with building blocks as a child? Do you remember what shapes they were? Squares, rectangles, circles, and triangles. These are the four basic shapes that can fit around anything and everything. As you begin outlining objects every day, start to notice which one of these four basic shapes your object fits into. It may be a blatant match like a rectangle for a door, but others may be more abstract. Look up at trees and figure out whether they are triangular, circular, or rectangular. This is so important because shape recognition is one of the first visual cue your brain determines when you look at an object. Your deep memory bank categorizes objects into different shape and color classifications. This way you can almost immediately eliminate all the improbable options and narrow down the most probable option of what that object is.

Hopefully you are now beginning to see how centralization is something that you can start accessing all day long, not just when doing specific vision practices. Just keep reminding yourself to see parts of the whole, to see best where you are looking, or to see worse where you are not looking. Shapes, counting, and colors will also help you centralize in your blurry zones, because no matter how blurry your vision is, you can likely still tell what color that blurry object is, or what general shape that blurry object is, or how many blurry objects there are.

Peripheral Expansion

Purpose:

- To loosen the muscles around the eyes.
- To distinguish between central and peripheral vision.
- To explore and expand your visual field.
- To stimulate rods in peripheral field through movement.
- To activate cones in central field through peripheral stimulation.

Directions:

1) Either standing or seated, gaze straight ahead in a relaxed way, without staring.
2) Wiggle your fingers as your hands trace the far edges of your peripheral field.
3) Move your hands as far out as you can until you can just barely see them peripherally.
4) Go all the way around in an oval, see how far you can go before losing sight of fingers.
5) Try it with a post-it note attached to your forehead blocking your central vision.

Time: 2 to 4 minutes.

Description:

Sometimes when people begin practicing centralization, they forget about their peripheral vision and end up with a feeling of tunnel vision. The goal of centralization is not to ignore the periphery, but rather to become more aware of the difference between the central and peripheral parts of your visual field. Perfect vision is a balance between a small area of central clarity and a wide area of peripheral awareness. You can still see things in your periphery, but not as clearly as you can in the center. Central and peripheral must coexist simultaneously, and it is important to work with both respectively.

This peripheral expansion practice can help you better understand the difference between peripheral and central vision, as well as the different layers of your peripheral field. Your central vision has capacity for 100% clarity. Your near-peripheral vision is closest to your central vision and has capacity for 90-99% clarity. Your mid-peripheral vision is farther from your central vision and has capacity for 70-90% clarity. Your far-peripheral vision stretches out to the far edges of your visual field and has capacity for 50-70% clarity.

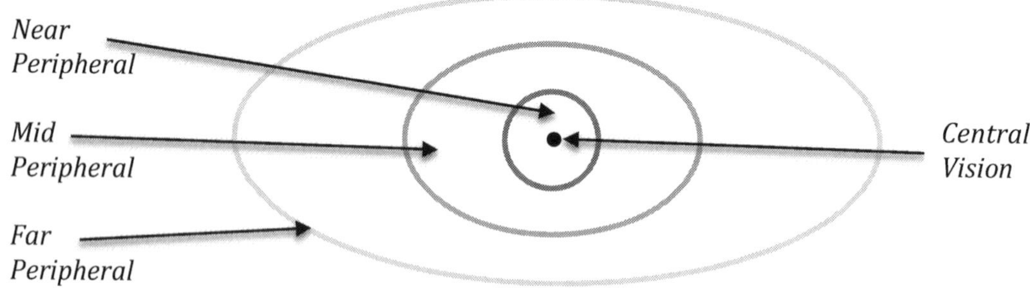

In this practice, you will be exploring your peripheral visual fields to stimulate and expand your peripheral awareness. Gazing straight ahead, begin wiggling your fingers in your near periphery, and slowly expand out into your mid and far periphery. Since your central vision is straight ahead, your fingers in the periphery will not be clear or distinct, but you can remain aware of their movement. Remember, the rods sense movement, not details. Raising peripheral awareness in turn helps heighten your central awareness.

At first you can perform this drill with both eyes open looking gently straight ahead. Once you try that, you can stick a post-it note or tape an index card to your forehead to block the central vision of both eyes while keeping the peripheral vision available. This can really raise peripheral awareness and boost the clarity of your central vision after removing the temporary obstruction.

Centralization of the Mind - Meditation

Just like the eyes cannot see two things equally clearly at once, the mind cannot think two things equally clearly at once. Physical centralization of the eyes is seeing one thing best. Mental centralization of the mind is thinking one thing best. At any given moment your mind may be speeding through dozens or even hundreds of different things one after the other. You may experience constant chatter in your mind or a sense of restlessness or mental exhaustion from over-thinking or multi-tasking in your mind. Multi-tasking is the opposite of centralization. It is decentralization, fragmentation of your thoughts, unfocused and diffused attention. Try applying this idea of centralization to your mind by only focusing on one task or one thought at a time and let the other thoughts remain in the periphery of your mind, less distinct than the one you are contemplating. Give one thought your absolute attention until it is satisfied and then move onto the next one. Do not try to juggle multiple thoughts at once.

Applying the idea of physical centralization to the mind may remind you of meditation. Meditation, put simply, is the practice of focusing your mind on one object or thought. The longer you are able to concentrate on that one object, the closer you get to actual meditation on that object, where your mind no longer wanders or loses concentration.

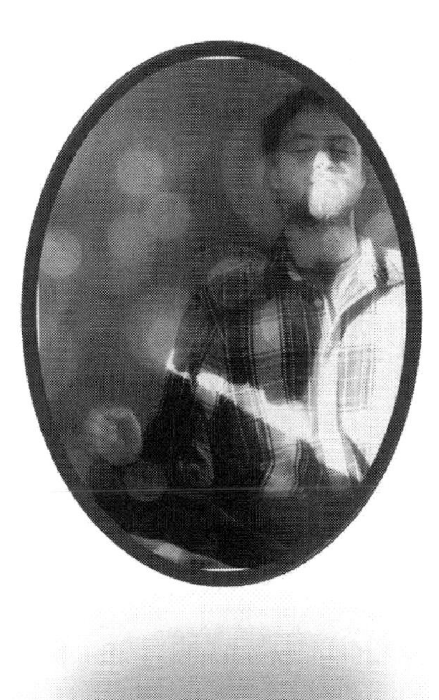

At first, meditation begins with sensory withdrawal. Instead of sending your senses out into the world, you turn them inward. Gently close your eyes and begin listening to what's going on inside, listening to your breath, feeling the sensations in your body, looking at the mental pictures that arise from your third eye. The next step is concentration. With your eyes closed and your senses withdrawn from the outer world, choose something simple to focus your mind upon, like your breath, a part of your body, a mental image, or a mantra. When your mind wanders from your one thing, gently bring your attention back to it. You will inevitably have to repeat this refocusing process several times, since the mind naturally wants to move and travel about. However, the more you practice concentration the longer you will be able to hold your mental focus on a single thing without your mind wandering.

Once your concentration upon an object is unwavering, you have achieved meditation. Meditation is the state of maintaining mental focus on one object without distraction. Meditation is achieving centralization of the mind. All of your mental focus hones onto one simple thing and all other things dissipate into the less-distinct peripheral awareness.

Practice focusing your mind every day on one thing for as long as you can. Even if it is only for one minute, this will greatly enhance the mental focus of your mind, which will help you enhance the physical focus of your eyes. Forgivingly bring your focus back to your meditation when your mind wanders. The more you centralize with your mind, the more you will centralize with your eyes. The more you centralize with your eyes, the more you will centralize with your mind.

See Here Now – Beware of the Stare

Perfectly clear vision is only possible in the present moment. When you begin to think about the past or the future you leave the present moment, begin daydreaming, start staring into space, and the quality of your vision declines. Remaining in the present moment is highly dependent upon a higher state of focus, awareness, and attention on both the physical and mental levels. So much of this vision practice comes down to awareness. Focusing on the present moment enhances your eyesight and insight. It also heightens and lengthens your attention span. In this way, all of the holistic vision practices can be used as pathways to enter into the present moment and to stay there. If you are not used to spending so much time in the present moment with this higher state of attention and consciousness, it may feel exhausting or tiring at first. That is why it is so necessary to balance the time spent using your eyes looking outward with an equal amount of time spent withdrawing your senses inward and allowing your eyes and entire visual system to rest, relax, and heal.

There is nothing wrong with daydreaming about the past or the future. It only becomes detrimental to your vision if your eyes stay open and end up getting locked in a stare. Instead, do your daydreaming and visualizing with your eyes closed or, better yet, while palming so you actually turn it into a mental focus practice. Not only will this help you uproot the bad habit of staring, but it will also enhance your visualization skills. You can connect with your thoughts and visualize what you are thinking about even better when your eyes are closed compared to when your eyes are open and staring. Greater mental focus leads to greater physical focus.

Often the habit of staring is such a deeply engrained habit that it can take a while to break it. Many children learned to stare in school when their teachers forced them to keep their eyes on their books or on the board instead of looking out the window or elsewhere in the classroom. Many people establish the staring habit as an escape mechanism to avoid the present moment. If the present moment seems uncomfortable, unpleasant, or uninteresting, then you may desire to leave it behind by staring. It may feel more comfortable to park your eyes while your mind goes off on a journey into the past or the future. Other times, people end up staring due to boredom or fatigue.

There are two types of staring, just like there are two types of relaxation: passive and active. Passive staring is described above where your eyes lock in on something while your mind wanders. Active staring is when you hold your focus at the same focal distance for long periods of time, like when performing up close tasks such as reading, writing, watching television, or using a computer, tablet, or smart phone. Your eyes are not motionless like in a passive stare, but they are being held at the same focal distance for too long. Your mind is not wandering like in a passive stare either, but it can quickly become fatigued if you do not give your eyes a break. If you are an active starer, use the 5-10-15 rule to avoid eyestrain and fatigue. Every 5 minutes, look up at something 10 feet away or farther for 15 seconds or longer. Staring is usually a sign that you have worked your eyes well beyond their comfort level and they need a rest.

The simplest remedy for staring is closing or palming your eyes. At once the stare is gone and your eyes are free to relax and shift. Establishing a rhythmic blinking habit helps break the stare too, because each blink is like a mini-rest period for your eyes. Your eyes move subtly each time you blink as well. Your eyes really do not want to be held still. Your eyes were designed to be in regular motion all the time. Contrary to what you may think, your eyes are only in a state of rest when in motion. It is only when they stop moving and begin staring that strain starts to take hold.

Become more aware of your staring habit. Catch yourself staring. Ask yourself, “Why am I staring?” or “What am I staring at?” By investigating the habit of staring you may pick up on patterns of when, what, and why you stare at things. Eyeglasses constrict the range of motion of your eyes, which can lead to habitual staring. And so, your vision practice becomes a strategy to simultaneously strengthen your mental focus, attain higher states of awareness, and deepen your presence in the continually unfolding present moment, all while providing your entire body the opportunity to come back into harmony by letting go of unnecessary tensions, strains, worries, and fears.

Mental Focus #5: Alphabet Categories

Since mental centralization is defined as thinking of one thing best, and since the nature of the mind is to move, you are going to accomplish mental centralization amidst constant change through practicing the alphabet categories. While palming your eyes, slowly make your way through the alphabet. Pick a theme like foods, animals, geography, or celebrities. Think of a different person, place, or thing that begins with that letter of the alphabet. See how long you can focus your mind on that object until it feels ready to move onto the next letter. Start small, only visualizing each letter's object for 5 to 10 seconds. With practice, draw out the length of time you spend on each letter, to 15 seconds, 30 seconds, or a full minute. Do not stare at the mental picture, think about the object moving or rotating.

For example, starting with the letter A you can visualize an apple. Picture yourself picking a ripe apple off a low hanging branch of an apple tree in an apple orchard. What color is the apple you picked? What size is it? Rotate the apple in your hand to picture all sides of it. Maybe you can even imagine taking a bite of the apple and think about what it sounds like and tastes like. Once your mind has had enough of the apple and feels ready to move on you can think of an object that starts with the letter B. Maybe you decide to visualize a blueberry. Do you see one blueberry or a bunch of blueberries? How do those blueberries taste? After a few seconds, move onto a food that starts with the letter C. Slowly make your way all the way to Z to complete the mental focusing practice. Sometimes you have to get creative on some of the harder letters. Observe whether your mind is able to stay concentrated on the letter you are on, or if it has a tendency to jump ahead and start thinking of objects that start with the next letter while you're still on the last letter.

A B C D E F G H I J K L M N O P Q R S T U V W X Y Z

Vision Work #5:

Incorporate centralization both into your daily vision routine and into your everyday activities. Apply the concept of centralization to all your vision practices simply by noticing the difference between your central vision and your peripheral vision while practicing them. Stop trying to focus on too much at once. Remind yourself all day long to keep shrinking your central focus and mental attention down to a smaller area and see best only where you are looking and think one thing best at a time. Try meditating for one minute.

Daily Practice Checklist Week 5

M Tu W Th F S Su		Activity	Time
☐☐☐☐☐☐☐		Morning Relaxation Routine	3-6 minutes
☐☐☐☐☐☐☐		Swinging	2-6 minutes
☐☐☐☐☐☐☐		Sunning	1-4 minutes
☐☐☐☐☐☐☐		Palming & Mental Drill	2-8 minutes
☐☐☐☐☐☐☐		Picket Fence Shifter	1-4 minutes
☐☐☐☐☐☐☐		Centralization	2-4 minutes
		Daily Target:	***12-24 mins***

Vision Journal: ____

____

____

____

____

____

____

"You should use your eyes correctly all day long, no matter what you may be doing. Practice blinking, shifting, central fixation, and imagining stationary objects to be moving opposite to the movement of your head and eyes. Wearing glasses for any purpose whatever retards your progress and lowers your vision."

-Dr. William H. Bates

Chapter 6

Phase 2:
Fusion Warm Ups
Connecting Your Eyes and Mind

"Since we have two eyes, it is obvious that in the act of sight two pictures must be formed; and in order that these two pictures shall be fused into one by the mind, it is necessary that there shall be perfect harmony of action between the two organs of vision. In looking at a distant object the two visual axes must be parallel, and in looking at an object at a less distance than infinity, which for practical purposes is less than twenty feet, they must converge to exactly the same degree."

-Dr. William H. Bates

"Fusion is the ability for your two eyes to point at the same point, at the same time, at the same rate."

-Dr. Jerriann J. Taber

Brain Balancing

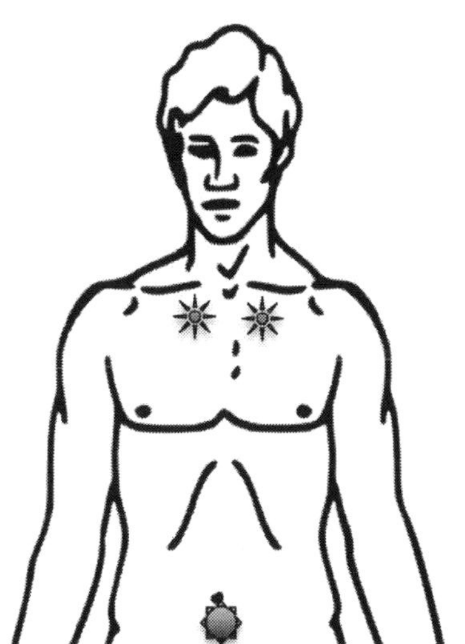

Purpose:

- Balance the left and right brain hemispheres.
- Balance the left and right eyes.
- Improve physical and mental coordination.
- Relax and reset the nervous system.
- Center the body, calm the mind.
- Prepare for fusion practices.

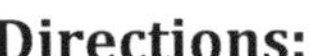

Directions:

Hydrate

1) Drink 8 to 12 ounces of fresh filtered water to hydrate your cells, eyes, and brain.

Brain Buttons

1) Firmly massage both K 27 points with your left hand, resting right hand on navel.
2) Gently press tongue to roof of mouth as you take 3 to 6 big breaths.
3) Firmly massage both K 27 points with your right hand, resting left hand on navel.
4) Gently press tongue to roof of mouth as you take 3 to 6 big breaths.

Cross Crawl

1) Lift your left knee and tap it with your right hand.
2) Lift your right knee and tap it with your left hand.
3) March in place, tapping left knee with right hand and right knee with left hand.
4) Rotate your upper body as you cross crawl to turn it into a long swing.
5) Rotate left when tapping left knee, rotate right when tapping right knee.
6) Notice oppositional movement with eyes open, then try it with eyes closed.

Hook-Ups

1) Extend both arms straight in front of you with back of hands facing each other.
2) Reach your right arm over your left arm and interlace your fingers.
3) Bend your elbows, curl your hands through to rest on your chest.
4) Cross your right leg over your left leg with both feet planted on the ground.
5) Gently press tongue to roof of mouth as you take 3 to 6 big breaths.
6) Repeat steps 1-5 with left arm over right arm and left leg over right leg.
7) Uncross your arms and legs and press all five fingertips together.
8) Gently press tongue to roof of mouth as you take 3 to 6 big breaths.

Time: 1 to 4 minutes.

Description:

Brain balancing practices are designed to harmonize your left and right brain hemispheres. Since your eyes are extensions of your brain and made up of brain tissue, these practices may also harmonize your left and right eyes if you experience an imbalance or have one dominant or one weaker eye. Brain balancing practices are sourced from things like Brain Gym, Applied Kinesiology, Brain Training, Energy Medicine and more.

Since the left brain hemisphere controls the right side of the body and the right brain hemisphere controls the left side of the body, the energies of the body are supposed to cross over through the center like an X. Your energies can get unbalanced however, in which case you get into what is called a 'homolateral' state, where your energies run up and down parallel without crossing like this: | | When in the homolateral state, you may feel unbalanced, ungrounded, and unclear.

Luckily there are easy and effective ways to balance the energies of your brain and eyes including hydrating, brain buttons, cross crawl, and hook-ups. Hydrating is the simplest, so start by drinking eight to twelve ounces of fresh, filtered water. Not only does water help conduct energy and assist in communication between the cells and systems of the body, but it is also crucial for optimal eye health. The vitreous fluid inside the eyes consists of 99% water, so make sure you are drinking about half your body weight in ounces each day. For example, if you weigh 160 pounds, drink about 80 ounces of water a day.

Next, locate your brain buttons, which are actually the Kidney 27 acupuncture points, which are located below your collarbones towards the center of your chest. If there is stagnation of energy or lymph in this area, it may feel sore or tender. Firmly massage your brain buttons with the thumb and first two fingers of your left hand while resting your right palm right below your belly button. Breathe deeply for about 20 to 30 seconds with the tip of your tongue pressed to the roof of your mouth. Then switch your hands and firmly massage your brain buttons with the thumb and first two fingers of your right hand while resting your left palm right below your belly button. Breathe deeply for about 20 or 30 seconds with the tip of your tongue pressed to the roof of your mouth.

Cross crawling or cross marching can be performed seated or standing. Lift your left leg off the ground and tap your left knee with the palm of your right hand. Lower your left leg, lift your right leg off the ground and tap your right knee with the palm of your left hand. Find a rhythm and march in place as you continue breathing deeply and blinking regularly.

If you tap the wrong knee with the wrong hand, just laugh and start over. To turn it more into a Bates Method practice, you can rotate your upper body as you cross crawl and observe the oppositional movement happening around you. Swing to the left and tap your left knee with your right hand. Swing to the right and tap your right knee with your left hand. Try the cross crawl long swing with your eyes open a few times and then with your eyes closed, remembering the oppositional movement in your mind. It may be a challenge to stay balanced while doing the cross crawl long swing with your eyes closed, so go nice and slow or do it while seated.

Once you master the basic cross crawl, try adding in some more brain training challenges. Can you clap your hands in between your knee taps on each side? If you mess up, just laugh and reset. Once you master clapping in between, try tapping your opposite ear with the free hand that is not tapping your knee. So, as your right hand taps your left knee, your left hand taps your right ear. Then clap. Then as your left hand taps your right knee, your right hand taps your left ear. If you mess up, laugh and start again. Once you master this, try adding an additional challenge of saying things out loud in perfect timing with your knee taps, like reciting the alphabet backwards, doing multiplication tables, singing a song, humming a tune, or reading your eye chart staying on pace by saying one letter every time you tap your knee.

The hook-ups can also be performed seated or standing. First you cross your right arm and right leg over your left arm and left leg. Whether seated or standing, both feet should be planted on the floor. Your fingers intertwine and you pull your hands through to rest them on your chest. Hold this position and breathe for 20 to 30 seconds with the tip of your tongue pressed to the roof of your mouth. Uncross your arms and legs and repeat on the other side. Cross your left arm over your right arm with the palms of your hands facing away from each other, intertwine your fingers, and pull your hands through the space your arms make to rest on your chest. Cross your left leg over your right leg and plant both feet on the floor. Hold this position and breathe for 20 to 30 seconds with the tip of your tongue pressed to the roof of your mouth. Finally, uncross your arms and legs and press all your fingertips together. Either rest your hands on your lap or lift them up and press your thumbs into the center of your forehead. Close your eyes and breathe for 20 to 30 seconds with the tip of your tongue pressed to the roof of your mouth.

Your brain is now balanced. Notice any changes like feeling more grounded or centered, clearer thinking, or more coordination between left and right eye. Use the brain balancing techniques as a way to prepare your eyes and mind for the following fusion practices.

Gateposts

Purpose:

- Align the eyes.
- Establish fusion.
- Differentiate central and peripheral vision.
- Clear up objects in between gateposts.

Directions:

1) Hold one finger, pen, pencil, or pointer 3 to 12 inches from your nose.
2) Centralize on your finger to see one finger up close and two objects in the background.
3) Centralize on the distant object to see one object in the background and two fingers in the foreground, framing the distant object.
4) Swing the distant object in between your gateposts by pivoting your head side to side.

Time: 1 to 3 minutes.

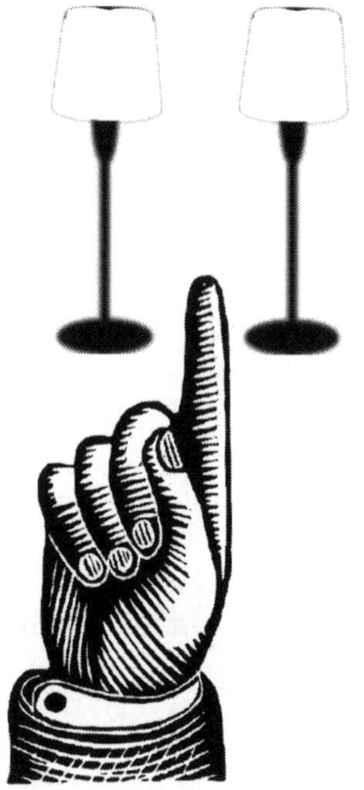

Looking at finger in foreground
Two lamps in the background

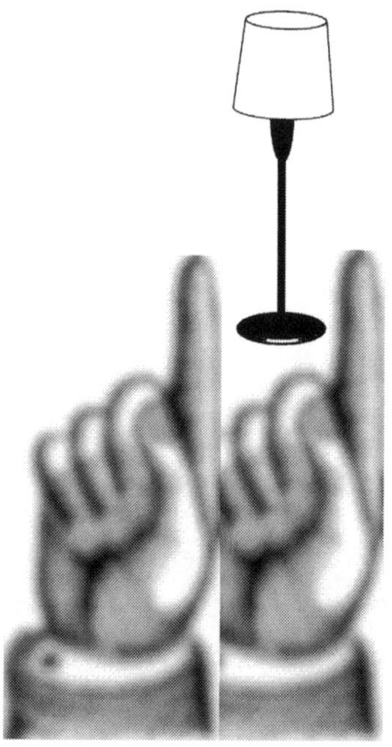

Looking at lamp in background
Two fingers in foreground = gateposts

Description:

The gateposts will be the beginning of a series of vision warm ups that seem almost like optical illusions. These warm ups are dealing with fusion and depth perception. Practicing these warm ups will help you become much more aware of your entire visual field as well as the noticeable difference between your central vision and your peripheral vision.

Holding a finger, a pen, a pencil, or a pointer vertically in front of your nose while you look at something in the distance will form 'gateposts.' Your finger will split into two and it ought to look like you are gazing at an object in the distance through two gateposts, one to the left of the object and one to the right of the object. The gateposts will not be clear or distinct because you are not looking at them with your central vision - they are in your peripheral field. You cannot see clearly with your peripheral vision. You can only see things clearly with your central vision. The gateposts help you centralize because anything that lands in between the gateposts is your clear central vision, and anything that lands beyond the gateposts is your peripheral vision that you don't need to see with as much detail. The gatepost phenomenon happens because of the overlapping fields of vision of each eye.

Swinging near or distant objects in between your gateposts can help clear those blurry objects up. If you turn your head to the right slightly you will be able to touch the right side of the object with your right gatepost. If you turn your head to the left slightly you will be able to touch the left side of the object with your left gatepost. Do not let the object go beyond the edge of the gatepost. Continue pivoting your head side-to-side keeping your near or distant object in between your two gateposts and breathe and blink to watch the object start to clear up. If you are nearsighted, swing your eye chart in the distance between your gateposts to see it more clearly. If you are farsighted, swing text up close between your gateposts to see it more clearly. You can swing anything between your gateposts. Typically, narrower objects are easier to swing between your gateposts. See how many things you can swing in between your gateposts throughout the day.

Without gateposts, your eyes and brain may not know exactly where to focus. If you are nearsighted and you look in the distance your eyes are still focused up close. If you are farsighted and you look up close your eyes are still focused far away. When you hold gateposts up in between your eyes and the object you're looking at, you are essentially telling your brain, "Don't focus here." So once your brain is able to see the gateposts split, it knows to focus elsewhere, either on the near object in your hand, or on the far object in the distance.

Near to Far Shifting

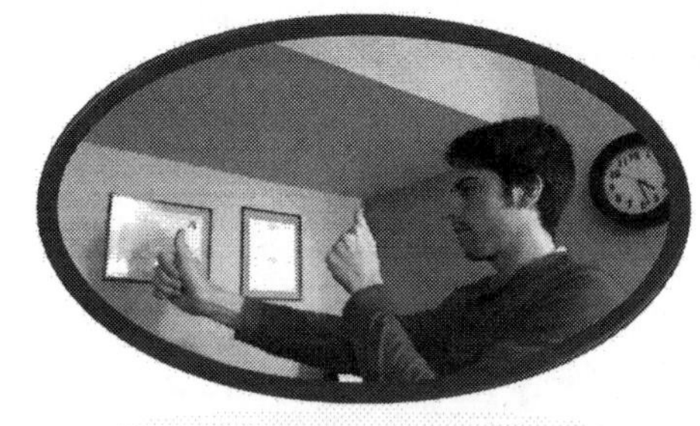

Purpose:

- Loosen tight extrinsic eye muscles.
- Enhance the peripheral vision.
- Break the habit of staring.
- Encourage fusion and teamwork between both eyes.
- Retrain the eye muscles to converge and diverge properly.
- Encourage the good vision habit of regular shifting during near work.

Directions:

1) Sit or stand in front of a window or facing a distant object.
2) Hold one thumb close and the other thumb at arm's length, aiming at a distant object.
3) Centralize on your near thumb to see one thumb near and two thumbs far.
4) Centralize on your far thumb to see one thumb far and two thumbs near.
5) Centralize on the distant object to see four thumbs in the foreground.
6) Bring your attention back to your far thumb, and then back to your near thumb.
7) Repeat steps 3-7 a few times, then pick a different distant object to shift out to.
8) Close your eyes and repeat the practice mentally.

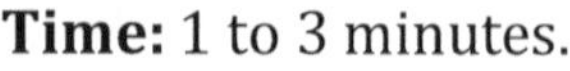

Time: 1 to 3 minutes.

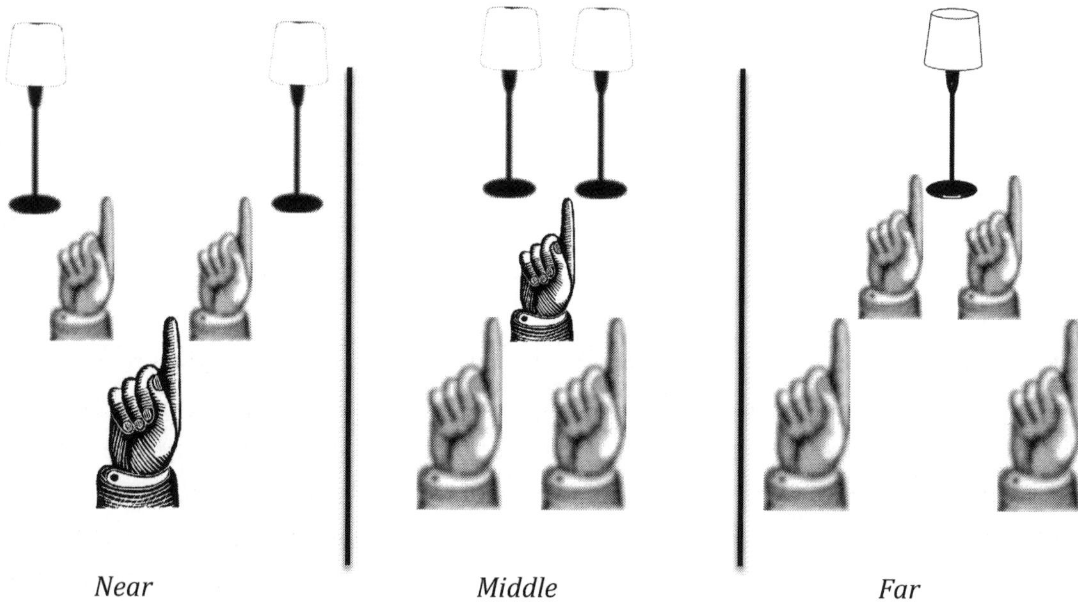

Description:

To practice near to far shifting, you can either use your thumbs or two different colored pens or pencils. Hold one thumb just a few inches from the tip of your nose and the other out at arm's length. Align your thumbs and aim them at an object in the distance, like a picture on the wall or a tree if you are outside. Converge your eyes to look at your near thumb. Notice that your near thumb is singular and it appears that there are two far thumbs and two distant objects. Diverge your eyes a little to look at your far thumb. Notice that your far thumb is singular and it appears that there are two near thumbs and two distant objects. Diverge your eyes even more to look at the distant object. Notice that the distant object is singular and it appears that there are two near thumbs and two far thumbs. So, whatever you are looking at, or centralizing on, appears single and whatever you are not looking at, or lands in your peripheral field, appears doubled. The diagram roughly demonstrates what you are meant to see during near to far shifting. It is just like the gateposts except you have two sets of gateposts up now, one up close and one farther away. The close gateposts will be wider and the far gateposts will be narrower.

It is important to repeat near to far shifting mentally with your eyes closed after you practice it a few times with your eyes open. If either one of your thumbs or your distant object was blurry when your eyes were open, this is your opportunity to picture them all perfectly clearly with your eyes closed. Remember the object you are thinking about is single and the objects you are not thinking about are double. Even though your eyelids are closed when you practice mentally, your eyes ought to still be responding as if they were open. They need to cross when your mental focus is on your near thumb, uncross slightly when your mental focus is on your far thumb, and totally relax and diverge when your mental focus is out on your distant object. Use your eye chart as your distant object for near to far shifting to get more clarity on the letters.

Your eyes always want to be adjusting their focal distance. Your eyes hate to be held at one distance for too long, like reading a book or staring at a screen. Near to far shifting helps replace the bad vision habit of staring with the good vision habit of shifting. It is very important to look up and away from any near material if you must focus up close for an extended period of time. Any type of up-close work, whether it is reading a book, writing or typing, working at a computer, using your cell phone, or even watching a movie, is an excellent opportunity to practice near to far shifting. If you need to, set a timer to go off every five minutes to remind you to look up at an object at least 10 feet away for at least 15 seconds. This is called the 5-10-15 Rule and it is imperative to integrate into up-close work.

Lens Flexor

Purpose:

- Keep your lens young and flexible.
- Loosen tight eye muscles.
- Improve convergence, divergence, and fusion skills.
- Retrain the ciliary muscles to change the shape of the lens.
- Stretch vision in to improve near vision, stretch vision out to improve distance vision.

Directions:

1) Palm or patch your right eye.
2) Hold your left thumb or flexing card at arm's length directly in front of your nose.
3) Watch your thumb slowly come toward the tip of your nose and say, "Larger."
4) Watch your thumb slowly move away from your nose and say, "Smaller."
5) Travel in and out 5-10 times with eyes open, repeat 5-10 times with eyes closed.
6) Palm or patch your left eye and repeat steps 2-5 with your right eye.
7) Repeat steps 2-5 with both eyes open.
8) Palm both eyes and repeat mentally, continuing to say "Larger" and "Smaller."

Time: 2 to 5 minutes.

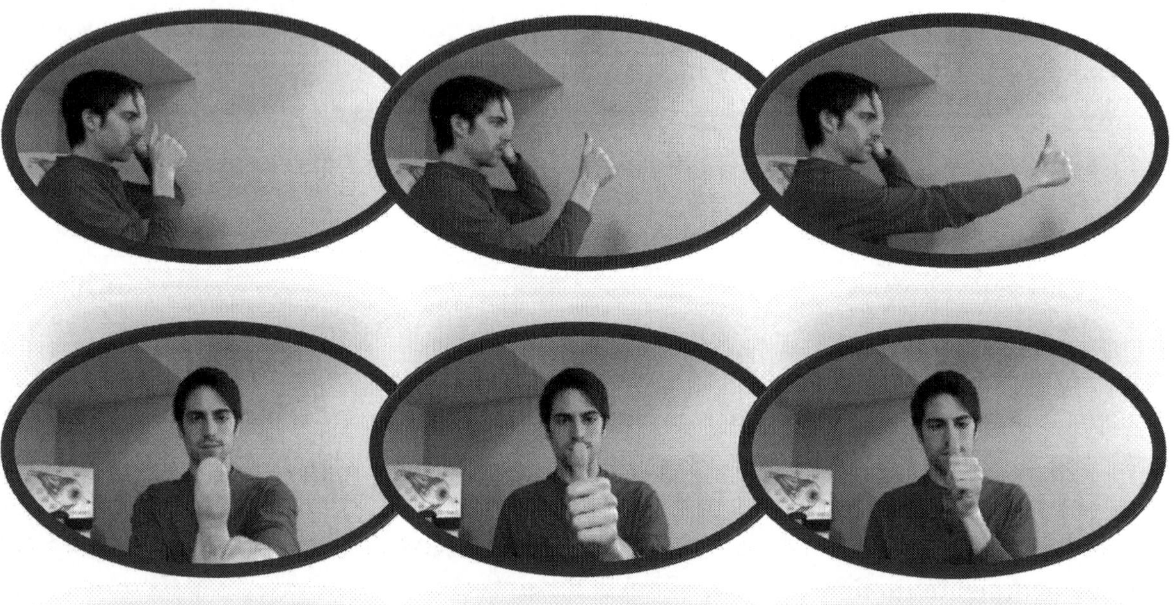

Description:

You may have heard that your lens hardens and become opaque as a natural byproduct of aging. This degradation is only a natural byproduct of aging if you do absolutely nothing to prevent it from happening. Flexing your lens regularly can keep it young, flexible, and functional for much longer in life. Flexing also works your extrinsic eye muscles, improving your ability to converge, or cross, your eyes so they are able to point at the same exact point at the same exact time at the same exact rate.

Flexing refers to watching an object come in toward your nose and then out away from your nose. You can use your thumb, a flexing card, a book, a cell phone, a photograph, etc. Using your thumb is very versatile because you always have your thumb handy. The alphabet cards *(Page 312)* are preferred though because it will be easier for you to tell where your 'edge' is, or where the letters just start to blur. Refer back to *Page 30* to see where your edge is.

Honor your edge and don't go too far beyond where it starts to blur. If you are nearsighted, flex the object out until it just starts to blur, then bring it back in to where it is clearer and easier. If you are farsighted, flex the object in until it just starts to blur, then send it back out to where it is clearer and easier. If you are farsighted so that the alphabet card never looks totally clear within arm's length, try doing this with your large eye chart in the distance. Stand beyond arm's length where the chart looks clear and then lean in closer until the letters just start to lose focus. Lean back to where they are clear and repeat. In both instances of nearsightedness and farsightedness, the letters will go from clear to blurry and back to clear.

When you repeat this practice with your eyes closed, you want to begin imagining that the letters never become blurry, even when they reach the distances where they looked blurry with your eyes open. Use your imagination to begin picturing what the clarity will eventually look like at those challenging distances. Keep thinking or saying, "Larger", "Smaller" in accordance to where the imaginary alphabet card is. Even though your eyelids are closed, your eyes ought to still be responding as if they were open - crossing as your mental thumb comes in and uncrossing as your mental thumb goes out. With time and practice, your edge can start to stretch out or in or both. Therefore, the lens flexor is an extremely powerful way to both improve near vision for farsighted people and improve far vision for nearsighted people. It is also one of the most pertinent practices to prevent or reverse cataracts, or opacities of the lens, by increasing flexibility of the lens.

Alignment is important here, so whatever object you flex with, make sure it travels directly in front of your nose instead of in front of your left eye or right eye. When you flex with one eye palmed or patched, your flexing object ought to look a little off center. When you flex with both eyes open, your flexing object ought to look like it is right in the center.

In order to focus on anything about 20 feet or closer the lenses inside your eyes must thicken like magnifying glasses. This happens by action of the ciliary muscles and suspensory ligaments that change the shape of your lens. To focus near your eyeballs must also elongate by way of your four recti muscles relaxing and your two oblique muscles contracting, squeezing the eye across the middle. In addition to those accommodative actions, your extrinsic eye muscles must also coordinate to cross, or converge, perfectly together so your eyes can both point at the near object in harmony. This convergence also stimulates accommodation. In a lot of cases of farsightedness *(presbyopia and hypermetropia)* the internal and external eye muscles do not function properly, which manifests as convergence insufficiency, or the eyes not crossing in equally or crossing at all. Luckily these muscles can be retrained with the lens flexor, which helps retrain your ciliary muscles and extra-ocular muscles to work in harmony and encourage fusion and focus.

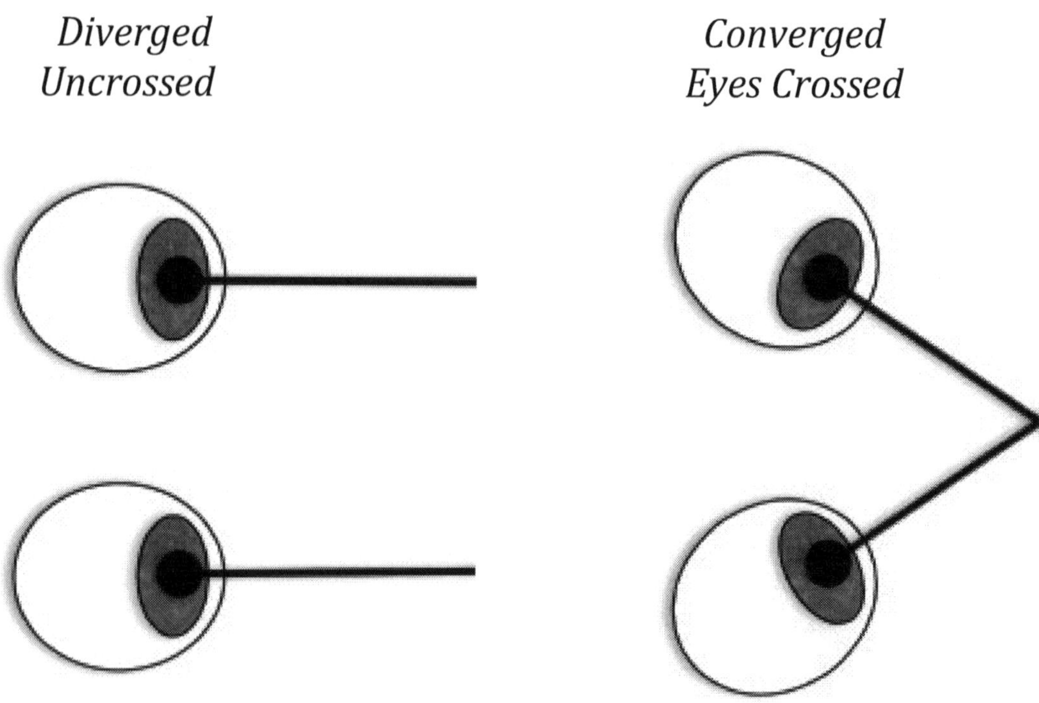

Rope Fusion

Purpose:

- Encourage teamwork between your two eyes.
- Stretch focus in and out.
- Retrain the eye muscles to converge and diverge properly.
- Raise awareness of peripheral vision.
- Establish stronger eye-mind connection.

Directions:

1) Attach one end of a rope to a doorknob or hold a short rope in outstretched hand.
2) Hold the other end of the rope directly in front of your nose, a few inches out.
3) Palm or patch your right eye and track up and down the rope with your left eye.
4) Repeat mentally with eyes closed for a few trips up and down the memory rope.
5) Palm or patch your left eye and track up and down the rope with your right eye.
6) Repeat mentally with eyes closed for a few trips up and down the memory rope.
7) Track up and down the rope with both eyes together.
8) Notice that the rope makes a V up close, an X in the middle, an A in the distance.
9) Repeat mentally with eyes closed for a few trips up and down the memory rope.

Time: 2 to 4 minutes.

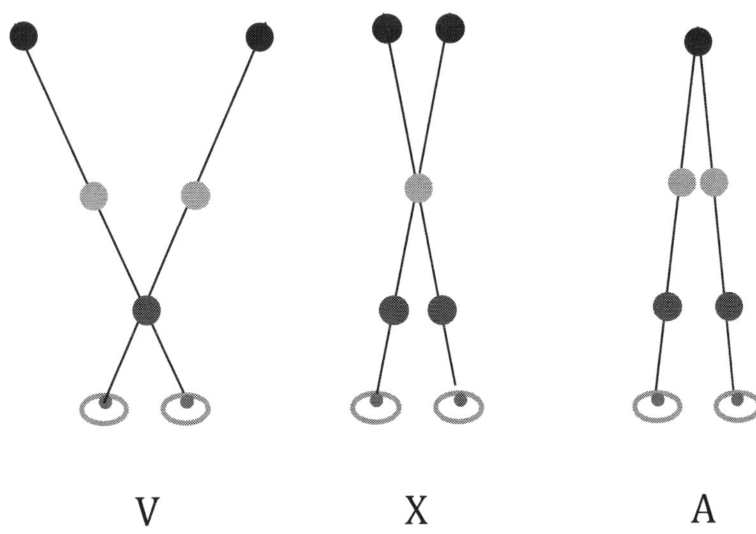

Description:

Having two eyes gives you three-dimensional, binocular, or stereoscopic vision. Your left eye sees one image and your right eye sees another image. Your mind must fuse the two images together into one perfectly overlapped image through fusion to avoid double vision.

The definition of fusion is the eyes' ability to look at the same exact point at the same exact time at the same exact rate. If there is any lack of fusion, focus will be compromised and you may experience blur, overlapping, doubling, shadows, lack of depth perception, or two-dimensional vision. Tracking your eyes up and down a rope or string helps to bring back and strengthen fusion. It helps your eyes learn how to work together as a team and realign with each other, while also improving focus. Some vision therapists refer to this as the Brock String, which is a string with colored beads on it. You can use a bare rope or add beads, washers, or knots to your rope to give your eyes and mind something more to fuse together and rest on as you track the rope. You can use a short 1 to 2 foot rope that you can hold with both hands or use a long 10 to 20 foot rope to work on fusion farther away.

Hold your end of the rope 3 to 12 inches in front of your nose so that you can easily look at the close end without straining. Either work with a partner who holds the other end of the rope in front of their nose or tie the other end to something in the distance at about eye level like a doorknob, a tree, or a coatrack. Alignment is important, so make sure you hold the rope directly in front of your nose, not off center closer to one eye or the other. Also try to pull the rope taut and hold the rope parallel with the floor.

Palm or patch your right eye and begin tracking up and down the rope with your left eye only. Keep the rope right in front of your nose so that the rope looks a little off-center and your left eye has to cross or turn in when your gaze comes up close. Remember to breathe and blink as you travel up and down the rope. Close your eyes and track up and down the rope in your mind a few times. Then palm or patch your left eye and begin tracking up and down the rope with your right eye only. Keep the rope right in front of your nose so you can feel your right eye turning in when you centralize up close. Close your eyes and track up and down the rope in your mind. Then begin tracking up and down the rope with both eyes together. When tracking with both eyes you will see the appearance of two ropes that intersect each other. Whichever point along the rope your gaze lands, or where you are centralizing, will be where those two ropes intersect and everywhere else along the rope will appear doubled because that is your peripheral vision in the foreground or background where you are not centralizing.

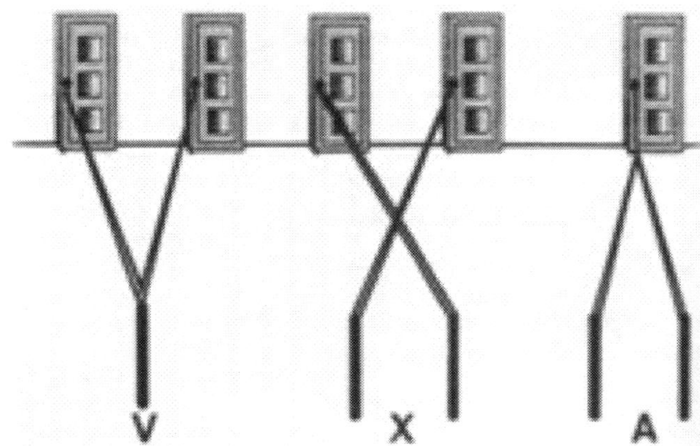

When looking up close the intersection will be at the very beginning and the two ropes will split off out into opposite directions creating a V shape. As you diverge and track out along the rope, the intersection will move farther out and create an X shape. As you get about halfway along the rope and beyond, the intersection will create an A shape. Say each letter out loud as they appear, "V, X, A, X, V, X, A, X, V, X, A, X, V, X, A" etc. If it helps, tilt your chin up as you track out from V to X to A and then tilt your chin down as you track in from A to X to V, rather than keeping your head still and just moving your eyes.

Just like with the gateposts, one rope may appear more solid or more transparent than the other. This is an indication of a weaker eye or a dominant eye. See if you can mentally move your attention from the left rope to the right rope as you track to see if you can make one more solid and then the other more solid.

Even if the rope gets blurry near in the case of farsightedness or it gets blurry far in the case of nearsightedness, keep tracking up and down and saying the letters out loud. Think about the texture of the rope and project that clarity onto the blurry parts. If your rope has beads on it notice that when you look at the closest bead it fuses into one and the other beads in the background appear to split in two. When you look at the middle bead, that one fuses together while the bead in the foreground and the bead in the background appear to split in two. When you gaze at the farthest bead that one fuses together and the other two beads in the foreground appear to split in two. Help this establish your eye-mind connection even more of making sure your eyes and your mind are both traveling together and looking at the same point on the rope at the same time at the same rate, without your eyes or your mind getting ahead of the other.

Convergence and Divergence Games

Purpose:

- Stimulate accommodation, see more clearly.
- Retrain the eye muscles to turn the eyes in and out properly.
- Enhance the peripheral vision.
- Strengthen fusion and cultivate clear flashes.

Directions:

Convergence Game

1) Hold 2 pencils or a fusion card 12 inches in front of your nose about ½ inch apart.
2) Gently cross (converge) your eyes slightly until you see three pencils.
3) If you see 4 pencils, your eyes are either too converged or not converged enough.
4) Once you get the third pencil, relax your gaze on it and allow it to come into focus.
5) Hold the third pencil as you move the pencils farther apart, side to side, or in and out.
6) Blink regularly and look at a distant object after holding the third image.
7) Follow with palming to relax your eye muscles.

Divergence Game

1) Hold two pencils or a fusion card 6 inches in front of your nose about ½ inch apart.
2) Gently uncross (diverge) your eyes slightly until you see three pencils.
3) If you see four pencils, your eyes are either too diverged or not diverged enough.
4) Once you get the third pencil, relax your gaze on it and allow it to come into focus.
5) Hold the third pencil as you move the pencils farther apart, side to side, or in and out.
6) Blink regularly and look at a distant object after holding the third image.
7) Follow with palming to relax your eye muscles.

Time: 1 to 4 minutes.

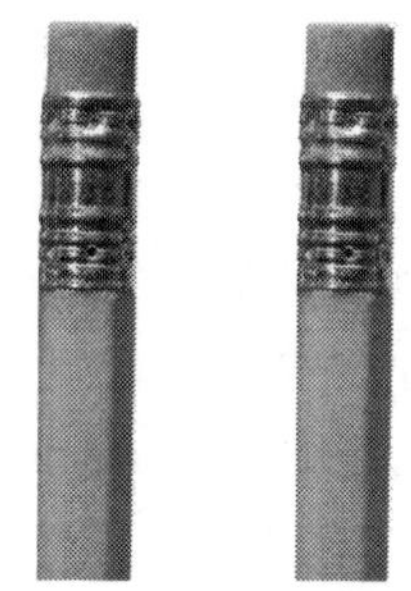

Focusing on pencils

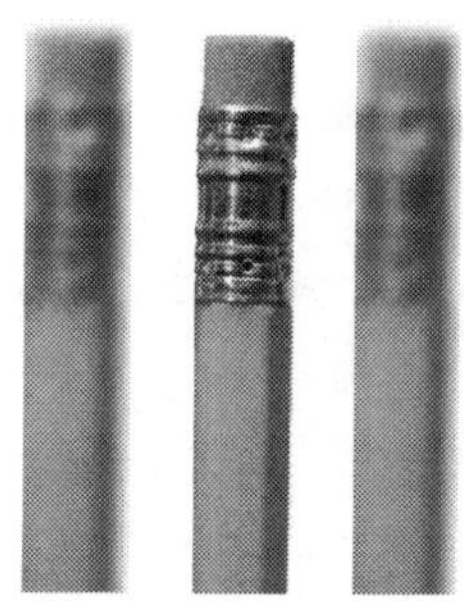

Focusing beyond or in front of pencils

Description:

Convergence and divergence games are more advanced fusion drills than gateposts and rope fusion. Any two identical objects, whether your two thumbnails, two pencils, two traffic lights, two taillights of a car, two identical eye charts side by side, or the fusion cards *(Page 313)* may be used. Make sure that your two objects are well lit so they are very easy to see. It may also help to have a plain background to avoid peripheral distractions. If using your thumbs or pencils it is very important to hold them perfectly parallel with each other and that your head is straight up and not tilted off-center. The way to see a 'third' object when there are really only two is to focus either at a closer or farther point than the two objects.

To get the third pencil using convergence, start by holding two pencils fairly close together. Gently cross your eyes and bring your focus somewhere between your pencils and your nose until you see a third pencil in between the two pencils. To get the third pencil using divergence, gently send your focus off into the distance beyond the two pencils until you see a third pencil in between the two pencils. In both cases, the third pencil will pop out into very 3D clarity and the other two pencils will become less clear. If you see four pencils you are either converging or diverging your eyes too much or not enough. It is much easier to adjust the pencils than it is to adjust your eyes, so make it easy for yourself by relaxing your gaze up close or far away and moving your pencils closer and farther from each other or closer and farther from your nose, until you can easily see the third image appear without trying too hard. Once you can get the third image to appear, see how long you can hold it without staring, remembering to breathe, blink, and stay relaxed. The harder you try the harder it gets, so keep it fun and playful. When you release your convergence or divergence, notice how things in general appear clearer than before.

To use your fusion cards, cut out the 7 pairs of two objects side by side. Some of the objects are identical, some objects are split in two, and some objects are slightly different. In all cases, you can either converge or diverge to get the third image to appear in the middle. If you need help converging, hold a pen, pencil, or pointer halfway between your nose and the card. Move the pen closer or farther from your nose until you can start to see the third object appear in the background behind the pen. It may take some practice to be able to diverge and 'look through' the card keeping your eyes relaxed in the distance. Often the divergence feels more relaxing than the convergence because it is like you are gazing in the distance, whereas the convergence involves muscular control to cross your eyes. It is possible to converge two objects that are farther apart than your two eyes, but it is only possible to diverge two objects that are as close together as your two eyes or closer.

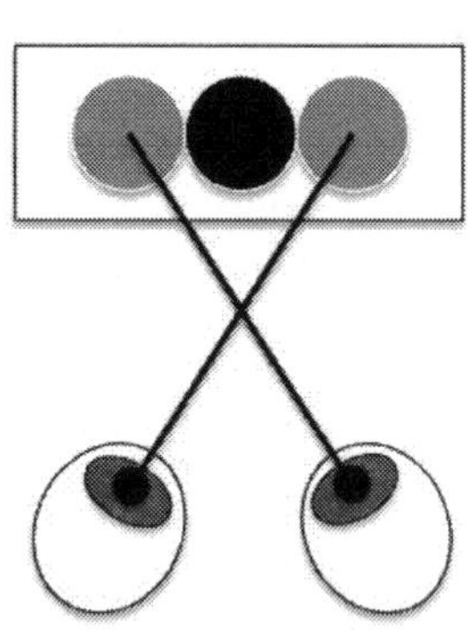

Converged
Eyes are Crossed
Looking closer than card
Left Eye sees Right Dot
Right Eye sees Left Dot
See 3 Dots

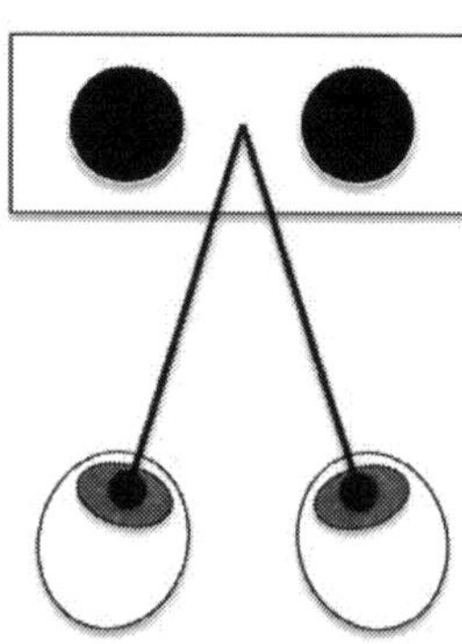

Normal
Focused
Looking at card
Both eyes point in
between two dots
See 2 Dots

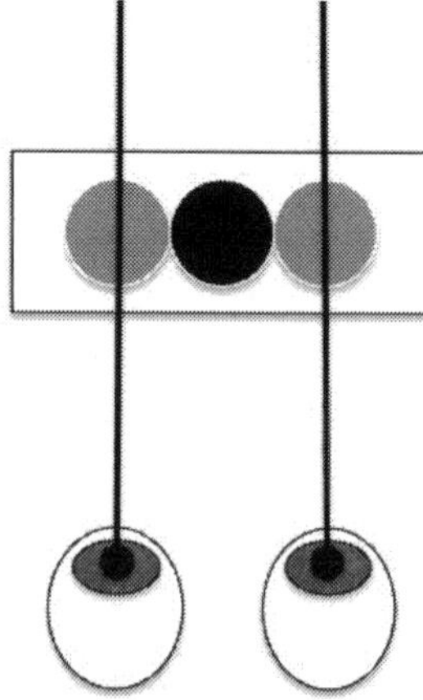

Diverged
Eyes are Uncrossed
Looking farther than card
Left Eye sees Left Dot
Right Eye sees Right Dot
See 3 Dots

The first goal of these advanced fusion games is simply to get the third image to appear and hold it without losing it. The second goal is to accommodate or focus on the third image so that it appears clearly, and maybe even three-dimensionally. The third goal is to hold the clear third image as you move it in and out, up and down, side to side, or around in a circle. Can you hold the clear third image while swinging? Can you easily go back and forth between converging and diverging to get the third object?

The most important thing to understand about this practice is that convergence and divergence can both stimulate accommodation, or focus. Essentially, they are training your eye muscles to learn how to focus and see clearly again. If you can get the third image to appear but it does not come into focus, keep practicing until it begins to appear clearer. This may take several days or weeks of practice before the focusing muscles reactivate. The convergence game tends to be more beneficial for farsightedness because it trains the eyes to turn in and focus up close. The divergence game tends to be more beneficial for nearsightedness because it trains the eyes to turn out and focus far away. If you cannot get the third object, there may be a basic fusion issue, and you need to spend more time working with gateposts, near to far shifting, lens flexor, and rope fusion before trying these.

Mental Focus #6: Teeter Totter / See Saw

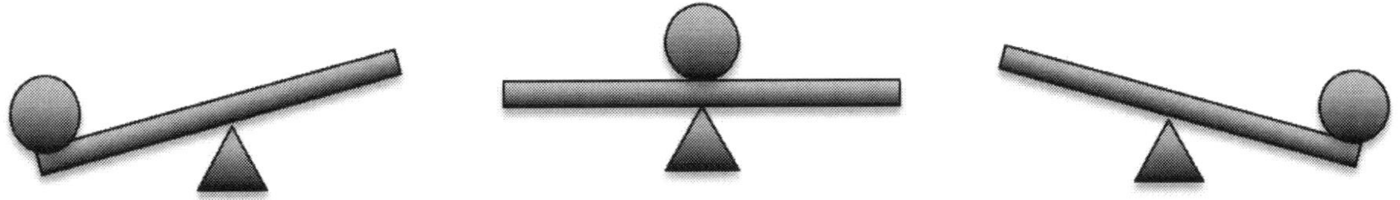

While palming, picture watching a heavy black ball roll from side to side on a teeter-totter. First picture the ball balanced right on the middle of an even board. Then imagine the board tilting to one side and watch as gravity slowly pulls the ball toward the lower side. Imagine the board lifts up and tilts to the other side. Watch as gravity slowly pulls the ball through the center and down the other side. Keep watching the teeter-totter rise and fall with your breath. You may even want to tilt your body left and right in the direction the board tilts. Notice how the ball almost creates the shape of an infinity sign as you watch it fall down to the right, up to the left, down to the left, up to the right, etc.

If you are nearsighted, try picturing a tiny teeter-totter far off in the distance with a small ball rolling on it. If you are farsighted, try picturing a tiny teeter-totter up close. Either way, picture the teeter-totter and the ball perfectly clearly. Another version of this mental focusing practice is actually picturing yourself and a friend having fun on a seesaw. So sit on an imaginary seesaw with someone you love sitting across from you. Watch their face smile and laugh as you press off the ground and float into the air. Then your friend presses into the ground and you sink down toward the ground. Get into a rhythm and enjoy the rising and falling feeling of being weightless and playful.

Vision Work #6

Add the brain balancing and fusion practices to your current daily routine of relaxing, swinging, sunning, palming, and mental focusing practices. Try to notice how centralization plays a part in the fusion practices. Remain aware of your peripheral vision while performing fusion practices as well. You do not necessarily have to do every single fusion practice every single day. Try rotating them to keep it fun and interesting. For example, today you could do swinging, sunning, palming, and then the picket fence shifter and lens flexor. Tomorrow you could do swinging, sunning, palming, and then the rope fusion and convergence/divergence. Do not overwhelm yourself with too many practices to do each day. Take your time and stay relaxed.

Daily Practice Checklist Week 6

M Tu W Th F S Su		Practice	Time
☐☐☐☐☐☐☐	♥	Morning Relaxation Routine	3-6 minutes
☐☐☐☐☐☐☐	◀◀ ▶▶	Swinging	2-6 minutes
☐☐☐☐☐☐☐	☼	Sunning	1-4 minutes
☐☐☐☐☐☐☐		Palming & Mental Drill	2-8 minutes
☐☐☐☐☐☐☐	|||||	Picket Fence Shifter	1-4 minutes
☐☐☐☐☐☐☐	⊙	Centralization	2-4 minutes
☐☐☐☐☐☐☐	※	Brain Balancing	1-3 minutes
☐☐☐☐☐☐☐	VXA	Fusion Practices	2-8 minutes
☐☐☐☐☐☐☐	☺	Convergence/Divergence	2-4 minutes
		Daily Target:	***15-30 mins***

Vision Journal: ____________________________________

"So if you read in a textbook that something is not possible, it ain't necessarily so. With a great deal of self-awareness, a lot of hard work and the right training, many of you may be able to accomplish what was once thought to be impossible."

-Sue Barry

Chapter 7

Phase 3:
Vision Building
Seeing Clearer Near and Far

"Reading is to the mind what exercise is to the body. As by the one, health is preserved, strengthened and invigorated; by the other, sight, imagination and mental efficiency are enormously improved."

-Dr. William H. Bates

"People with short sight are afraid of distance, afraid mentally even to look at something far away. This mental strain immediately tightens the eye muscles, the obliques, and prevents far vision. It is this fear of the inability to see what the mind says ought to be seen that makes a blockage to the object before the eyes, therefore a blockage to interpretation by the mind."

-Margaret D. Corbett

"It rests the eyes to read the Snellen test card with good vision. To fail to read it perfectly requires a strain or an effort."

–Dr. William H. Bates

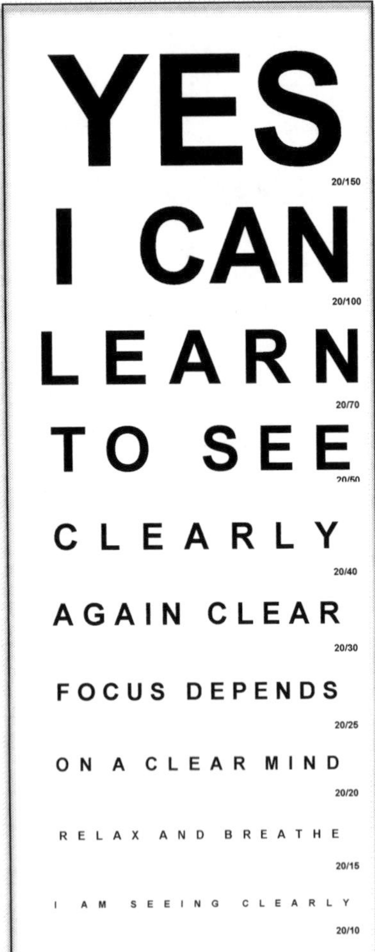

YES
20/150
I CAN
20/100
LEARN
20/70
TO SEE
20/50
CLEARLY
20/40
AGAIN CLEAR
20/30
FOCUS DEPENDS
20/25
ON A CLEAR MIND
20/20
RELAX AND BREATHE
20/15
I AM SEEING CLEARLY
20/10

Eye Chart for
Vision Building Far
Read beyond arm's length
(Pages 325 & 327)

A	B	C	D
E	F	G	H
I	J	K	L
M	N	O	P
Q	R	S	T
U	V	W	X
Y	Z		

Integral Eyesight Improvement LLC
www.integraleyesight.com

Alphabet Card for
Near to Far Matching
(Page 311)

Fundamentals of Eye Training

By Dr. William H. Bates MD

1. Vision can be improved by natural methods.

2. Tension causes eye strain and impairs vision. Relaxation relieves tension.

3. Relaxed eyes are normal eyes. When eyes lose their relaxation and become tense, they strain and stare and the vision becomes poor.

4. Vision can be improved only by education in proper seeing. Proper seeing is relaxed seeing. Normal eyes shift rapidly and continuously. Eyes with defective vision are fixed and staring. When staring eyes learn to shift, vision is improved.

5. The eyeball is like the camera, and changes in focal length. To focus the camera, you must adjust the distance from the negative to the front of the camera.

6. To focus the eye, the distance between the retina at the back and the cornea in the front must be increased for close vision and decreased for the distant view.

7. Six muscles on the outside of the eyeball control its shape; four, reaching from front to back, flatten the eye; two, belting it around the middle, squeeze it long from front to back.

8. When the eyes are relaxed, these six muscles are flexible and cooperate automatically, adjusting the focal length so eyes may see both near and far.

9. Just as dependence on crutches weakens leg muscles, so dependence on glasses weakens eye muscles by relieving them of responsibility. But muscles can be reeducated to do their duties.

10. Relaxation of the eyes and mind brings relaxation of the entire body. This general relaxation increases circulation and brings improved physical, visual and mental health.

Reading Card for
Vision Building Near
Read within arm's length
(Page 323)

Vision Building

Everything you have learned up until this point has been preparing you for the third phase of vision training, called Vision Building. The first phase, called Relaxation Foundations, was all about encouraging physical relaxation of the eyes and mental relaxation of the mind. The relaxation techniques include swinging, sunning, palming, visualizing, breathing, blinking, and stretching. The second phase, called Vision Warm Ups, was all about encouraging proper use and coordination of the eyes. The vision warm up techniques include centralizing, brain balancing, and the various fusion practices like gateposts, near to far shifting, lens flexor, rope fusion, and convergence divergence games.

Now the third phase, called Vision Building, is all about applying the principles of relaxation, centralization, and fusion to the act of reading with the goal of transforming blurry text into clearer text. At first this manifests in the form of temporary clear flashes, which may only last a few seconds. Maybe you have already begun experiencing some clear flashes as a result of applying the practices from the first two phases. The third phase of vision training is typically where the clear flashes begin to multiply and amplify, until they begin to become more permanent and long-lasting.

You may be able to easily relax your eyes while sunning or palming, but are you able to keep your eyes relaxed while reading? Only once you master the art of relaxed reading may you begin to master the art of relaxed seeing. Then, you can take the new clarity you achieve on reading cards and eye charts out into the world of three-dimensional objects.

Vision building consists of incorporating reading cards and eye charts into the various techniques you have already learned up to this point, and then following a new sequence of techniques summarized into a 6-Step Chart Clearing Formula to cultivate more clarity and hone your skills of both near and far vision.

Eye charts are not only for testing your vision. If used correctly, they can also be used for building and developing your vision. These pieces of paper with varying sized print will act as your vision training-ground and playground. They become the arenas for practicing applying the good vision habits you've been learning like breathing, blinking, stretching, shifting, swinging, balancing, flexing, fusing, visualizing, remembering, imagining, and most importantly relaxing. Do not let all the things you have been learning go right out the window once you begin reading. The vast majority of people realize that once they begin concentrating on reading, they totally forget about blinking and breathing.

Try to eliminate any preconceived notions you may have about these eye charts. Do not associate the eye charts with going to the eye doctor and getting your vision tested. That thought alone may induce stress, strain, or anxiety, which will negatively affect your vision and keep the charts blurry. Instead, think of vision building as one big fun experiment. You will be experimenting with various physical and mental techniques to see whether or not they have a positive effect on your vision. If you are able to access and maintain the good vision habits listed above, you will start to see the letters and words of the print more clearly. If you try too hard, treat this as a test, or take it too seriously, you will find yourself holding your breath or breathing shallow, holding your eyes open too long or staring, stiffening your body, constricting your eyes, squinting, squeezing, stressing, and straining. When your eyes and mind are in that state, the print will remain blurry. Relaxation is required to see the charts clearly. This is not 'vision testing', this is 'vision building.'

Vision building near is for accessing more clarity up close and involves using reading cards with different sized text within arm's length where some of the letters look slightly blurry. Vision building far is for accessing more clarity in the distance and involves using eye charts with different sized text beyond arm's length where some of the letters look slightly blurry. The main purpose of vision building near is to see how close you can hold the reading card and which size print you can read down to. The main purpose of vision building far is to see how far you can stand from the eye chart and which size print you can read down to. Even if the letters are blurry, you may still be able to make them out. You want the letters to start a little blurry so you can notice when you get a clear flash and you are able to see the letters more distinctly, or possibly see the next line down.

Whether working near or far or both, you will be applying essentially the same techniques, and this chapter explains how to adapt these techniques to fit your specific vision. Keep in mind you may have to adjust the distance between your eyes and your charts in order to be able to comfortably read the different sized text. If you are highly presbyopic you may need to begin the near vision building farther out beyond arm's length. If you are highly myopic you may need to begin the far vision building closer in within arm's length. It all comes down to your comfort level and finding the perfect distance where you are challenging your eyes and mind just enough without compromising your physical and mental relaxation.

You will obtain the best results by practicing vision building near your edge of clarity. *(Page 30)*. Your edge of clarity is the distance where the print on the reading card or eye chart begins to change from being clear to being blurry. That way, you will still be able to easily make out the letters and words but they will not be perfectly clear. You will be practicing clearing the print by relaxing rather than by straining. You are learning a totally new way to focus. Go back and reference the distances you wrote down when you first created your starting point. That will most likely be the best distance for you to start.

If you are farsighted, hold your reading card at arm's length. Are the letters clear or blurry? If they are a little blurry, that is where you will begin. If they are clear, slowly bring the card closer until the letters start to get blurry. That is where you will begin. If you are nearsighted, sit or stand 1 foot from your eye chart. Are the letters clear or blurry? If they are a little blurry, that is where you will begin. If they are clear, slowly move away from your eye chart until the letters start to get blurry. That is where you will begin.

If you are farsighted you may want to spend more time using your reading cards with the intention of stretching your vision closer in. If you are nearsighted you may want to spend more time using your eye charts with the intention of stretching your vision farther out. In either case you will still want to do both vision building near and far because the two different versions complement each other. Not only will the vision building far be easier for farsighted people and vision building near be easier for nearsighted people, but the developments you get in the clearer parts of your visual field will begin to infuse more developments into the blurrier parts of your visual field. Instead of obsessing about the blurry parts of your vision where you can't see as well, notice what happens when you direct your energy toward the clearer parts of your vision where you already can see better and build on that.

Ideally, vision building is meant to be performed one eye at a time and then with both eyes together. If you are vision building for 15 minutes, start with an eye patch covering your right eye for 5 minutes, then spend 5 minutes with the eye patch covering your left eye, and then finish with 5 minutes of vision building without the eye patch using both eyes simultaneously. You may also want to palm your eyes in between vision building with your left eye, vision building with your right eye, and vision building with both eyes.

Try your best to apply the 50/50 vision building rule, which is equally balancing the amount of time you spend with your eyes open with the amount of time you spend with your eyes closed. One of the biggest mistakes people make when it comes to reading eye charts, and when it comes to seeing in general, is spending too much time with their eyes open and not enough time with their eyes closed. The human population is chronically overworking their eyes and neglecting the sizeable amount of rest they need to function optimally. Sometimes seeing more clearly is simply a matter of closing one's eyes more to rest them and focus the mind. It may seem paradoxical at first, but the more you close your eyes, the more you'll see when they are open.

"In order to improve your eyesight, you must improve your insight."
-Nathan T. Oxenfeld

Eventually the reading cards and eye charts may encompass the majority of your vision practice. As you will see, there are ways to incorporate the eye charts and reading cards into nearly all the practices from phases one and two, which is what you will learn first. Then you will learn a more specific sequence of techniques specific to the vision building process that tend to yield the most development and increased clarity with repetition.

In general, a good structure for your vision practice moving forward is spending 5 to 15 minutes warming up in preparation for vision building (any combination of swinging, sunning, palming, breathing, blinking, stretching, centralizing, fusing, etc.) followed by 10 to 30 minutes of actual vision building near and/or far. It would take you hours to do every single practice every single day. Instead, try cycling and rotating through your practices and varying your daily routine occasionally to keep it fun and interesting. So maybe today you will spend 10 minutes swinging, sunning, and palming leading into 20 minutes of vision building. Tomorrow you might spend 10 minutes brain balancing and the rope fusion leading into 20 minutes of vision building. The next day you might spend 10 minutes doing tapping, acupressure points, and converging/diverging leading into 20 minutes of vision building.

Do not overdo vision building. If you were to painstakingly go through every single vision building technique on your left eye, then your right eye, then both eyes, it would take half a day. Start small and only go for as long as you are engaged and relaxed. Allow your vision building practice to grow organically over time and have fun with it.

Clear Flashes

Clear flashes are moments of clarity that you begin experiencing when regularly practicing the vision building techniques near and far. You may have already experienced some clear flashes so far while practicing your relaxation foundations and vision warm ups. Achieving these clear flashes is a glimpse of where your vision is headed and they only occur when your eyes and mind are relaxed. At first, your clear flashes may be temporary in nature and only last for an instant. Many times, the excitement of seeing perfectly clearly without glasses makes you lose the flash and start straining or staring again. Sometimes your eye muscles have been chronically straining for so long that they quickly retreat back to their old patterns of constriction. So, what can you do to make these flashes last longer?

There are two things you can do when you experience a clear flash. Option one is to take in as much clarity as you can by pivoting your head and letting your eyes travel all around the space you are in while breathing and blinking easily. State a verbal confirmation to solidify the flash such as, "I am seeing clearly" or "My vision is clear." Option two is to close your eyes and 'deposit' the clear flash into your recent memory bank. The more recent memories of clarity you 'deposit', the more clarity you will be able to 'withdraw' from your memory bank in the future.

With continued practice you will get more comfortable with this new state of clear vision, which will enable you to maintain your flashes longer. Eventually, your flashes will stick around for 30 seconds, a full minute, five minutes, all afternoon, or even all day. The overall goal of this entire natural vision improvement process is achieving a permanent clear flash that doesn't go away. That will be your new vision, or your new baseline.

Keep in mind that clear flashes can be quite subtle at first. Since the cones in your macula are best equipped for seeing details, try noticing flashes in a small area within your central visual field. Your clear flash may only be on one leaf of a tree, one blade of grass, one petal of a flower, one word on a page, or one letter on an eye chart. Your entire visual field may not pop out into complete clarity at first. However, even if just one piece of the picture pops out into clarity that is still considered a flash and is a very good sign that you are reactivating your focusing muscles and relearning how to see clearly again with your naked eyes. Over time, the flashes will expand and multiply. It helps to keep track of your clear flashes by writing them down in your vision journal.

Incorporating Eye Charts Into Your Vision Practices

Swinging the Charts

Standing or sitting, do a few long swings or gentle body sways to encourage relaxation, increase saccadic eye movements, activate your involuntary system, and get the chart to move in the opposite direction. Try swinging or swaying both side-to-side to see the oppositional movement and forward-to-back to see the larger-smaller effect. Constant movement during your vision building practice will prevent staring and help you maintain rhythmic motion, which will clear the chart.

Swing facing the chart, watching the chart swing in the opposite direction. Instead of looking at your thumb in the second step of the long swing, look at your alphabet card and observe everything in the background sliding by smoothly in the opposite direction. Swing with the eye chart off to your left so your eyes land on a different part of the chart each time you swing to the left. Swing with the chart off to your right so your eyes land on a different part of the chart each time you swing to the right. Swing with the chart directly behind you so your eyes land on a different part of the chart as you glance over each shoulder. Swing with your eyes closed and remember the oppositional movement mentally. A gently swinging chart will clear up much more than a stationary chart.

A constant theme of all the different vision building techniques is motion. Avoid staring by keeping your head in constant gentle motion. Pivot your head left to right as you underline the letters of the chart with your nose. This is the most important habit to maintain while reading near and far. Never stop moving your head or you may end up staring, straining, or trying too hard. Keep it moving!

Sunning the Charts

If possible, bring your reading cards outside and hang your eye chart outdoors where the sun can shine on them at an angle without producing glare. Not only will the full-spectrum sunlight increase the contrast of the letters against the background and help you see the text more clearly, but you can also easily sun your eyes to refresh them whenever they feel tired during reading. The charts usually sharpen up after sunning. If indoors, use a bright light or lamp to replace the sun.

Palming the Charts

Close your eyes and palm your eyes often to avoid overworking them or trying too hard. Remember and visualize the letters and words on your reading cards and eye charts. Nose draw them and imagine them perfectly clearly. Maintain clear thoughts while palming to rest your eyes and focus your mind. Keep your mind attentive with mental focusing practices while palming and you will see more clearly when you come back out of palming. Recall pleasant happy memories, picture the darkest black or a black dot, visualize parts of objects while going through alphabet categories, occupy your mind with the rhythm of the teeter totter, memorize the letter classifications, or employ other mental centralizations. Whatever you decide to think of while palming, try to think of that one thing best.

Breathing the Charts

Take long, deep, slow, rhythmic breaths while reading. Contract your abdomen on your exhale and relax and expand your abdomen on your inhale. Oxygenating your eyes and brain will help clear up your vision. Holding your breath will lower your vision. Try taking five or ten big yawns in a row and watch the print clear up before your lubricated eyes. Observe any effect that the yogic breathing practices from Chapter 8 have on your vision. Allow your rhythmic breaths to instill a deep state of physical and mental relaxation. When you slow down your breath, your body and your mind also slow down and you can access deeper states of relaxation. Notice when you've lost connection with your breath or you hold your breath, and restart your deep 2:1 ratio belly breathing. The harder you try to see, the less you breathe.

Blinking the Charts

Avoid staring by blinking regularly, every 2 to 5 seconds while reading. Keep your blinks soft and effortless and notice that the chart jumps slightly each time you blink. Remember that blinking ought not to interfere with your clear flashes. When you get a clear flash, keep the faith that it will still be there even after you blink. Every once in a while, do some rapid yet gentle butterfly blinks to jumpstart your focusing muscles. The harder you try to see, the less you blink.

Stretching the Charts

If your body is tense, your eyes will be tense. Stretch out your head, neck, shoulders, and back with some simple stretches and movements. Notice if the print clears during or after the body stretches. Explore the connection between your eyes and the rest of your body, all the way down to your hips, legs, and toes. Your posture can affect your clarity. If you slouch, jut your chin out, or some other misalignment, your nervous system cannot communicate totally effectively. Whether you are sitting or standing, remain aware of the position of your head, shoulders, and spine. Pay attention to all the muscles in your face and ensure that you are not clenching your jaw, scrunching your brow, or tensing your eyelids. Stretch out your eye muscles with the yogic eye movements. Notice if the print clears during or after the eye stretches. The harder you try, the tighter your muscles get.

Centralizing the Charts

See whichever letter or word you are looking at more distinctly than the rest. Realize that all the rest of the letters or words in your peripheral vision are less distinct and less black than the one you are looking at. Look at the left side of each letter, then the right side, then the top and bottom, and remind yourself that whatever part you are looking at is the most clear compared to the areas you are not looking at. Practice outlining, counting, and shape recognition on the charts. Do some peripheral stimulation by wiggling your fingers or moving your picket fence shifter around in your peripheral field while centralizing on your charts. The harder you try to see, the less you centralize.

Balancing the Chart

Make sure you are hydrated before reading. Massage or tap your brain buttons, or kidney 27 points and notice if the print clears during or after. Try different variations of the cross crawl or cross march and notice if the print clears during or after. Try both versions of the hook-ups and notice if the print clears while holding the positions or after you release. Try the brain balancing practices with eyes open and with eyes closed. In addition to the specific brain balancing practices, balancing your body can sometimes stimulate vision. Your ocular and vestibular systems are linked, and your vestibular system deals with your balance. Try reading while balancing on one foot or while balancing a book on your head.

Shifting the Charts

Hold one finger, pen, pencil, or pointer in front of your nose when reading your cards and charts with both eyes open. Look at the text through the gateposts and swing the letters or words between the gateposts. Then try the near to far shifting by holding up two alphabet cards, one in each hand, one near your nose and one at arm's length, aiming at your eye chart. Gaze at the near alphabet card, then the far alphabet card, then out to the eye chart, then back to your far alphabet card and back to your near alphabet card. Repeat several times with your eyes open and eyes closed.

You can also use your picket fence shifter with your chart in the background. Slowly move the pickets horizontally, vertically, or diagonally in front of your eyes and glance at the chart once the pickets get out of the way. Move the picket fence shifter vertically in front of your left eye as you read the text with your right eye. Move the picket fence shifter vertically in front of your right eye as you read the text with your left eye.

In addition to the gateposts, near to far shifting, and picket fence shifting, try to maintain constant short shifts or short swings on the card or chart you're looking at. Short shifting means moving your attention from one part of a word or letter to another. Remember that your eyes attend your thoughts, so allow your mind lead the way and let your eyes and head follow.

As you shift your mental attention on and around letters and text, bring your attention to the subtle oppositional movement that happens. When you look from the top of a letter to the bottom of a letter, observe how the letter shifts up slightly. When you look from the bottom of a letter to the top of the letter, observe how the letter shifts down slightly. When you look from left to right the letter jumps left. When you look right to left the letter jumps right. This is very subtle but very valuable because according to Dr. Bates, the shorter the shift the greater the relaxation.

"It has always been demonstrated that the continuous memory, imagination, or vision of one thing for any length of time is impossible. To see one letter of the Snellen test card continuously, it is necessary to shift from one part of the letter to another."

–Dr. William H. Bates

Flexing the Charts

Hold up one thumb or alphabet card a few inches in front of your nose and perform the lens flexor. Gaze at your thumb or card as you slowly send it out to arm's length. Watch it get smaller and smaller and then send your gaze out to the chart. Bring your gaze back to your thumb or card and watch it slowly return to your nose getting larger and larger. Repeat several times with your eyes open and closed. To get the flexing action using your distance eye chart, stagger your feet with one foot in front of the other. Shift your weight from your left foot to your right foot and begin rocking forward and back, getting closer and farther from the chart. As you get closer the letters grow larger and as you move farther the letters shrink smaller. Repeat with eyes open and eyes closed.

Fusing the Charts

Hold your short rope up in front of your nose and point it out toward the chart or attach a longer rope to the chart. Track up and down the rope and notice the chart separating and coming closer together in the background. Watch the rope create a V up close, an X in the middle, an A in the distance, gaze at the chart for a moment and call out a letter, then come back to the rope to watch the A turn into the X turn into the V. Even without a rope you can simply cross your eyes to see the chart split into two in the background and then diverge your eyes to see the chart and all the letters fuse back into one. It is almost like you are tracking up and down an imaginary or invisible rope from the chart to your nose and back.

Defocusing and Refocusing the Charts

If the print up close or far away appears blurry, can you try making the print even blurrier temporarily? As you breathe in, strain your eyes in a way that makes your vision worse for a moment, whether that means diffusing your focus out into the periphery, retracting your focus closer in, or temporarily straining your eyes in some way. As you breathe out, fully release that strain and watch as your vision gets relatively better. Even if it does not become perfectly clear, it looks better compared to when you were straining. This helps you reorganize your visual system to associate blur with strain and clarity with relaxation. Some people find this easier to do with just one eye at a time while others find it easier to do with both eyes together. When defocusing with both eyes you may be converging to make the text blurrier, which will result in double vision. When you exhale and diverge the image becomes single again, which will make it easier to see and read as opposed to seeing two images.

Tensing and Releasing the Charts

Similar to the defocusing and refocusing, tensing and releasing involves temporarily straining your facial muscles as you inhale and then fully relaxing on the exhale. Whereas in the defocus refocus you keep your eyes open the whole time, in the tense and release you actually squeeze your eyes shut as you inhale and open them as you exhale. You do not have to squeeze very hard, especially if you have glaucoma or high eye pressure. A gentle squeeze is fine. You can either just squeeze your eyes, or you can squeeze all the muscles in your face toward the tip of your nose. Pair the release of the squeezed muscles with a big exhale, sigh, or yawn and you may notice a flash of clarity upon opening your eyes.

Remembering the Charts:

Memory brings vision. Using your memory is not 'cheating.' The point is to memorize your charts and reading cards. You are supposed to already know exactly what the vision building charts say. Remind yourself often that this is not a test. While you are first rehabilitating your vision, you will need to use your memory as an aid to help your eyes see more. Once you see start seeing more clearly more often, you will not need to rely on your memory quite as much. But until then, do not suppress your memory. That will only put you at a disadvantage and make it harder for yourself. Perfect memory of anything leads to more perfect vision. Close your eyes and remember any letter of the alphabet perfectly clear and perfectly black. Keep that image in your mind as you exhale and open your eyes back up looking out at the chart for a flash of clarity. Even when your eyes are open, keep your memory active and keep thinking about that clear mental picture. 'Fish for flashes' by repeating this dozens of times in a row with an open mind. Close and remember the chart, breathe and open, and repeat. You can also remember or visualize any pleasant object or person as long as you can remember it perfectly and effortlessly.

"Memory of imperfect vision or a blur will make the vision still more imperfect so do not let your mind indulge in memories of astigmatic aberrations. Instead, close your eyes and remember something formerly seen that was clear and sharply defined. Incline your mind to the memory of perfect sight."

–Dr. William H. Bates

Converging and Diverging the Charts

Convergence stimulates accommodation. Therefore, when you converge on your fusion cards the third image that appears in the middle will become very clear. After holding that clear third image for a few breaths, diverge your eyes and look at your reading card or eye chart to see if the accommodation carries over. You can also use the 3D eye charts on *Pages 315 and 317* to get more clarity near and far.

If you are farsighted, hold the convergence 3D reading card *(Page 315)* or the divergence 3D reading card *(Page 317)* up close at a distance where it would normally be blurry. Cross your eyes or diverge your eyes to get the third dot and chart to appear in the middle and you ought to be able to see smaller text more clearly.

If you are nearsighted, hang the convergence 3D eye chart *(Page 315)* on a wall at a distance where it would normally be blurry. Cross your eyes to get the third eye chart to appear in the middle and you ought to be able to see smaller text more clearly. Not only will you experience more clarity on the middle column that appears, but you will also experience some interesting three-dimensional depth perception illusions. Certain lines and certain black dots will appear to pop out of the page and seem closer to you than others. This is only possible through relaxation; so do not try too hard. Make sure you keep breathing and blinking while converging. If your eyes or mind ever start to feel tired or strained, take a palming break to rest and rejuvenate.

You may also hang two identical YES I CAN or standard Snellen eye charts side by side on a wall and cross your eyes to get a third eye chart to appear. The bigger the text, the farther away you may be able to stand and stimulate better accommodation through convergence.

Smiling and Laughing at your Charts:

This is great to do when you catch yourself trying too hard or taking your vision building practice too seriously. It is nearly impossible to strain when you are smiling or laughing. Keep it light by putting a smile on your face and chuckling, giggling, or laughing out loud while reading. Show your teeth to your charts. Realize how simple reading is and how you don't have to do a single thing to see the charts. Even if you fake your smile or laugh, your brain doesn't know the difference and will initiate relaxation and enjoyment regardless. Just laugh and feel how joyful this process can be!

6-Step Chart Clearing Formula *(Vision Building Far)*

Purpose:

- Build distance vision by reading smaller and smaller print farther and farther away.
- Provide an opportunity to apply all the relaxation and focusing principles in practice.
- Keep track of your progress as your vision continues to improve.

A similar formula will be applied for both near reading cards and far eye charts. First you will learn how to apply it to your big YES I CAN eye chart *(Page 325 and 327)*. This version is more specific for nearsightedness, but will also benefit farsighted eyes. Standing or sitting at a comfortable distance from your well-lit eye chart where the letters are easily readable but slightly blurry, place an eye patch over one eye and spend between 10 and 60 seconds in each of the following steps on the top line of the eye chart.

Directions:

1) Space Riding
2) Centralizing and Verbalizing
3) Near to Far Matching
4) Closing and Visualizing
5) Breathing and Opening
6) Fishing for Flashes

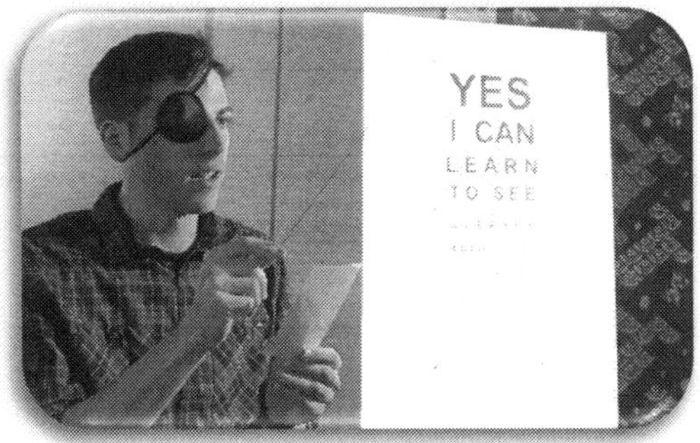

Either repeat 6-step formula on the same line again or move down to the next smaller line down and repeat. Gradually make your way down the eye chart as far as you can with one eye then continue space riding all the way down to the very bottom line, even if you cannot read it. Take a short palming break and then place the eye patch over your other eye to begin the 6-step formula back up on the top line. You may stand farther or closer if needed to get at the perfect distance where the letters are easily readable but slightly blurry with your other eye. Repeat some or all of the six steps on as many lines of the eye chart as you can with your other eye and then continue to space ride all the way to the very bottom line, even if you cannot read it. Take a short palming break and finish by repeating the 6-step formula on as many lines of the eye chart as you can with both eyes open and then space ride all the way to the bottom. The distance may change for reading the chart with just your left eye, just your right eye, and then both eyes together.

Time: 3 to 6 minutes with the left eye, 3 to 6 minutes with the right eye, 3 to 6 minutes with both eyes together, 10 to 20 minutes total.

Description:

Begin with **Step 1: Space Riding**. Keep your attention on the white areas of the eye chart as you underline the top line with your finger, a pen, pencil, or pointer. Follow the movement of your pointer with your nose, pivoting your head left to right as you ride beneath the letters from the left margin to the right margin and pivoting your head right to left as you ride beneath the letters from the right margin to the left margin. Essentially you will be moving your head throughout your entire vision building practice. Ride horizontally back and forth through the space above the letters. Ride vertically up and down in the white space to the left of the first letter and to the right of the last letter. Ride through the spaces in between, inside, and around the letters. Imagine that the white part of the chart you are riding on is brighter white than the rest of the chart you are not looking at. When space riding with an eye patch on, your pointer will appear single, helping you centralize. When space riding with both eyes open, your pointer will double, so use your pointer as gateposts and swing the entire line or individual letters in between your left and right gateposts as your eyes explore the white spaces.

Second, move to **Step 2: Centralizing and Verbalizing**. You will now be space riding around one letter at a time instead of the whole line of letters. You may also begin glancing directly at the black letters themselves. As you explore a smaller area tune into your centralization and realize that the other peripheral letters are not as distinct or dark as the one you are looking directly at. Say each letter out loud as you centralize on it. You may want to even trace the letters with your pointer and nose draw them. Pay attention to how you are verbalizing the letters. Call out the letters with a confident downward inflection at the end rather than inflecting upward at the end, making each letter sound like a question. Remember that constant shifting is necessary to maintain centralization, so keep breathing, blinking, and shifting to avoid the possibility of staring and diffusing out to try and see the other words on the eye chart that you are not centralizing on.

Third, move to **Step 3: Near to Far Matching**. Hold your alphabet card *(Page 311)* in your hand at a distance where the letters look best. Find the first letter of the eye chart on the alphabet card. Nose draw the close letter as you say, "Y near". Match the close letter with the far letter by nose drawing the far letter as you say, "Y far". Go back and forth from looking at the close clear version of the letter to looking at the far less-clear version of the letter two or three times before matching the next letter on the eye chart. When matching with both eyes open, swing the close letter between your gateposts as you call it out and then swing the far letter between your gateposts as you call it out.

Fourth, move to **Step 4: Closing and Visualizing**. Close your eyes and nose draw the letters of the eye chart in your mind at approximately the same size and distance that they actually are on the chart. Say the letters out loud as you draw them and picture them perfectly clearly. Activate your memory, imagination, and visualization to 'see' the letters using your insight or your inner vision. Even if the letters appeared blurry with your eyes open, you know what a Y looks like and an E looks like and an S looks like. You just saw them clearly on your alphabet card up close. So simply remember what you just saw. Do not suppress your memory; use it to help you see more clearly. Once you have drawn the word YES in your mind, imagine drawing a bright white line beneath the word YES. As you trace that white line back and forth your head will pivot gently side to side.

Keep that head movement going and maintain the clear memory as you transition into **Step 5: Breathing and Opening**. With your eyes still closed and your head still pivoting, tracing that imaginary white line beneath the perfect nose drawing of the letters, inhale deeply through your nose. As you exhale with an audible breath, sigh, or yawn, open your eyes back up onto the eye chart to either trace the white line under the letters or nose draw the letters with your eyes open. In other words, keep some sort of movement going as you open your eyes instead of freezing and staring. Notice if you see a clear flash upon opening.

Step 6: Fishing for Flashes is simply repeating steps 4 and 5 a handful of times. Consider this fishing analogy. If you don't catch a fish the first time you cast your line out, you don't just give up and go back to shore. You cast your line back out again a second time, a third time, a fourth time, until you catch a fish. Maybe the fish aren't biting today, so then you go back to shore, but at least you tried. Maybe you catch enough fish to feed the whole town. Think about clear flashes like fish. If you don't get a clear flash the first time you do your chart formula, don't just give up. Repeat it as many times as you can until you catch a flash. Some days you won't get any flashes, but other days you'll get enough flashes to see the whole town! So close your eyes again visualize the letters perfectly in your mind. Breathe and open your eyes back onto the chart with a big exhale. Maintain diaphragmatic or belly breathing to increase the chances of catching a flash and to avoid holding your breath. Pay attention to the clear flashes that come by noticing when the print becomes clearer. Remember that clear flashes are primarily found in your central vision, not your peripheral vision. Know that they can be partial clear flashes too, so even if your vision only gets 50% clearer instead of 100% clearer, that still counts as a clear flash. Observe and allow the fluctuations to happen, and experiment with different ways to stretch the clear flashes out to last longer by maintaining centralization and dynamic relaxation.

Once you complete the 6 steps on the top line of the eye chart you can either repeat them again on the top line or begin the 6-step formula on the second line. Take your time and try not to rush through the eye chart. Make your way down the chart that way as far as you can until you can no longer read the print. You can either get closer in order to be able to easily perform all 6 steps, or you can stay at the same distance and simply space ride the remaining lines all the way to the bottom. Once you reach the bottom of the eye chart with one eye, you can switch the eye patch to cover your other eye and start over from the top. Take your time and make your way gradually down the chart with your other eye until you can't read the print any more. Either get closer to keep doing all 6 steps or simply space ride to the bottom. Once you reach the bottom of the chart with your other eye, you can remove the eye patch and start over from the top using both eyes together. Notice that if you try to use a pointer with both eyes you will see two pointers when looking at the chart in the distance. You can use your gateposts instead to fix this dilemma. Instead of pointing at individual letters, you will swing those letters in between your two gateposts. You can also do it without gateposts, but the gateposts often lead to more development and flashes.

Never squint, strain, or stare at your eye chart. The chart will only clear when you are in a state of relaxation. Close your eyes often and look away from the chart often. Try to customize your chart practice by figuring out which practices seem to clear the print more and spend more time repeating those. Once you begin noticing more flashes of clarity and more development in your vision at one distance, try standing a little farther away from your eye chart to continue stretching your vision farther away. Let's say this week you can read down to the 5th line standing at 5 feet. With daily practice, next month you may be able to read down to the 6th line at 10 feet. Maybe in two months you'll be able to read down to the 7th line at 15 feet. You will be approaching 20/20 vision when you can clearly read the 8th line at 20 feet.

"One of the best methods to improve the vision is to regard a letter of the Snellen test card with the eyes open, then close the eyes and remember or imagine the letter better for about ten seconds, open the eyes and regard the letter while testing the imagination of the letter for a moment. By alternately regarding the letter with the eyes open and closed, the imagination of the letter improves in flashes. By continuing to alternate the flashes improve and last longer until the vision becomes continuously improved." *-Dr. William H. Bates*

Number Charts, Picture Charts, Real World Charts

This new way to read eye charts will be different than how you may be used to using eye charts. Instead of just reading through it for a few moments to see how far down you can go, you will be spending lots more time playing with your eye chart to practice developing and building your vision, as evidenced by the appearance of clear flashes. Instead of 30 seconds, you may spend 30 minutes with your eye chart. How could you possibly fill 30 minutes with one simple eye chart? Let's say it takes you one minute to go through the 6-step chart clearing formula on one line of the eye chart. Since there are ten lines on the eye chart, it would take you ten minutes to go through the entire chart. And that's only with one eye.

You would then switch your eye patch over and it might take you another five or ten minutes to go through all ten lines on the eye chart with your other eye. Once you have gone through the 6-step chart clearing formula with each eye separately, you'll want to balance it out by repeating the same thing without an eye patch using both eyes together, which may take another five to ten minutes. That right there brings you to about the thirty-minute mark, and that's not even including any of the other ways you can incorporate your eye charts into the relaxation, centralization, and fusion practices you already know.

Do not get overwhelmed with the chart practice and do not overwork your eyes. At first 30 minutes might be way too long. You may only be able to keep your eyes relaxed for 2 or 3 minutes of vision building before you need to take a palming break. These reading vision building practices are the true test of your dynamic relaxation, or your ability to maintain relaxed eyes while in use. Do not forget all the good vision habits you have learned up until this point. The test is whether or not you can stay physically and mentally relaxed while looking at slightly blurry print. Do not stress too much about the quality or clarity of the print at first. Do not let the blur disturb your peace of mind, relaxation, or memory of clarity. Practice keeping the memory of perfect vision in your mind with your eyes closed, and with your eyes open. Think more about the clear mental version of the letter or word in your mind than the blurry physical version you see when your eyes are open.

At the end of the book you will also find two additional charts to practice with: a number chart *(Page 329)* and a picture chart *(Page 331).* The number chart goes in order from 0 to 9 all the way down to the very bottom, which will make reading the chart even easier because you already know what the next number is. Do not suppress your memory. Allow your memory to bring your vision through even clearer. The chart practice is not supposed to be a surprise. You are supposed to be very familiar with what the charts say at first, so that you can use your memory to help you. Eventually, you will be able to see clearly without relying on your memory, but for now it is a necessary step to get the first glimpses of clarity. There is also a picture chart that has 10 different pictures that repeat randomly going down to the bottom. Instead of saying numbers or letters out loud, you would say, "Sun near, Sun far… Bike near, Bike far… Pepper near, Pepper far… Candle near, Candle far… Magnifying Glass near, Magnifying Glass far… Hourglass near, Hourglass far…"

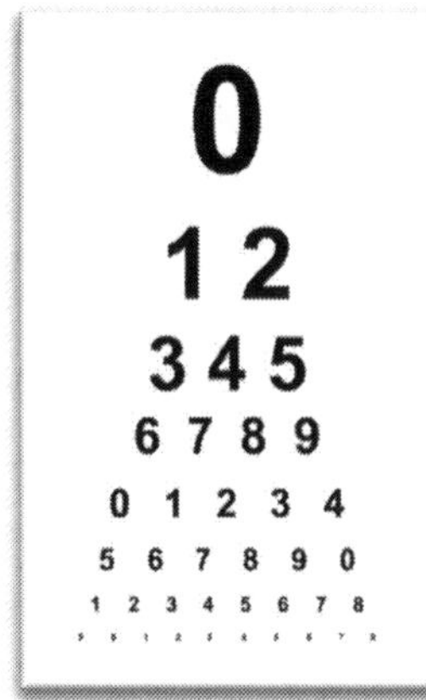

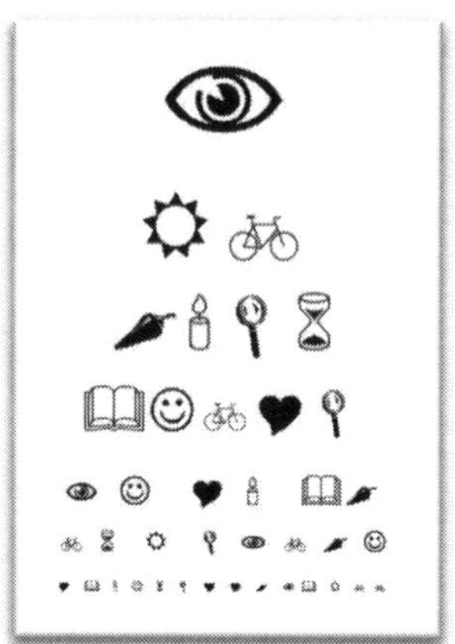

The purpose of the eye chart practice is to gradually introduce yourself to smaller and smaller print at farther and farther distances to stretch your focus out. You may not be able to get all the way down to the bottom line at the distance you started reading the top line. You can either stay at that distance and just do some space riding, or you can get closer to the chart to make it easier to read the smaller letters. You never want to be so far from the chart that it creates strain, effort, confusion, or frustration. This is supposed to be fun and relaxing so don't make it a boring chore for yourself.

Also try not to get stuck at any given distance. Dr. Bates found that some people obtain the best results 1 foot from the chart, while others obtain the best results 5 feet from the chart, while still others obtain the best results all the way at 20 feet from the chart. And they did not necessarily align with the degree of their nearsightedness. He first thought very nearsighted people would only get results very close to the chart but was surprised to find that sometimes they would get better results standing farther away. So certainly pay attention to your edge of clarity, but don't get stuck there. Incorporate a lot of movement into your chart practice, not just swinging or swaying side-to-side, but getting closer to your chart and farther from your chart to experiment with lots of distances.

Once you learn how to stay relaxed while reading your eye charts, you can carry that sensation over into general sight, reading signs on the street, billboards, license plates, and recognizing faces.

Take your chart techniques out into the real world with you. Do not only apply Vision Building to eye charts. Build your distance vision outdoors on three-dimensional objects and on moving objects. Space ride around and nose draw on trees, clouds, cars, and buildings. Shift from a near object to a far object and back and forth. Centralize on one part of the distant object, then another part. Close your eyes and visualize that distant object clearly, open your eyes with a big exhale to look for a flash of clarity.

Next you will learn how to apply that same 6 Step Chart Clearing Formula to your up close reading charts in order to build your near vision. One big difference between your big distance eye chart and your up close reading chart is that your reading chart has a lot more letters and words on it. Your big eye chart only has between three and sixteen letters per line, whereas your small reading chart has between a sentence and a paragraph per line. That is why it will be important for you to differentiate between 'regular reading' and 'vision building' reading. Regular reading refers to the normal type of reading you are used to, where you read entire sentences and draw meaning from the words you read. There is a logical, linear order to it, moving from left to right across the page. If you are farsighted, regular reading may require using reading glasses.

What you are about to learn is a different type of reading called 'vision building reading'. Vision building reading is performed with either weak reading glasses or no glasses. It is not about reading entire sentences and making sense of the words you read. It is about experimenting with various vision building techniques to encourage a flash of clarity on the word or letter, to make it transform from blurry to clear, or relatively clearer. You may only be working with one word or letter per sentence or paragraph for a while, and then moving on to a new random word or letter in a different sentence or paragraph.

Once your near vision improves more, vision building reading will become regular reading, and just the act of reading normally will become a way to preserve clear near vision. Until then though, it will be helpful for you to keep the two different types of reading separate and understand which type of reading you are performing at what times of the day. Most times you will be regular reading. But when you take your glasses off and spend time doing conscious vision practices, you are doing 'vision building reading'.

6 Step Chart Clearing Formula *(Vision Building Near)*

Purpose:

- Build near vision by reading smaller and smaller print closer and closer in.
- Provide an opportunity to apply all the relaxation and focusing principles in practice.
- Keep track of your progress as your vision continues to improve.

Vision Building Near involves a very similar sequence that is more specific for farsightedness, but will also benefit myopic eyes as well. Instead of using the big YES I CAN eye chart, you will hold a smaller eye chart *(Page 323)*, alphabet card *(Page 311)*, or reading card *(Page 321)* in your hand. Once again you will begin with an eye patch covering one eye and hold your well-lit reading card at a comfortable distance within arm's length where the letters are easily readable but slightly blurry. You can also attach the reading card to a surface and sit or stand within arm's length to be more hands-free. Spend about 10 to 60 seconds in each of the following steps on the top line of the reading card.

Directions:

1) Space Riding
2) Centralizing and Verbalizing
3) Near to Far Matching
4) Closing and Visualizing
5) Breathing and Opening
6) Fishing for Flashes

Either repeat the 6-step formula on the same line again or move down to the next smaller line. Gradually make your way down the reading card as far as you can with one eye then continue space riding all the way to the microprint. Take a short palming break and then place the eye patch over your other eye to begin the 6-step formula on the top line. You may need to hold the reading card farther or closer if needed to get at the perfect distance where the letters are easily readable but slightly blurry with your other eye. Repeat all 6 steps on as many lines of the reading card as you can with your other eye and then continue to space ride all the way to the microprint. Take a short palming break and finish by repeating the 6-step formula on as many lines of the reading card as you can with both eyes open and then space ride all the way to the microprint.

Time: 3 to 6 minutes with the left eye, 3 to 6 minutes with the right eye, 3 to 6 minutes with both eyes together, 10 to 20 minutes total.

Description:

The difference between the eye charts and the reading cards is that the reading cards have a lot more letters and words on them than the big eye charts do. Instead of reading the entire line on your reading card, just pick one, two, or three words to do the 6-step formula on per line. For example, just use the word 'Vision' instead of the whole sentence 'Vision can be improved by natural methods.'

Begin with **Step 1: Space Riding**. Keep your attention on the white areas of the reading card as you underline the word 'Vision' with your finger, a pen, pencil, or pointer. Follow the movement of your pointer with your nose, pivoting your head left to right as you ride beneath the letters from the 'V' to 'n' and pivoting your head right to left as you ride beneath the letters from 'n' to 'V'. Ride horizontally back and forth through the space above the letters. Ride vertically up and down in the white space to the left of the 'V' and to the right of the 'n'. Ride through the spaces in between, inside, and around the letters. Imagine that the white part of the chart you are riding on is brighter white than the rest of the chart you are not looking at. This will feel like a lot more head movement than you are used to when doing regular reading. When space riding with one eye, your pointer will appear single and will help you centralize. When space riding with both eyes open, your pointer will appear double so use your pointer as gateposts and swing the word 'Vision' in between your left and right gateposts as your eyes explore the white spaces.

Second, move to **Step 2: Centralizing and Verbalizing**. You will now be space riding around one letter at a time instead of the whole word. You may also begin glancing directly at the black letters themselves. As you explore a smaller area tune into your centralization and realize that the other peripheral letters and words on the reading card are not as distinct or dark as the one you are looking directly at. Say each letter out loud as you centralize on it one at a time. You may want to even trace the letters with your pointer and nose draw them. Pay attention to how you are verbalizing the letters. Call out the letters with a confident downward inflection at the end rather than inflecting upward at the end, making each letter sound like a question. Remember that constant shifting is necessary to maintain centralization, so keep breathing, blinking, and shifting to avoid the possibility of staring and diffusing out to try and see more than the word 'Vision'.

Third, move to **Step 3: Near to Far Matching**. Point your nose and pointer at the 'V' and shift around on it as you say, "V near." Point your nose and pointer up at the distance eye chart in the background and scan the chart to see if you can find a 'V'. If you can find one, shift around on it as you say, "V far.", whether it is lowercase or capital. If you cannot find that letter on the eye chart you can say, "No V far." or you can search for a distant object that starts with the letter V like a vase or vacuum. Go back and forth from shifting on your reading card to shifting on your eye chart or a distant object two or three times before matching the next letter 'i'. Then you say, "I near.", "I far.", or "I near.", "Instrument far.". When matching with one eye, your pointer will appear single so use it to point directly at the near and far objects. When matching with both eyes, your pointer will appear double so swing the close letter between your gateposts as you call it out and then swing the far letter or distant object between your gateposts as you call it out.

Fourth, move to **Step 4: Closing and Visualizing**. Close your eyes and nose draw the letters of your chosen word or words in your mind. Say the letters out loud as you draw them and picture them perfectly clearly. Activate your memory, imagination, and visualization to 'see' the letters using your insight, your inner vision. Even if the letters appeared blurry with your eyes open, you know what a 'V' looks like and an 'i' looks like and an 's' and an 'o' and an 'n' looks like. So simply remember what those letters look like and picture them perfectly in your mind. Do not suppress your memory; use it to help you see more clearly. Once you have drawn the word 'Vision' in your mind, imagine drawing a bright white line beneath the word 'Vision'. As you trace that white line back and forth your head will pivot gently side to side.

Keep that movement going and maintain the clear memory as you transition into **Step 5: Breathing and Opening**. With your eyes still closed and your head still pivoting, tracing that imaginary white line beneath the perfect nose drawing of the letters, inhale deeply through your nose. As you exhale with an audible breath, sigh, or yawn, open your eyes back up on the reading card to either trace the white line under the letters or nose draw the letters with your eyes open. In other words, keep some sort of movement going as you open your eyes instead of freezing and staring. Notice if you experience a clear flash upon opening.

Step 6: Fishing for Flashes is simply repeating steps 4 and 5 a handful of times. So close your eyes again visualize the letters perfectly in your mind. Breathe and open your eyes back onto the reading card with a big exhale. Instead of a belly breath, you may want to try opening your eyes with an audible sigh or a great big yawn. Maintain diaphragmatic or belly breathing to increase the chances of catching a flash and to avoid holding your breath. Pay attention to the clear flashes that come by noticing when the print becomes clearer. Remember that clear flashes are primarily found in your central vision, not your peripheral vision. Know that they can be partial clear flashes too, so even if your vision only gets 50% clearer instead of 100% clearer, that still counts as a clear flash. Observe and allow the fluctuations to happen, and experiment with different ways to stretch the clear flashes out to last longer by maintaining centralization and dynamic relaxation.

Once you complete the 6 steps on the large line at the top of the reading card you can either repeat them again on the top line or begin the 6-step formula on the second line, choosing another one, two, or three words instead of the whole sentence. Take your time and try not to rush through the reading card. Make your way down the card that way as far as you can until you can no longer read the print. You can either hold the chart farther away in order to be able to easily perform all 6 steps, or you can stay at the same distance and simply space ride the remaining lines all the way to the microprint at the bottom. Do not try to read the text of the microprint, just see how much white space you can see in between the lines of text.

Once you reach the microprint with one eye, you can switch the eye patch to cover your other eye and start over from the top of the reading card. Take your time and make your way gradually down the card with your other eye until you can't read the print any more. Either hold the chart farther away to keep doing all 6 steps or simply space ride to the microprint at the bottom. Once you reach the microprint with your other eye, you can remove the eye patch and start over from the top using both eyes together.

Anytime you achieve a flash of clarity with one eye or both eyes, say a positive affirmation out loud like, "I am seeing clearly and I love it!", "I can read the letters easily and effortlessly.", "My vision is clearing, my vision is improving.", "I can see clearer now than when I began." etc. Feel free to make up your own too. It is essential to confirm that your vision is improving when you observe it happening to solidify it and make the improvements last with more permanence instead of fading away after a few seconds. The more your subconscious mind hears you say these confirmations and affirmations, the more conditioned and comfortable it will become with maintaining clear vision more often.

Once you start noticing more flashes of clarity and more development in your vision at one distance, try holding your reading card a little closer to continue stretching your vision closer in. Let's say this week you can read down to the 3rd line at 24 inches. With daily practice, next month you may be able to read down to the 5th line at 20 inches. Maybe in a few months you'll be able to read down to the 8th line at 12 inches.

A New Way to Read Books

Now that you know a new way to use reading cards and eye charts to invite more flashes of clarity on individual letters and words at a time, you will now want to apply these concepts to reading books in general to obtain and maintain clarity on entire paragraphs and pages. Dr. Bates developed a new way to read called 'Thin White Line' reading or 'Strain Proof' reading that involves centralizing on the bright white line that appears beneath the print you are reading rather than directly at the print. The following pages will help you prepare for more reading and offer you some guidance of how to perform this new way of reading. See pages 12-13 for a summary of this relaxed way of reading.

Reading Strategies

- Close your eyes briefly at the end of every sentence or every other sentence.
- Visualize the last word or letter seen, and the punctuation mark after it.
- Open your eyes back up on that word or letter and see it more distinctly.
- Palm your eyes for a moment at the end of every page or every other page.
- Look up at a distant eye chart or object out a window in between pages.
- Space ride on tiny micro-print in between pages to accustom the eyes to tiny text, which will make regular size text seem bigger and easier in comparison.
- Read through a slot-reader, or a piece of black construction paper with a long thin rectangular slot cut out of it. The slot-reader will cover the rest of the page you are not reading, exposing only the sentence you are reading through the slot.

Reading Reminders

- Do some vision warm ups before reading (sunning, palming, space riding).
- Sun and palm often. Short, frequent rests will prevent exhaustion. Rest before you become weary.
- Provide yourself with the best light possible shining over your shoulder. If reading outside in the sunlight, tilt the page to avoid glare.
- Carry a small LED light with you in case of reading emergencies.
- Blink your eyes often for rest and lubrication and to break the stare.
- Breathe deeply, frequently, and rhythmically while performing close work.
- Keep your eyelids and eyebrows loose and pressure-free.
- Close your eyes often to check for and restore softness.
- Alternate and balance near and far gazing while performing close work.
- Do not try to see the print. If your vision declines, you are trying too hard.
- Do not resort to trick vision (squinting or straining). Such tricks of pressure or distortion are physically unhealthy to the eyes. They defeat improvement and prevent permanently good vision.
- Memory of imperfect vision or blurring will make vision even more imperfect. Do not let your mind indulge in memories of blurry vision. Close your eyes and remember or imagine seeing something clearly and sharply defined. Incline your mind to the memory of perfect sight.
- Use mental focusing practices between paragraphs to loosen tense muscles and relax your mind.
- Sit in a way that allows your head to pivot freely and comfortably. Do not hold your head still and only move your eyes.
- Keep your attention in the white spaces in between the lines rather than on the lines themselves.
- Use a book prop like a stand, pillow, or other books to achieve the best angle and height for reading.
- If farsighted, hold your reading material close enough that it is readable, but blurry and practice thin white line reading at that distance. Find your edge and slowly stretch it closer in toward your nose.
- If nearsighted, hold your reading material far enough that it is readable but blurry and practice thin white line reading at that distance. Find your edge and slowly stretch it farther out away from your nose.

Space Riding

Purpose:

- Prepare the eyes and mind for reading.
- Create a rhythmic pivot in the head to free the eyes.
- Practice sliding through the white spaces at the foot of the letters.

Directions:

1) Gently pivot your head as your nose, eyes, and mind follow your pointer as you slide from left margin to right margin in the white spaces between the lines of print.

2) Space ride for a few pages without necessarily reading the words to establish the rhythm of the head pivoting and your eyes, mind, nose, and pointer traveling together.

Time: 1 to 3 minutes.

Anfangen ist leicht, Beharren eine Kunst. Übung macht den
Meister. Wer zwei Hansen auf einmal jagt bekommt keinen.
Anfangen ist leicht, Beharren eine Kunst. Übung macht den
Meister. Wer zwei Hansen auf einmal jagt bekommt keinen.
Anfangen ist leicht, Beharren eine Kunst. Übung macht den
Meister. Wer zwei Hansen auf einmal jagt bekommt keinen.

Description:

Space riding helps prepare your eyes and mind for thin white line reading. It helps establish a gentle pivot in your head that helps build the habit of reading with your nose instead of your eyes. When you hold your head still and only move your eyes it can be very exhausting since you are using your voluntary eye muscles. When you pivot your head and point your nose as you slide across the page, your eyes will move involuntarily, which can be sustained longer and more effortlessly.

Since the point of space riding is not to read or understand any of the words, it may help to use text in another language, like the German paragraph on the previous page, or turn your reading material upside down so you will not be as tempted to try and read.

Always keep your pointer, your nose, your eyes, and your mind traveling together. Slide your pointer, nose, eyes, and mind from left margin to the right margin in the white spaces between the lines of print on the first line, then the second line, and so forth all the way down the page. Find a nice rhythm and speed and always remember to breathe and blink as you go.

Tune into the oppositional movement of the letters, words, and paragraphs. As you swing your head right, the text swings left. As you swing your head left, the text swings right. Imagine that the letters are like the pickets of the picket fence shifter. Instead of vertical black and white lines, they are differently shaped letters, but they can create the same saccadic shifting that the pickets do.

Practice space riding for a few pages before turning your material right side up again to begin the actual thin white line reading.

Thin White Line Reading

Purpose:

- To use reading as a way to improve your eyesight.
- To stretch your vision further in or further out and see the print more clearly.
- To reduce eyestrain and fatigue while reading.
- To allow you to read faster and longer without straining.
- To eventually encourage speed reading.
- To keep the eyes and mind moving and avoid staring.

Directions:

1) Hold your reading material where it is readable, but blurry.
2) Use your pointer and have your eyes, nose, and mind follow the pointer.
3) Slide from margin to margin in the white space under the letters at an swift rate.
4) If you jump up to the letters, gently bring your gaze back down to the white space.
5) At the end of each paragraph close eyes and nose draw last word seen.
6) Trace a thin white line at the foot of your nose drawing, inhale, pivot your head as you exhale and open your eyes, landing back on the word that your pointer is still resting under.

Time: 5 to 10 minutes as vision building reading. No time limit for regular reading.

"We see very largely with the mind, and only partly with the eyes. The phenomenon of vision depends upon the mind's interpretation of the impression upon the retina. What we see is not that impression, but our own interpretation of it."

Dr. William H. Bates

Description:

It takes little to no effort to focus on a plain white background. Only when you try to focus on black print on top of the white background is there any chance of strain. Therefore, in thin white line reading you always look at the white spaces between the lines instead of at the lines themselves, as if you were following the black line that underlines the quote on the previous page, except imagining it being bright white instead of dark black.

Just like space riding, you slide your pointer, nose, eyes, and mind through the white space beneath the line of print. Instead of just using the letters like pickets and noticing the words moving in the opposite direction like in space riding, while thin white line reading you will actually be reading and comprehending the words you are sliding beneath. Eventually you will not need a pointer, but it is necessary while learning to make sure you are not getting ahead of yourself and that you are truly looking down in the white spaces.

This new way to read is called thin white line reading because with practice you may begin to perceive the illusion of a thin white line appearing at the foot of the words. If it does not appear right away, keep in mind that the more you imagine and visualize the white line mentally with your eyes closed, the more it will appear for you with your eyes open. Following this thin white line helps prevent fatigue and allows you to read much longer and more effortlessly. Dr. Bates also called this, "Strain proof reading." because it is a way to read in a more relaxed way than looking directly at the words and letters.

Thin white line reading is much different than you may have been taught to read as a child. It takes practice to stay in the white spaces between the lines and you will almost certainly catch yourself jumping back up to look directly at the print like you are used to. Using a pointer is necessary at first to help stay on track. At first your speed may be fairly slow and your comprehension levels may be fairly low. However, with practice you will be able to stay in the white spaces easily and increase your speed as thin white line reading turns into speed-reading.

It is better to rest your eyes before they feel tired, so it is very important to close your eyes and nose draw the last word you saw every so often. At first, try closing your eyes at the end of every sentence and nose draw the last word you just read. Then you can try closing your eyes at the end of every other sentence and nose draw the last word you just read. Once your endurance grows, you can stop at the end of each paragraph and nose draw the last word of the paragraph. After a few paragraphs you can increase your reading time and close your eyes and nose draw the last word of every other paragraph. Once you are more warmed up you can read an entire page and close your eyes and nose draw the last word of every page, and eventually nose draw the last word of every other page.

While practicing thin white line reading, hold your material just beyond your own edge of clarity so the print is readable but blurry. If you are farsighted, you'll start out towards arm's length and gradually hold your reading material closer and closer. If you are nearsighted, you'll start closer to your nose and gradually hold your reading material farther and farther. Notice any changes or improvements and slowly begin to stretch your edge closer in or farther out depending on your vision.

Begin by practicing thin white line reading on the Art of Reading card *(Pages 319 and 320).* The print is large and the spaces between the lines are wide. Slide in the white space under the line of text from the left margin over to the right margin. Try reading out loud while going nice and slow. Once you get better on the big print you can graduate to thin white line reading on smaller print with less space in between the lines, like the Fundamentals of Eye Training card.

"In the early stages of visual re-education, clear and effortless reading cannot be accomplished without plenty of rest and relaxation. In other words, relaxation is one of the principal means whereby we can achieve our end, which is to see as much print as possible, in the shortest possible time, with the least possible fatigue and the highest degree of intellectual efficiency."

-Aldous Huxley

Writing to Improve Near Vision

Not only can reading be used as a way to help improve your near vision, but writing can too. On the blank lines below, write the phrase, 'I can see clearly when I relax.' ten times. As you write, follow the tip of your pen or pencil with your nose, eyes, and mind. Nose draw the words as they appear on the paper. This is a good habit to practice when writing anything because it prevents staring. Instead of holding your head still and rigid as you write, let your head pivot freely and easily to relax the involuntary muscles that control accommodation.

Write the phrase in print and cursive. Once you have written the phrase, go back over and nose draw the phrase several times with eyes open. Then close your eyes and nose draw the phrase several times with eyes closed, picturing the words you wrote perfectly clear. Incorporate lots of movement in your head as you write or perform up close tasks like knitting, sewing, drawing, painting, etc. to turn as many up close activities into vision building practices as you can.

1. ______________________________

2. ______________________________

3. ______________________________

4. ______________________________

5. ______________________________

6. ______________________________

7. ______________________________

8. ______________________________

9. ______________________________

10. ______________________________

Vision Stretching

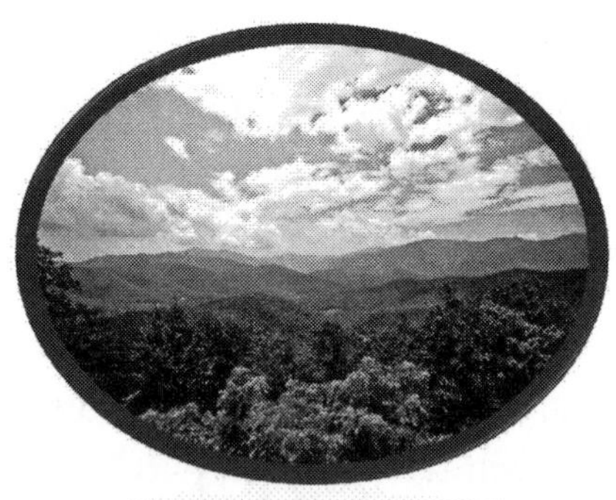

Purpose:

- Keep eyes relaxed and prevent staring amidst blur.
- Stretch the vision farther out into the distance.
- Stretch the vision closer in at the near point.
- Retrain four rectus muscles to loosen and encourage focus up close.
- Retrain two oblique eye muscles to loosen and encourage focus far away.

Directions:

1) Find a place outdoors with something very far away to look at.
2) Let your eyes scan the horizon, following the contours of the landscape.
3) Belly breathe, blink often, keep your head moving and do not stare.
4) Bring your attention to an object up close or in your hand.
5) Belly breathe and blink at the near point.
6) Stretch your vision in and out for at least seven minutes.
7) Palm your eyes and remember what you saw in complete clarity.

Time: 7 to 10 minutes.

Description:

This is an extremely simple yet powerful relaxation practice that helps stretch vision out to improve distance vision and in to improve near vision. Your eyes were designed to easily see up close, far off into the distance, and everywhere in between. Vision problems are functional in that they are based on how you use your eyes. If you primarily use your eyes to focus up close on books, cell phones, computers, etc. your eyes never get the chance to focus far away. Vision stretching counteracts all the time spent focusing up close. Find a vista where your eyes can relax and look as far away into the distance as possible. Depending on where you live this location may be standing on the beach gazing out over the ocean, hiking up a mountain to gaze out over the hills, riding an elevator up to an observation deck to gaze out over the city skyline, or just in a park to gaze out across an open field. Even just gazing up at clouds or the moon counts. Wherever you are, what is the farthest object you can observe, even if it's not clear? Every so often, bring your vision closer in and breathe and blink on close objects. Spend several minutes stretching your vision in and out to make sure your muscles truly relax. Breathe, blink, relax, shift, centralize, fuse, or do any of the techniques you've learned so far.

Night Walking

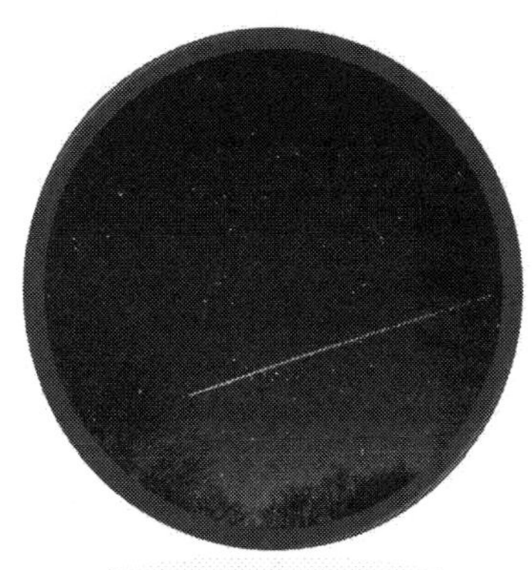

Purpose:

- Improve night vision and peripheral vision.
- Stimulate rods in the retina.

Directions:

1. Go on a stroll at night without your glasses on.
2. Allow your eyes to adjust to the darkness as you walk, tune into your peripheral field.
3. Breathe deeply, blink often, keep your head moving and do not stare.
4. Outline objects with your nose, read street signs, gaze at stars or moon, stay relaxed.
5. Palm your eyes and picture what you saw in dark clarity.

Time: 7 to 10 minutes.

Description:

Many vision students only practice improving their vision during daylight hours since light brings sight. However, the vision practices ought to occasionally be practiced in the dark to make sure you have well-rounded daytime and nighttime vision. Try some swinging with the lights off. Do some fusion practices in dim light. Try vision building near or far by reading cards or eye charts by candlelight. Avoid any type of eyestrain or squinting in the darkness. Most of us lack actual darkness in these modern times because when the sun goes down the lights come on, extending our daytime vision well beyond sunset. Over time and lack of use, our night vision can diminish.

Like vision stretching, night walking is a very simple way to help your eyes and mind relearn how to see in the dark. Start small and eventually make your walks longer. Walk somewhere that you know your way around and you feel comfortable in. Feel free to bring your glasses with you on your walk just in case. Remember that your rods are active in the dark, not your cones. So use your peripheral vision to sense movement. Do not rely on your central vision quite as much and do not try too hard to focus or see things clearly at first. Look up into outer space often and then come back to earth. Remind yourself how far away the moon and the stars are. You can see them, so it ought to be no problem to see things here on earth. For best results, walk in the darkest place you can find, free from streetlights or headlights.

Mental Focus #7: Letter Classifications

While palming, nose draw all the letters of the alphabet in the five different letter classification categories: straight line letters, round letters, combination letters, boxy letters, and diagonal letters. The more you memorize how capital letters look mentally, the easier you will see them physically on your chart with your eyes open. When the letters get too small on your eye chart or reading card to read, see if you can tell which shape classification the letter is. Are the lines that make up that letter straight, round, both, or diagonal? The process of elimination will decrease the possible answers from 26 to 4 or 5.

Straight Line	**I F E L T**
Round	**C G O Q S**
Combo	**B D J P R**
Boxy	**H M N U**
Diagonal	**A K V W X Y Z**

Vision Work #7

Add the vision building techniques and thin white line reading into your daily vision routine. Structure your vision practice like this: spend 5 to 15 minutes warming up and then spend 10 to 30 minutes doing vision building or reading or both. You ought to be reading your cards or charts every single day, even if you only have a few minutes. Apply the good habits and techniques you have learned so far from other practices into the act of reading. Carry these vision building techniques out into the world with you. Apply the good vision habits when viewing actual 3D objects and not just while reading flat 2D things. Use the tables below to keep track of your own progress. Make some copies of these blank tables so you have plenty of tables to fill in over the next several weeks and months of home vision training.

Track Your Personal Progress

Make some copies of the next page so that you can record the status of your vision as you continue to improve. Every few weeks record the results of your vision building practice, writing not only how far down you could read but also how it looked. Be as detailed as possible in explaining how the letters and words look because sometimes the changes and improvements you experience can be very subtle.

To better understand this, let's say you are the parent of a three-year-old daughter. Over the span of one year your child grows six inches. You don't really notice her growth though, because you spend every single day with her and she only grows approximately 0.0165 inches a day. But when your parents come to visit their granddaughter once a year, the first thing they proclaim is, "My goodness, you've grown so much! You're so much taller than when we saw you last year!"

So it is with your eyes. You may not notice the tiny improvements your vision makes as much because you look through your eyes every single day. So let's say your vision improves slowly over time and your prescription drops from -7.0 to -1.0 diopters over the span of one year. Spaced over 365 days, that's only a 0.0164 diopter improvement each day. So the little baby steps you take might not be that pronounced, but by the end of one year you will be seeing so much more clearly than when you began.

Example:

Date: 5/20/2018	**Reading Card Distance: 24"**	**Far Chart Distance: 12'**
Left Eye:	*Read down to line 8* *Starts to lose focus & double*	*Read down to line 3* *Looks fuzzy and not very black*
Right Eye:	*Read down to line 7* *Blurrier than L eye, more shadows*	*Read down to line 4* *Clearer than L eye,* *but still see double letters*
Both Eyes:	*Read down to line 9* *Clearer than L & R eyes, but still a little blurry*	*Read down to line 6* *Much better with both eyes, but bottom lines are not very*

Date:	Near Card Distance: _________	Far Chart Distance: _________
Left Eye:		
Right Eye:		
Both Eyes:		

Date:	Near Card Distance: _________	Far Chart Distance: _________
Left Eye:		
Right Eye:		
Both Eyes:		

Date:	Near Card Distance: _________	Far Chart Distance: _________
Left Eye:		
Right Eye:		
Both Eyes:		

Date:	Near Card Distance: __________	Far Chart Distance: _________
Left Eye:		
Right Eye:		
Both Eyes:		

Date:	Near Card Distance: __________	Far Chart Distance: _________
Left Eye:		
Right Eye:		
Both Eyes:		

Date:	Near Card Distance: __________	Far Chart Distance: _________
Left Eye:		
Right Eye:		
Both Eyes:		

Daily Practice Checklist Week 7

M Tu W Th F S Su			
☐☐☐☐☐☐☐		Morning Relaxation Routine	3-6 minutes
☐☐☐☐☐☐☐		Swinging	2-6 minutes
☐☐☐☐☐☐☐		Sunning	1-4 minutes
☐☐☐☐☐☐☐		Palming & Mental Drill	2-8 minutes
☐☐☐☐☐☐☐		Picket Fence Shifter	1-4 minutes
☐☐☐☐☐☐☐		Centralization	2-4 minutes
☐☐☐☐☐☐☐		Brain Balancing	1-3 minutes
☐☐☐☐☐☐☐	VXA	Fusion Practices	2-10 minutes
☐☐☐☐☐☐☐		Vision Building	15-30 minutes
☐☐☐☐☐☐☐		TWL Reading	5-15 minutes
		Daily Target:	***15-45 mins***

Vision Journal: ______________________________

____

____

____

____

____

"Memory brings vision. Boredom kills vision."

-Dr. Jerriann J. Taber

Chapter 8

Phase ॐ:
Yoga for the Eyes
Beyond the Bates Method

"We cannot relax the eyes without, at the same time, relaxing the entire nervous system. This, in turn, improves the condition of every organ and every part of the body by freeing the circulatory channels from tension, thus speeding the circulation. Conversely, the body affects the eyes... A person with slack muscles in the rest of the body, will have poor muscle tone in the eyes... When the... muscle tone improve[s], a marked step up in vision can be noticed. Eyes, however, can be affected even more violently by the emotions than by the physical condition. The physical condition is likewise affected by emotions, since mental strain creates tension throughout the system."

-Margaret D. Corbett

Integral Eyesight Improvement integrates several paths toward the achievement of improved vision. The holistic approach of Integral Eyesight Improvement is represented by its symbol of an eye atop a geometric figure, known as the seed of life, which is a harmonious arrangement of seven overlapping circles. The way the circles precisely overlap equidistantly creates six petals emanating from the central dot (the pupil of the eye). The six circles that create the petals represent the six branches of yoga and vision: *Hatha, Raja, Jnana, Bhakti, Japa, and Karma.* The seventh bold circle (the iris of the eye) represents the unification of all the branches of Integral Eyesight Improvement working together simultaneously to achieve the unification of eyes, body, and mind required for perfectly clear eyesight and insight.

The Six Branches of Integral Eyesight Improvement

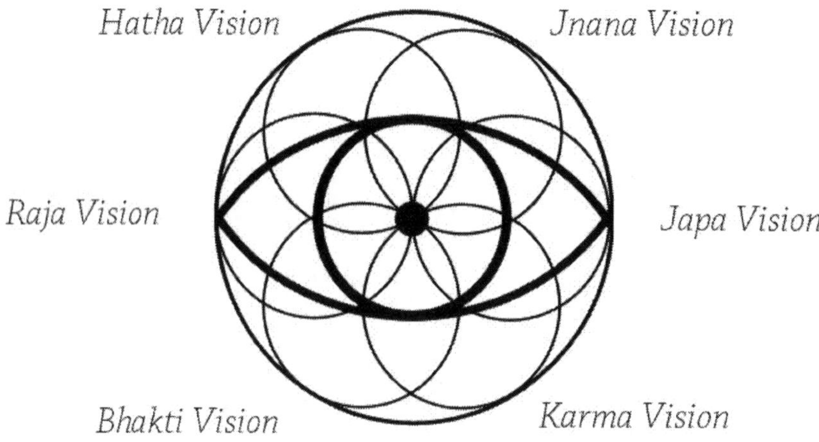

For a 15 minute video guiding you through a series of yoga poses, breathing practices, and meditation, visit:
www.integraleyesight.com/yoga

Yoga is a Sanskrit word that means, 'yoke' or 'union.' Yoga is a lifestyle that connects mind, body, and vision through various practices. These practices are categorized into six branches: *hatha, raja, jnana, karma, bhakti,* and *japa*. In the scope of yoga, the six branches involve the entire body and energy field. In the scope of Integral Eyesight Improvement these same six branches can each be applied to the eyes and the miracle of vision.

	YOGA	VISION
Hatha *The Physical Branch*	*Asanas, pranayamas, kriyas* Yoga poses, breathing practices, internal & external purity	Physical relaxation and focusing practices performed with eyes open, diet, nutrition & supplementation ***Eyesight, Outer Vision***
Raja *The Royal Branch*	Study of sacred scriptures Path to bliss through sensory withdrawal and meditation	Study of Bates Method writings Path to clarity through relaxation ***Theory, Philosophy, Physiology, Anatomy, Knowledge, Understanding***
Jnana *The Mental Branch*	Intellectual understanding, inner exploration & deep self-inquiry	Mental relaxation and focusing drills performed with the eyes closed Transformation of identity ***Insight, Inner Vision***
Bhakti *The Love & Devotion Branch*	Heart-opening practices with dedication and conviction	Strengthening intuition and practicing with dedication and conviction ***Loving Practices and Having Fun!***
Japa *The Vibrational Branch*	Repetition of sacred mantras	Daily vision routine, maintaining good vision habits 24/7 ***Frequency, Repetition***
Karma *The Action & Intention Branch*	Selfless service with no attachment to the fruits of your labors	Non-attachment to the results of your vision practice ***Not expecting, forcing, or judging***

Yoga and the Bates Method share much in common. Yoga is designed to increase the overall health of the body and mind. The Bates Method is designed to increase the overall health of the eyes and mind. The following pages explore what more we can learn by looking at vision through the lens of yoga.

हठ

The word 'hatha' is a Sanskrit word, which is broken down into two parts: 'ha' means sun and 'tha' means moon. Putting these two opposites together insinuates balance. The branch of hatha yoga refers to the physical path, consisting of *Asanas* (yoga poses or postures), *Pranayama* (breath control and manipulation), and *Kriyas* (purity through proper diet and cleansing practices). Hatha yoga is the most widely known branch and is generally the first thing most people associate with the word 'yoga'. An image of a group of people stretching around in a room together for an hour or so is an approximation of hatha yoga. Hatha is just one out of six paths and both yoga and the Bates Method run deeper.

"Yoga Asanas are not exercise. The word exercise tends to give the idea of a practice done with quick movement and with a measure of strain involved. 'Asana' simply means posture. The definition of a posture, or pose, means one that gives steadiness and comfort. The different asanas are aimed at achieving one pose comfortably. All the other asanas make your body more flexible, more easeful, so that you can sit comfortably and steadily in one pose. That is the aim behind Hatha Yoga. If you achieve that one pose without any movement at all, then automatically you go on to the other controls—control of the breath, the senses, the mind. So the main purpose behind all the Yoga practices is control of the mind." -Sri Swami Satchidananda

The entire goal of learning and practicing all of the hatha yoga *Asanas* (poses) is to be able to sit comfortably with your eyes closed and see clearly internally. Therefore, the entire goal of learning and practicing all of the physical vision practices is to be able to stay relaxed with your eyes open and see clearly externally. Once you can sit comfortably in meditation without discomfort, it is no longer necessary to do *asanas* every day. However, it won't hurt to keep up your practice for maintenance. Likewise, once you can maintain a state of dynamic relaxation and see clearly without glasses, it is no longer necessary to do vision practices every day. It doesn't hurt to keep up your practice to maintain sharp vision.

Hatha vision is the physical path of the Bates Method. It includes all of the Bates Method relaxation practices that enhance eyesight like swinging, sunning, palming, shifting, centralizing, etc. Anything regarding the physical body can be categorized under hatha vision. Just like *Pranayamas* are a huge part of yoga, breathing is of utmost importance in vision because it is the primary vehicle to relaxation of the body and mind. Reestablishing the habit of deep, rhythmic breathing calms the entire nervous system and helps the involuntary systems of the body to release, including the smooth muscles around each eye that hold chronic strain. Shallow breath leads to shallow vision.

Since the goal of hatha is balance, the Bates Method strives to achieve balance in several respects. We first distinguish the clearer eye and blurrier eye and work to balance them more. Hatha vision, or 'sun-moon' vision, uses light (sunning) and darkness (palming) to reactivate the lens and ciliary muscles in order harmonize central and peripheral, or daytime and nighttime vision. Another important balance to establish is near and far vision. This is accomplished by frequently glancing at an object at least fifteen feet away while performing up-close tasks such as reading, writing, or while using computers or cell phones. If the eyes are only used for up-close tasks and are rarely used for looking in the distance, then near and far vision become unbalanced and the eyes lose their flexibility.

Hatha vision also brings more awareness to the diet and emphasizes the intake of vitamins, minerals, and nutrients necessary for sufficient eye health. Balancing your diet and increasing levels of Vitamins A, B complex, C, D3, E, and K, as well as lutein and zeaxanthin can help keep your eyes young and resilient. Classical Chinese Medicine has perfected the use of herbal blends to sharpen eyesight for thousands of years and has established the connection between certain organs, like the liver and kidneys, with the eye organs. Meridian tapping and acupressure points are also practices of hatha vision that help release fears deeply embedded in the limbic system and reduce levels of the stress hormone, cortisol. In addition to a clean diet, hatha vision also includes cleansing and purifying the eyes themselves. Using a neti pot to cleanse the nasal passage indirectly benefits the eyes. The daily hygiene practice of rinsing your nasal passages with distilled water or a saline solution can improve the health of your olfactory system, which in turn improves the health of your visual system, since all the senses are intricately linked. Rinsing with a neti pot can also decrease inflammation of the sinuses and possibly decrease the intraocular pressure of the eyes. Rinsing your eyes with an eye bath is also an important cleansing practice to keep your eyes clean and clear. Detailed directions for using a neti pot and eye bath are explained later in this chapter.

Visual blur is a sign that something is out of balance. Glasses and contacts trick the mind into thinking everything is fine, but underneath the surface the imbalance grows further out of alignment and the blur becomes worse. By removing your lenses and performing the various physical practices of Yoga and the Bates Method, you begin the process of coming back into balance physically, mentally, emotionally, and spiritually. Like in yoga, hatha vision is usually the first experience people have with the Bates Method, which opens the doorway into the subtler paths of *raja, jnana, bhakti, japa, and karma,* vision.

राजन्

The word 'raja' is Sanskrit for: royal. Raja yoga is the royal path of yoga. The royal path is an eightfold path of attaining enlightenment or bliss. The eight limbs of yoga are detailed in the *Yoga Sutras* by Patanjali. The eight limbs in order are *yamas* (non-violence, truthfulness, non-stealing, moderation, non-greed), *niyamas* (purity, contentment, austerity, study of sacred texts, surrender), *asanas* (physical poses), *pranayamas* (breath restraints), *pratyahara* (sensory withdrawal), *dharana* (concentration), *dhyana* (meditation) and sa*madhi* (bliss). Many people in the Western world skip the first two steps and begin their yoga practice by going to a yoga class and going through a series of asanas or physical stretches and poses. Some benefits may certainly be experienced this way, but the *yamas* and *niyamas* act as the foundation of the yoga practice. If they are overlooked then the entire practice will be less sturdy. The eight-limbed path is a sure-fire way to achieve the desired end goal of a calmer mind.

"Your true nature, the Self, is like a radiant Light that is always shining within you. The mind is like a mirror. The Self is reflected on the mirror of the mind. If the mirror gets distorted or disturbed, you see a disturbed image. You identify with the image and feel that you are disturbed. So, even though the true you, the Self, is always the same, you appear to be distorted or mixed up with the mind. The aim of Raja Yoga is to make the mind clean and calm. When that is achieved, you feel that you have gone back, or you appear to have gone back, to your original state. You see a steady image and experience the Peace and Joy that is your true nature. Raja Yoga is a practical guide for gaining control over the mind." –Sri Swami Satchidananda

When we apply these concepts to vision improvement we get raja vision. Instead of the *Yoga Sutras* by Patanjali, we have *Perfect Eyesight Without Glasses* and other books, magazines, and articles by Dr. William H. Bates. His original research and publications outline the systematic process of attaining clear vision just like the yoga sutras laid out the systematic process of attaining a healthier life and mind. So, in addition to spending time doing hatha vision practices, it is also smart to spend time reading, re-reading, and reflecting upon the original works written by the creator of the method you are using to normalize your vision.

In my experience, just reading about vision improvement led to changes and improvements in my own vision because it was sinking deeper in on a mental level. The more I pondered it, the more it challenged my previously held beliefs and opened me up to new ideas and possibilities. It can also be quite inspiring to read case histories and success stories of people who have already walked the path and gone through the process you are going through now. Similar to how most people skip the first two foundational steps in yoga and go right to the physical level, many people also skip the foundational steps of vision improvement and begin their practice by only doing physical eye exercises that they found in a book or online. Some benefits may still be experienced this way, but the path of raja reminds us that there is a particular order to climb the ladder and achieve the end goal. If the mental, emotional, and other subtle steps are skipped and the physical approach is the only one taken, the results will not be as good. The higher levels of vision improvement cannot be accessed without the mastering of the lower levels. The habits and practices passed down from Dr. Bates in this book are the precise way to achieve the desired end goal of better eyesight.

The highest levels of raja yoga before enlightenment are sensory withdrawal, concentration, and meditation, which are much more mental than physical. Since vision is 90% mental and only 10% physical, those techniques are also a large part of raja vision. In raja vision, enlightenment can mean perfect vision. Attaining enlightenment requires lifting a veil of ignorance to uncover the underlying truth. Attaining perfect vision requires removing the veil of blur to uncover the underlying clarity within.

ज्ञान

The word 'jnana' (pronounced: yah-nah') is Sanskrit for: knowledge. Jnana yoga is the yoga of knowledge or the path of self-inquiry. One way to practice jnana yoga is to continually ask yourself, "Who am I?" It is an investigation of identity, an exploration of ego, a consideration of how you think of "I." Initially, your first few answers might sound like, "I am a man." "I am a woman." "I am 34 years old." "I am spiritual." "I am a Canadian." "I am nearsighted." "I am blind as a bat." "I am a carpenter." "I am a mother." etc. Those answers may be true on the surface, but they do not sufficiently answer the question. Material possessions, religions, nationalities, societal roles, genders, and all types of labels are things that we use, act, or do on the surface and certainly make everyday conversation easier. But on a more fundamental and deeper level they are not really who you truly are.

Repeating the simple question, "Who am I?" continually peels away surface layers until you eventually end up at your core - your true self. At the center of all beings is the pure light of oneness, a perfectly clear crystal, untainted by all the layers that cover it up through the hardships of life. Since change is the only constant, we cannot identify our true selves with transient objects, emotions, or people. This subtle shift is expressed in a simple change in phrasing. “I work as an electrical engineer.” is a less attached way to say, “I am an electrical engineer.” “I practice Islam.” is different than saying, “I am Muslim.” “I live in Canada.” is different than, “I am a Canadian.”

“Deep in the middle of the ocean of the mind there is no pollution. It is absolutely pure. That part is always contented. It never likes or dislikes. It accepts everything; it is not proud. And this is the real nature of your true Self. Only knowledge of this true nature will free you from the turmoil of this world. It will free you from the petty-mindedness, which divides humanity into thousands of names: ‘I am this; he is that. He is different from me.’ People kill each other because they group and divide themselves. They fail to see and know that they are above these differences.” –Sri Swami Satchidananda

When applied to the eyes, we end up with jnana vision. We use the same question: “Who am I?” Do you identify with your vision? Have you ever said, “I am nearsighted,” or “I am farsighted”? Instead, you can say, “I see best up close,” or “I am working on improving my distance vision.” Identifying yourself as someone with a visual defect is accepting it as the way you are and always will be. By separating your true self from a visual problem, you open up the door for change to occur. Instead of being a person with blurry vision who experiences flashes of clarity from time to time, shift your consciousness to become a person with clear vision who experiences temporary periods of blur from time to time. This is a subtle shift, but it can yield very powerful transformations.

Jnana vision is also called the mental branch. As opposed to hatha vision, which includes all the physical practices performed with the eyes open, jnana vision includes all the mental and closed-eye practices involving visualization, imagination, and memory. This includes anything that enhances insight like pleasant happy memories while palming, the bar and the dot, or nose drawing. Jnana vision is also activated through meditation and mental focus.

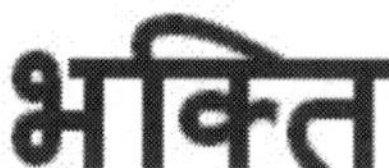

The word 'bhakti' is Sanskrit for: love or devotion. In yoga it is the path of the heart that is experienced through love, devotion, and worship of the divine. One popular way that bhakti yoga is practiced is through *kirtan*, which is the musically oriented call and response chanting of Sanskrit mantras and names of Hindu deities. Bhakti yogis also create shrines or altars with sacred objects and images, which creates a tangible focal point to pour loving energy into.

"Bhakti, or devotional Yoga, might seem even better than Jnana Yoga, the path of wisdom through self-analysis. But devotion without wisdom is not devotion at all." –Sri Swami Satchidananda

Bhakti vision can be thought of as the devotional aspect of vision improvement. Not many people are able to permanently fix their vision overnight, so you must be dedicated to a lengthy journey. Not only does it take time and energy, but it also requires a certain level of devotion, desire, and enthusiasm for it to work. You must want clarity very strongly to see the entire process through to completion. You must be totally committed to going without glasses or wearing training glasses, and totally committed to performing your practices regularly and selflessly. You must be absolutely driven to be able to make it all the way through. Your heart has to be involved, not just your eyes. Tune into how the vision practices make you feel, not just how they make you see. Notice the influence your emotions have on your vision.

Someone with Bhakti vision looks with love. The phrase, 'look with love' sounds nice, but what does it mean? Maybe it will help you to understand what it means by understanding the opposite. Looking with fear, doubt, judgment, concern, worry, confusion, resistance, effort, or strain leads to blurry vision. Looking with love, acceptance, allowance, excitement, embrace, joy, ease, and relaxation leads to clear vision.

You take information in through your eyes in the form of light. Instead of reaching out into the world with your eyes to pull the light in, just sit back, relax, and invite the information to enter on its own. Reaching outward from your eyes makes your head reach forward, which can compromise your posture and disrupt your nervous system. Looking with love in a receptive way encourages your head to naturally relax back into a more comfortable position, which will make you feel both cradled and confident simultaneously. You switch from reaching to receiving, from forcing to inviting.

Imagine how a baby uses his or her eyes and try to remember when you looked at the world for the first time. When you practice looking with love you will notice that your eyes soften, your muscles relax, and the corners of your mouth may curl up into a little smile. Keep in mind that it is nearly impossible to look with love with a frown upon your face. The art of receptive sight is seeing with your heart, instead of your head. Looking with love banishes all physical, mental, and emotional strain, therefore inducing clearer eyesight and insight. A good indicator that you are truly looking with love is that your eyes feel like they are smiling. They may tingle with the awakening sensation of eagerly allowing light to enter them. It almost tickles!

Tip #1: See if you can begin to actually feel the light entering your eyes, landing on your retinas, traveling through your optic nerves and stimulating your visual cortex in the very back of your brain.

By becoming more receptive, you may also become aware that vision is not just a one-way process. The art of receptive eyesight is both passive and active. Your eyes receive and your eyes give. By sending love and light out through your eyes, you are inviting more love and light to return through your eyes. If, on the other hand, you send out anger, confusion, fear, or blur, then that is what will return to you.

Tip #2: Use your eyes like expensive paintbrushes, gently painting a beautiful portrait in front of you. Become an artist by playing more of an active role in your vision. Even if the picture is blurry at first, accept it and love it as you practice.

One of the first steps to improving your eyesight is embracing the blur and working with the vision that you have at this moment. Resisting the blur will only bring more blur. Blurry eyesight is a message from within that something is out of balance. Resisting or covering up the blur with glasses, contacts, or surgery is ignoring that critical message from within. Removing your lenses and accepting the blur is receiving that message and initiating an investigation as to what is out of balance and why. As you dig deeper within, remember to look with love internally as well as externally.

जप

The word 'japa' is Sanskrit for: repeat. In yoga it is the vibrational path and those vibrations take the form of *mantras*, or prayers or thoughts, which are repeated mentally or verbally. Japa vision draws both from the repetitive and the vibrational nature of japa yoga. Japa vision is the daily repetition of the physical vision practices, which over time helps you release poor vision habits and establish good vision habits. The only way to successfully retrain your eyes and your mind is through repetition and frequency.

The vibrations made by saying positive affirmations also strengthen japa vision. The affirmations are the mantras of japa yoga. Whenever you verbalize something it sinks it down into the subconscious or unconscious mind. When you experience a flash of clarity or reach a point in your vision improvement where things are looking much clearer, it is very beneficial to say out loud to yourself or to another, "I am seeing clearly, and I love what I see!"

कर्म

The word 'karma' is Sanskrit for: action, work, or deed. Karma yoga is the yoga of action and intention. It is not just performing the action though; it is performing the action without expectation of anything in return or having no attachment to the fruits of one's labor. A random act of kindness is an example of karma yoga. It is performing an action for the sake of the action or for the sake of benefitting others rather than benefitting only yourself. Volunteering in your community, helping someone in need, or advising a friend are all examples of karma yoga. Do good deeds in the world, not to get rich or famous, but for the sake of making the world a better place. When you truly practice karma yoga, everyone benefits instead of just you. When you give ample gifts of your time and energy, have faith that you may receive equal amounts, if not more, in return in the future.

"People who act with their minds on the future benefits don't even think about what they're doing. They lose efficiency. If you think fast, you lose all your power. It's better to go slow and be steady, to do one thing at a time and concentrate your efforts. Don't even think about the fruits. If some fruit comes to you, you may certainly taste it, but don't reach for it." –Sri Swami Satchidananda

When we apply this notion to vision it becomes karma vision, which is a subtle and complex aspect of vision improvement. Just like volunteering at a homeless shelter for an afternoon without attachment to monetary reimbursement for the hours you worked, you must perform your vision practices without attachment to the results you obtain. The results will come in due time and you must have complete faith in that. Until they do come though, maintain an attachment-free mindset so that you don't feel frustrated or disappointed by the non-linear path of your improvement. Simply accept this practice as an ongoing process and continue investing your time and energy into it for the sake of making your eyes healthier for life. Relax for the sake of relaxing and you will be rewarded.

Karma vision can be a tricky concept to employ, since your original intentions of going through vision training were probably to obtain results. There is nothing wrong with that, and like Swami Satchidananda says, if some clarity comes to you, you may certainly enjoy it, but don't reach for it. You may find that the results you originally set out to achieve only come once you loosen your grip on those expectations, let go of attachment to those results, and simply sink into the relaxing rhythms of your practices. You can think of it like this: you aren't improving your vision simply for your own benefit, but rather for the benefit of all those around you including your friends, family, and co-workers, because you will be able to better serve them with healthier, stronger eyes.

"Many patients with imperfect sight are benefited by breathing.

One of the best methods is to separate the teeth while keeping the lips closed, breathe deeply as though one were yawning.

When done properly one can feel the air cold as it passes through the nose and down the throat.

This method of breathing secures a great amount of relaxation of the nose, throat, the body generally including the eyes and ears.

At one time I experimented with a number of patients, first having them hold their breath and test their vision, which was usually lower when they did not breathe. They became able to demonstrate that holding their breath was a strain and caused imperfect sight, double vision, dizziness and fatigue, while the deep breathing at once gave them relief.

By practicing the habit of frequently deep breathing one obtains a more permanent relaxation of the eyes with more constant good vision."

-Dr. William H. Bates

Breathing Practices

Pranayama is a Sanskrit word that refers to different types of breathing practices. *Prana* means the vital life force or breath that inhabits all living things. *Yama* means constraint, retention, or control. All of the *pranayamas* are designed to allow you to take in more *prana* and oxygen and increase your vital life force energy. When practiced regularly, they also help calm and clear the nervous system of stagnation and fatigue. The breathing practices are very important for vision because both your eyes and your brain need lots of oxygen to thrive. Without proper breathing, your visual system may not get the amount of oxygen it needs. If the breath shallows, the vision shallows. If the breath deepens, the vision deepens.

The breath is the primary vehicle to relaxation, and therefore the most direct way to clear vision. When you relax your body, your breath relaxes. When your breath relaxes, your mind relaxes. When your mind relaxes, your eyes relax. When your eyes and mind are relaxed, your vision relaxes and becomes clearer. Therefore, clear vision starts with the breath. You are about to learn three yogic breathing techniques. In addition to practicing these specific breathing techniques on their own or during your other vision practices, it is also very important to instill an ongoing deep and rhythmic breath pattern throughout your day and night. Many people unknowingly hold their breath while concentrating or performing a task. Even if they are breathing, it is often shallow and sporadic. Pay more attention to how you breathe during different activities. Deepening your breath can enrich any activity you do. Breathing rhythmically can invigorate and energize your exercises. Breathing while reading, writing, or typing can keep you focused and keep you blinking. Breathing while chewing can enhance your eating experience by extracting more flavor from the food. Explore and cultivate the connection between your breath and your vision.

Another interesting connection between the vision and the breath is the similarity between the eyes and the lungs, in that they are both voluntary and involuntary organs. Your lungs expand and contract involuntarily all day long whether you think about breathing or not. However, you can pay attention to your breath and consciously control your breath with specific breathing practices, with the intention of influencing the rhythm and depth of your unconscious breath when you're not thinking about it. Likewise, your eyes move and accommodate involuntarily all day long whether you think about seeing or not. However, you can pay attention to your vision and consciously control your vision with specific vision practices, with the intention of influencing the fluidity and focus of your unconscious vision when you're not thinking about it.

2:1 Belly Breathing

Purpose:

- Establish deep, rhythmic, diaphragmatic breath.
- Relax the body and mind.
- Take in up to 7 times as much oxygen and *prana.*
- Oxygenate the bloodstream, eyes, and brain.

Directions:

1) Find a comfortable place to sit or lie on your back.
2) Pull your belly in as you exhale through your nose for 2 seconds.
3) Let your belly relax and expand as you inhale through your nose for 1 second.
4) Repeat 2 second exhales and 1 second inhales a few times.
5) Pull your belly in as you exhale for 4 seconds.
6) Let your belly relax and expand as you inhale through your nose for 2 seconds.
7) Repeat 4 second exhales and 2 second inhales a few times.
8) Pull your belly in as you exhale through your nose for 6 seconds.
9) Let your belly relax and expand as you inhale through your nose for 3 seconds.
10) Repeat 6 second exhales and 3 second inhales a few times.
11) Continue increasing your 2:1 exhale to inhale ratio up to a comfortable length.

Time: 1 to 3 minutes.

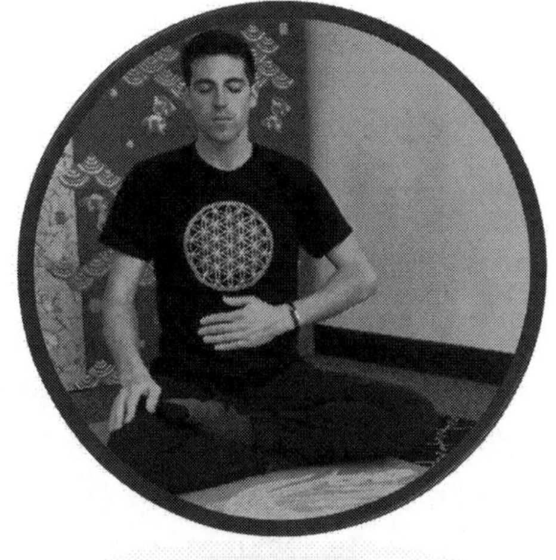

Description:

Many people have the bad habit of shallow breathing or chest breathing, where the shoulders lift up and down with the inhale and exhale. In correct belly breathing or diaphragmatic breathing, the shoulders remain level and the belly moves in and out with the exhale and inhale. If you study an infant or a pet dog or cat, you will notice the belly rising and falling with the breath. This is the natural way to breathe. You probably used to breathe with your belly at some point in your life, but somewhere along the line most people adopt the incorrect chest breathing instead. It may feel awkward at first, but with enough practice your breathing muscles will be retrained to contract and relax to assist your breath automatically without you making them move. Just like the clear vision you are working towards, you also want your deep breathing to become effortless and involuntary.

When you pull your belly in on the exhale it presses your diaphragm up to squeeze all the *stale* air out of your lungs. When you relax your belly out on the inhale it creates more space for your diaphragm to sink down, which allows your lungs to stretch open wider to receive more air. Belly breathing is the deepest breathing, the most oxygenating breath.

Some people find it difficult to expand their belly when they inhale, so instead try pulling your belly in first to squeeze all the air out of your lungs first, and then simply let your belly relax back out. When your belly relaxes back out it will automatically draw air back into your lungs. Then activate your abdominal muscles to pull your belly back in as you exhale for a few seconds and push out as much air as you can. Simply let your abdominal muscles relax and allow your belly to expand out as you inhale for a few seconds. Focusing more on contracting on the exhale will make expanding on the inhale easier and more relaxing. It may help to use your hand to press into your belly as you breathe out and squeeze your abdominal muscles, and then feel your belly fill up like a balloon when you relax your abdominal muscles and breathe in. All the while, your shoulders do not rise or fall because all the movement is happening in your abdomen.

Once you get your breathing muscles moving, begin a 2:1 breath ratio, exhaling about twice as long as you inhale. If you exhale for 4 seconds, inhale for 2 seconds. If you exhale for 10 seconds, inhale for 5 seconds. Do not exceed exhaling for 20 seconds and inhaling for 10 seconds. This pranayama can allow you to take in up to 7 times more oxygen than a regular breath, and since your eyes need a ton of oxygen it is very important to establish deeper and rhythmic breathing all day long.

Breath of Fire

Purpose:

- Increase circulation to the eyes and face.
- Cleanse the *nadis*, or energy pathways throughout the body.
- Build heat and energy.

Directions:

1) Take a full inhale through your nose followed by a full exhale.
2) Take a half an inhale and begin the first round of breath of fire.
3) Repeatedly contract your abdomen in with each exhale, let inhale come automatically.
4) Start at about one contraction/exhale per second and gradually speed it up.
5) After 10 exhales, take a long slow deep inhale to finish.
6) Rest and breathe for a few moments before beginning the second round of 15 exhales.
7) Rest and breathe for a few moments before beginning the third round of 20 exhales.
8) Allow your breath to return to a normal rhythm and observe effects.

Time: 1 to 3 minutes.

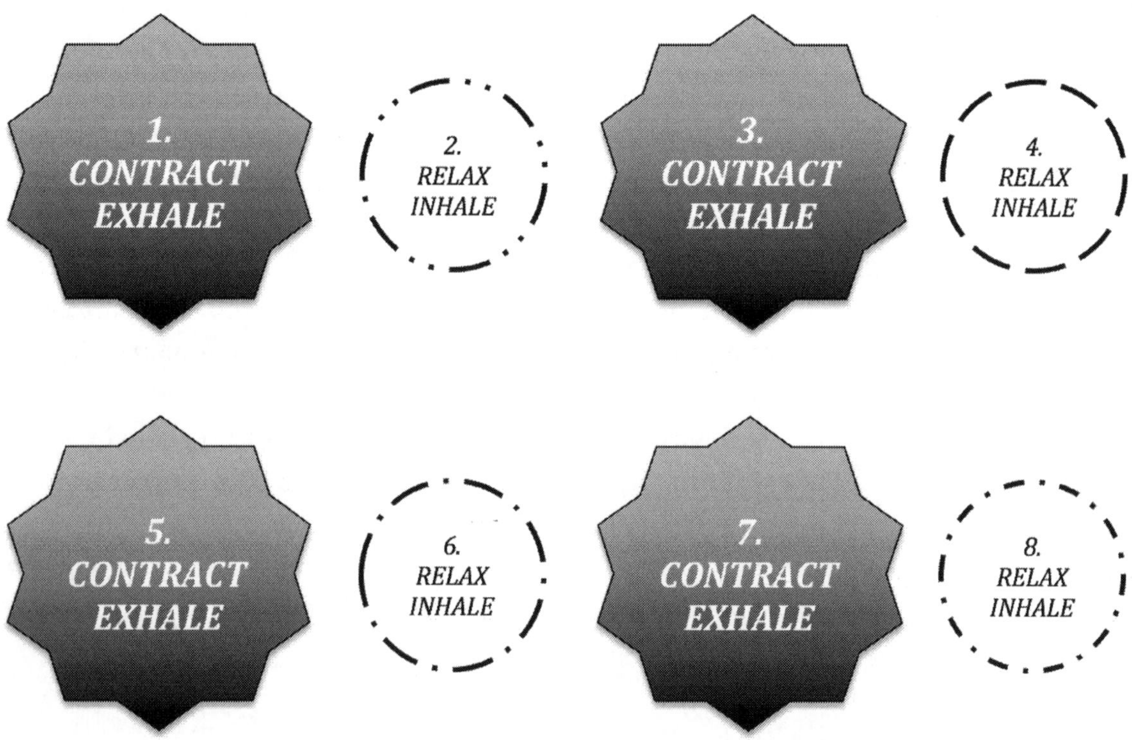

Description:

The 2:1 belly breathing taught you how to lengthen your breath by slowing it down and exhaling longer and longer as you breathe. The breath of fire utilizes the same abdominal breathing muscles but is more of a sped-up version. Instead of slowing down as you go, you speed up and breathe once per second, twice per second, and maybe even three times per second. It can be a very energizing and invigorating pranayama. It really gets the heart pumping and the blood circulating, while also breaking up stagnant energy and emptying the lungs of any stale air lingering. It is less about forcing air out of your nose and more about rapidly and continuously contracting your abdomen in and up, the force of which influences your diaphragm to squeeze more air out of your lungs. Try to keep your body relaxed and your breath easy.

Do not let the rapid exhales make your shoulders bounce or your eyes tense. The only movement ought to be the conscious contraction and automatic expansion of your abdomen. Focus only on the exhales. Do not worry about the inhales, for they will come automatically. Your attention will remain on the *'out... out... out...'* of your breath, while allowing your body to instinctively take in tiny sips of air in between your exhales. You will have time to catch your breath in between your rounds.

It is best to do the breath of fire in short rounds with breaks in between, for example three 30 seconds rounds with 30 second breaks in between, rather than doing the breath of fire for 3 minutes straight. You can perform the breath of fire as subtly or as intensely as you feel comfortable with. The slower and gentler form is more relaxing, while the faster and powerful form is more energizing.

Once you get comfortable with the rhythm and pattern of the breath of fire, you can take it to the next level and combine this breathing practice with a blinking practice. Try gently blinking your eyes in time with each contraction of your abdomen. Each time you exhale, you blink. The faster you breathe, the faster you blink. Take your time coordinating your body, breath, and eyes to make it very relaxing and aligning.

Alternate Nostril Breath

Purpose:

- Balance the left and right hemispheres of the brain.
- Balance the left and right eyes.
- Equalize the breath.
- Calm the mind.
- Increase focus and clarity.

Directions:

1) Make a gentle fist with your right hand.
2) Extend your right thumb, ring finger, and pinky finger.
3) Inhale deeply through both nostrils.
4) Block right nostril with your thumb, exhale out left nostril.
5) Inhale through your left nostril.
6) Switch, block your left nostril with your ring finger.
7) Exhale through your right nostril.
8) Inhale through your right nostril.
9) Repeat steps 4-8.

Time: 1 to 3 minutes.

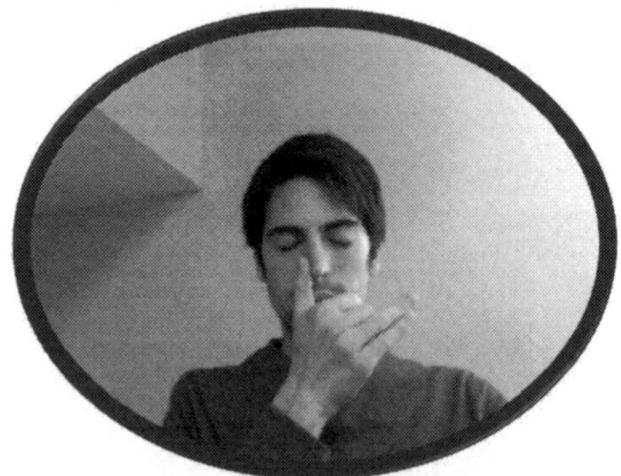

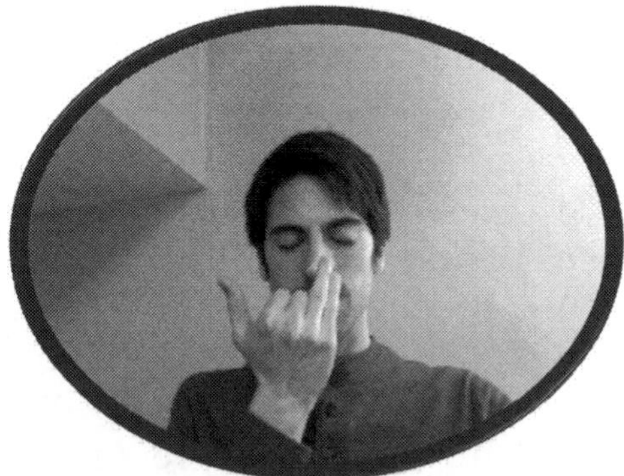

Pattern:
Exhale, Inhale, Switch... Exhale, Inhale, Switch... Exhale, Inhale, Switch...

Description:

This pranayama is very relaxing and helps to balance the left and right hemispheres of your brain. Since your eyes are extensions of your brain, it can also help balance your left and right eyes.

If possible, try to incorporate the 2:1 belly breathing into the alternate nostril breath to elongate and deepen your exhales. Start with a full inhale through both nostrils, then block your right nostril with your thumb and exhale for 4 seconds out your left nostril, pulling your belly in. Inhale for 2 seconds through your left nostril, letting your belly relax back out, then switch and cover your left nostril with your ring finger, exhale for 4 seconds out your right nostril, pulling your belly in, and then inhale for 2 seconds through your right nostril, letting your belly relax back out.

Continue at this rate and maintain the pattern of exhale left, inhale left, then switch and exhale right, inhale right, then switch. Eventually you can work your way up to 6 second exhales and 3 second inhales, 8 second exhales and 4 second inhales, etc. Try feeling or thinking about your right brain hemisphere when you breathe through your left nostril. Try feeling or thinking about your left brain hemisphere when you breathe through your right nostril.

Remember to keep contracting your abdomen on your exhales and expanding your abdomen on your inhales. This is an excellent pranayama to center your body, relax your mind, and prepare you for concentration or meditation.

Yogic Eye Movements

Purpose:

- Strengthen and tone voluntary eye muscles.
- Identify eyestrain and loosen tight eye muscles.
- Explore and expand visual field.

Directions:

1) Keep your entire body relaxed (shoulders, neck, face, brow).
2) Isolate movement to the six muscles around each eye.
3) Inhale and look as far up as is comfortable and hold for a few moments, then center.
4) Exhale and look as far down as is comfortable and hold for a moment, then center.
5) Repeat up and down 6 to 10 times then close your eyes to rest in the center.
6) Inhale and look as far right as is comfortable and hold for a moment, then center.
7) Exhale and look as far left as is comfortable and hold for a moment, then center.
8) Repeat right and left 6 to 10 times then close your eyes to rest in the center.
9) Imagine that there is a large clock in front of you.
10) Slowly make your way around clockwise 12, 1, 2, 3, etc. a few times.
11) Close your eyes to rest in the center.
12) Slowly make your way around counterclockwise 12, 11, 10, 9, etc.
13) Close your eyes to rest in the center.
14) Palm your eyes for the same amount of time you did the eye movements.

Time: 1 to 3 minutes.

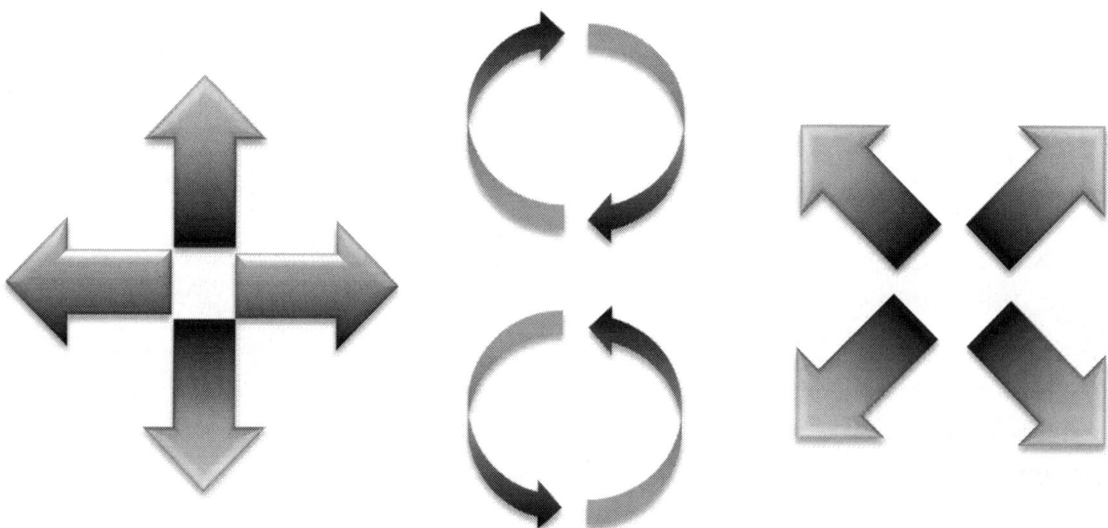

Description:

The yogic eye movements (or *Netra Vyayamam in Sanskrit)* are not a part of the Bates Method. First of all, they have been around for thousands of years as a part of the ancient practice of yoga. Secondly, they do not necessarily guarantee relaxation or the complete release of eyestrain. The main goal of the Bates Method is to replace strain with relaxation. These eye movements can be performed while still holding onto eyestrain or can even increase eyestrain if not done correctly. So, it is important to stay nice and relaxed as you move your eyes around in the different directions and avoid any type of strain.

Instead of thinking about pulling the muscle that is turning your eye, think about the opposite muscle that is releasing and allowing your eye to turn. In other words, when you look up, try to focus more on your lower rectus muscle releasing than your upper rectus muscle pulling. The greatest way to avoid eyestrain in this exercise is to always follow the eye movements with an equal amount of time palming. This way even if there is any strain discovered during the eye movements, it gets released immediately after. The horizontal and vertical eye movements help loosen the four recti muscles around each eye and the circular eye movements help loosen the two oblique muscles around each eye. You may also move your thumb and follow with your eyes, or do the eye movements while palming.

Even though the yogic eye movements are not necessarily a part of the Bates Method, they can still be beneficial, especially if you have particularly tight or tense eye muscles or if you have strabismus or astigmatism. The eye movements help you explore different areas of eyestrain around each eye and help equalize any muscular imbalances. The first few times you perform the eye movements you may experience interesting sensations when looking in particular directions. You are simply discovering an area of eyestrain. Spend more time looking in that direction until you no longer feel that sensation. After a few weeks, your yogic eye movements will become smoother and you will be able to look farther in all directions.

The figure on *Page 305*, called the Tibetan Wheel, can also be used to practice eye movements. Hold the page a few inches from your nose with your nose pointing at the central dot. Hold the page and your head still as you trace the outline of the shape with your eyes in one direction all the way around. Close your eyes to rest at any time to prevent overworking your eyes. Then trace the outline of the wheel in the opposite direction all the way around. Follow this exercise with palming as well to ensure adequate relaxation immediately after.

Body Looseners

Tightness and rigidity in the body can translate to tightness and rigidity in the eyes. Loosening up other muscle groups throughout the body can help influence the muscles of the eyes to loosen and relax. Most of these stretches can be performed standing or sitting. Look at your eye chart or reading card before, during, and after these body looseners and see the immediate difference they can make in the clarity of your vision.

Neck Stretches

Begin by looking straight ahead. Keep your head centered and look with your eyes to the right. This will initiate a movement in your head so slowly turn your head as far to the right as is comfortable and look over your right shoulder. Look as far to the right as you can as if you were trying to see something behind you. Turn your eyes back to the left as you slowly turn your head as far to the left as is comfortable and look behind you over your left shoulder. Repeat several times, allowing your eyes to initiate the movement of your head. End back in the center. Tilt your head back and look up toward the ceiling. Tilt your chin down toward your chest and look down at the floor. Repeat up and down head movements a few times and end back in the center.

Head Rolls

Gently lower your chin toward your chest keeping your neck relaxed. Slowly begin to roll your head to the right, bringing your right ear toward your right shoulder. Instead of continuing beyond your shoulder, begin rolling your head back down and bring your chin back to your chest, then over to the left, bringing your left ear toward your left shoulder. The head rolls are more of a semi-circle than a full circle, so that you do not tilt your head too far back, unless that is comfortable for you. Keep your eyes soft and allow them to shift naturally. Notice the oppositional movement that happens during the head rolls.

Shoulder Rolls

Shrug your shoulders up toward your ears. Keeping them raised, roll them as far back as you can and lower them back down to the relaxed position. Now shrug your shoulders up toward your ears and roll them as far forward as you can and lower them back to the relaxed position. Go back and forth between shrugging up and back and shrugging up and forward several times.

Arm Circles

Stand with your arms relaxed by your side. Inhale and slowly begin to raise your arms out and up overhead with your palms facing up as if you were tracing a large circle around your body. Exhale and slowly lower your arms with palms facing down back to the original position by your side. Really extend your arms far out to draw the biggest circle you can with your arms. Stretch and wiggle your fingertips out into the space around you. Gaze straight ahead and notice the movement of your fingers in the far edges of your peripheral visual field. Repeat several times.

Spine Stretch

Sit or stand up tall and take a deep breath in. As you exhale, hinge at your hips and slowly begin to fold forward. Let your arms hang like a rag doll. Breathe deeply while upside down and sway gently from side to side. Nod your head, 'Yes.' Shake your head, 'No.' When ready, roll back up to an upright position vertebra by vertebra with your head being the last to rise. Another great spinal stretch is to stand with your arms extended out to either side. Tilt your torso over to the right and look up toward your left hand. Rise back up to center and tilt your torso over to the left and look up toward your right hand. Go back and forth several times, coordinating with your breath and keeping your eyes soft. If you are more comfortable seated, sit on the very edge of a chair with your knees open. Elongate your spine upward and begin to fold your upper body forward into the space between your legs and relax.

Hip Circles

Stand with your hands on your hips. Begin rotating your hips in a clockwise direction, making as small or big circles as is comfortable. Repeat several times and then rotate your hips in a counterclockwise direction several times. This helps stimulate your liver and kidneys, which are the main organs associated with your eyes and vision.

Joint Looseners

Roll your wrists and ankles. Wiggle your fingers and toes. Bend your knees and elbows. Explore all the joints in your body and give them a little movement.

Bouncing

Stand comfortably. Begin quickly bending your knees and then pressing into the ground so that your shoulders begin to bounce up and down. Pretend that you are bouncing on a rebounder trampoline without your feet leaving the ground. If you have a trampoline to bounce on that is even better. This will greatly help dissipate any tension in your neck and shoulders.

30 Second Martini

For thirty seconds give every part of your body a vigorous shake. Shake your head, your arms, your legs, your hands, your feet, jump up and down, have fun! After thirty seconds, stand still and feel the wonderful effects of increased circulation and energy.

Vision and Posture

Which came first, poor vision or poor posture? Vision and posture are intricately linked. Since your eyes are extensions of your brain, they are a part of your central nervous system. When light lands on your retina in the back of your eye, it travels as an impulse through your optic nerve to the visual cortex in the back of your brain, which processes and interprets information to send down your spinal cord and onward throughout the rest of your body.

If your posture is poor and your body is slumped or hunched, these lightning-fast connections can be interrupted or skewed. Improper posture interferes with the visual system and over time can lead to shallow breathing, decreased circulation, lymph stagnation, physical fatigue, and blurred vision. Poor posture can lead to poor vision, and poor vision can lead to poor posture.

Blurred vision from poor posture often leads to worse posture by straining to see either a close or distant object, which is usually accompanied with reaching your neck forward or cranking it back. Vision and posture are intertwined and can either work together to spiral downward toward imbalance or spiral upward toward optimal functioning.

The neat thing about this subject is that better posture is often a natural side effect of practicing the Bates Method. Your body's intelligence will start to realize that clearer vision comes when in a comfortable and aligned posture, which encourages the new habit subconsciously. Do not stress too much about sitting up straight or forcing yourself into a posture that does not feel like you. Just stick with the vision improvement and your posture may re-adjust on its own.

There are also several other modalities that can help you improve your posture and release stored tension throughout the spine and body including exercise, massage, acupressure, acupuncture, reflexology, Alexander Technique, Feldenkrais, Network Spinal Analysis, yoga, qigong, tai chi, and even dance. I personally used to slouch significantly. Not only did I devote lots of time to poor-posture-promoting activities such as reading, writing, schoolwork, computer work, and video games, but also my tall height forced me to look down at other people and scrunch my spine to get on their level. As a tall person, I had to compromise my full posture potential to fit into an average sized world by bending down to reach low counters and see in 'average' height mirrors. Luckily, I recognized my bad habits early on and set an intention to improve my posture, stand with more confidence, relax my shoulders, and expand my heart out to allow for more breath to enter my system and to prevent ending up with a hunchback. It has been a long and steady process, but through daily mental reminders, practicing yoga, meditation, breathwork, and the other modalities listed above, my posture slowly transformed and further assisted my natural vision improvement process.

Tip: Try and see from your spine. Instead of reaching your eyes forward and straining or squinting to see something, try relaxing back into your center or your core, like you are seeing with the visual cortex in the very back of your brain instead of with the eyes on the front of your face. This practice encourages relaxed use of the eyes and takes the pressure off the need to see. It also allows for deep, rhythmic breathing and a gentle tuck of the chin to encourage a more natural curvature of the cervical spine.

Eat, Drink, and See Clearly

Diet and nutrition are crucial components of healing your eyes from within. Your eyes will respond to vision training even more if they get the nourishment they need from what you feed them every day. Research has proven the correlation between better nutrition and decreased risk of vision problems including glaucoma, cataracts, and even macular degeneration. If nutrition and supplementation can help with these more advanced vision problems, think of how much they can help the more basic vision problems. Below are some diet tips for optimal eye health. I am not a dietitian, but I did personally experience positive shifts when I modified my own diet for the sake of a healthier body and mind.

Oxygen

Before you eat or drink anything, take a deep breath. Keep breathing slowly and deeply as you eat. Breathe as you chew. Your eyes need oxygen. Your eyes literally breathe. The transparent part of your eyes, the corneas, have no blood vessels flowing through them. Without blood vessels, the corneas must literally absorb oxygen from the air. Oxygen dissolves in the tear fluids on the eye and spreads around the cornea to keep it healthy and transparent. A waste product of a healthy 'breathing' cornea is carbon dioxide, which diffuses out of the cornea in the opposite process. Contact lenses 'suffocate' your eyes by impeding this two-way exchange, which can affect the growth of the cornea and cause blood vessels grow into the cornea for survival. Each breath initiates circulation of freshly oxygenated blood to all the rest of the parts of the eyes that are nourished by blood vessels.

Liquids

Your body is primarily liquid. Different parts of your body are comprised of different concentrations of water. On the lower end of the scale are your teeth (1.8% water) and your bones (30% water). On the higher end of the scale are your brain (75% water), heart (79% water), and blood (90% water). However, at the very top of the list are your eyes. The part of your body that contains the most water is the vitreous humour, or the vitreous body, inside your eyes, which is 99% water. Your eyes need sufficient intake of fresh, clean water to remain moist and lubricated inside and out. Caffeine and alcohol both affect the eyes and ought to be moderated. Since the liver is the primary organ associated with the eyes according to Classical Chinese Medicine, limit the amount of alcohol you consume. The moment alcohol enters your body, your liver works in overdrive to filter it out. A toxic, poisoned liver can translate to sluggish, blurry vision.

Solids

Foods that are good for your brain and heart are also good for your eyes. As a general rule, eyes prefer fresh, whole foods like fruits and vegetables. Locally grown foods are often fresher than those packed and shipped to grocery stores far away. Organically grown foods are often safer and healthier without the use of harmful chemicals and pesticides in the growing process. Usually the more color and aroma a food has the more life it has. Eyes dislike 'dead' food, or highly processed foods with refined white sugars, artificial ingredients, colors, dyes, or flavors. Do your best to moderate your sugar intake, because increased levels of glucose can damage proteins, create free radicals, accelerate aging, and lead to macular degeneration and cataracts. Eyes prefer alkalizing, anti-inflammatory foods as opposed to acidic, inflammatory foods. The only foods that alkalize your body are fruits and vegetables. Dark leafy greens are the most important foods to eat for healthy eyes.

Nutrients

Lutein and zeaxanthin are two of the most commonly known nutrients specific to eye health. The antioxidant lutein and pigment zeaxanthin both protect and preserve the macula, which contains the fovea centralis in the middle of your retina that gives you your central, high definition vision. They also support your lens and optic nerve and aid your eyes ability to safely absorb light and improve night vision. Omega-3 fatty acids like DHA and EPA keep your eyes lubricated and your retinas functioning. Vitamin C is present in all eye tissues and supports the health of ocular blood vessels. Vitamin E supports eye health and better night vision.

Minerals

A wide range of trace minerals is necessary for the basic functions of the human body like bone growth, fluid regulation, muscle and nerve function, metabolism maintenance, connective tissue growth, and optimal eye health. Zinc transports vitamin A from your liver to your retina to produce the protective pigment melanin and deficiencies in zinc can lead to impaired vision, low night vision and cataracts. Some other vision-specific minerals include magnesium, zinc, selenium, chromium, potassium, sodium, phosphorus, iron, manganese, copper, and iodine. Once again, many of these trace minerals are accessible through raw fruits and vegetables.

Herbs

Eyebright has been used for hundreds of years across England and Europe. It has shown to reduce eye irritation and inflammation issues like conjunctivitis. Ginkgo increases circulation to the retina, protects nerve cells, and can help with glaucoma. Coleus, which contains forskolin, can also help with glaucoma by reducing intraocular pressure. The antioxidants in green tea help absorb free radicals that can lead to glaucoma, macular degeneration, and cataracts. Cannabis has long been used to treat glaucoma by significantly reducing eye pressure. Garlic and turmeric have both shown to help prevent cataracts. Saffron has shown to help prevent and reverse macular degeneration. Other eye herbs include nettle, dandelion, calendula, chrysanthemum, and lamb's quarters.

Foods to Eat

Dark leafy green vegetables (kale, spinach, arugula, collards, parsley, cilantro, etc.) eggs, broccoli, peas, and corn contain high concentrations of lutein and zeaxanthin. Citrus fruits (oranges, grapefruits, tangerines, lemons, etc.) and parsley provide high levels of vitamin C. Nuts and oils provide vitamin E. Fatty fish and flax seeds provide omega 3s. Bilberry and blueberry support blood vessels and capillaries, improve circulation to and within the eyes, and provide antioxidant support. Orange-colored foods like carrots, sweet potatoes, squashes, and turmeric provide beta-carotene, which the body converts into vitamin A, and helps to improve night vision. A few other great eye-foods include avocados, garlic, onions, peaches, and bananas.

Supplements

The best way to absorb vitamins, minerals, nutrients and phytonutrients is by consuming enough whole living foods every day. However, if your wallet or your watch won't allow for it, supplementation is a great way to fill in any gaps. There are several different supplements available designed specifically for eye health. However, you want to be careful about where you get them from to make sure they don't have any fillers or artificial colors.

Good Eating Habits

Avoiding chemicals, white sugar, and processed, refined, packaged foods will help you avoid disease. Chew carefully, slowly, and thoroughly before swallowing to improve digestion. Digestion begins in the mouth and the more you masticate, the easier the food is to digest.

Limit liquid intake during a meal. Drinking too much liquid with a meal dilutes your digestive fluids. Try to drink your liquids before or after eating. If possible, try to avoid eating cooked and raw foods at the same time since they digest at different rates.

Eat only when you are truly hungry and drink only when you are truly thirsty. As your intuition becomes clearer, you will know when you really need to eat or drink. The hunger sensation is a sign that you have fully digested your last meal and are ready for the next one. Sometimes the hunger sensation is actually a symptom of dehydration. Drink a glass of water and see if it still remains.

Try focusing more on eating instead of multitasking while you eat. Look at the meal you are eating or the people you are eating with instead of reading a newspaper or watching a television while you eat. Don't eat when you're angry, depressed, in a hurry, or before bed.

👁 *Are you still following the 13 Rules of Relaxed Reading from Page 12-13?* 👁

How is your posture? How are the muscles in your face, eyes, and brow? How is your breathing? How is your blinking? Are you stopping at the end of every few sentences to close your eyes and picture the last word you read clearly? Are you looking off into the distance every so often? Can you see an imaginary bright white line underlining the sentences as you read? Can you imagine a bright white line underlining these words with your eyes closed?

Foods to Eat

Primarily a plant-based alkaline diet

- **Vegetables** – *Spinach, Kale, Cabbage, Chard, Collards, Romaine Lettuce, Parsley, Cilantro, Tomatoes, Onions, Corn, Peppers, Sweet Potatoes, Brussels Sprouts, Beets, Asparagus, Mushrooms, Broccoli, Avocado, Carrots.*
- **Fruits** – *Apricots, Oranges, Tangerines, Grapefruits, Lemons, Limes, Strawberries, Blueberries, Cranberries, Raspberries, Blackberries, Currants, Goji Berries, Watermelon, Cantaloupe, Apples, Pears, Peaches, Bananas, Kiwis, Nectarines, Papayas, Pineapples, Mangoes, Pomegranates.*
- **Nuts and Seeds** – *Almonds, Cashews, Chestnuts, Hazelnuts, Peanuts, Pecans, Pine Nuts, Pistachios, Walnuts, Chia, Hemp, Pumpkin, Sunflower.*
- **Beans and Legumes** – *Black-Eyed Peas, Chickpeas, Edamame, Green Beans, Kidney Beans, Lentils, Lima Beans, Navy Beans, White Beans.*
- **Animal Protein** – *Salmon, Tuna, Trout, Catfish, Flounder, Haddock, Sole, Shrimp, Anchovies, Sardines, Chicken, Steak, Eggs.*
- **Grains** – *Brown Rice, Oatmeal, Farro, Flaxseed, Quinoa, Hemp, Amaranth, Spelt.*
- **Herbs and Spices** – *Mint, Basil, Saffron, Curry, Ginger, Garlic, Cinnamon, Turmeric.*

Foods to Avoid / Limit

- **Sugar** – *White, Brown, Cane, Powdered, Turbinado, Demerara, Fructose.*
- **Soda** – *Sugary beverages, High Fructose Corn Syrup, Aspartame, Phosphoric Acid, Fluoride.*
- **Processed Foods** – *Packaged Foods, Refined Sugars, Refined Flours, Hard to pronounce ingredients, Candy, Fast Food, Junk Food.*
- **Animal Products** – *Factory Farmed Animals, Red Meat, Ground Beef, Pork, Fish Oil*
- ***Dairy*** – *Milk, Yogurt, Ice Cream, Cheese.*
- **Alcohol and Caffeine** – *Beer, Wine, Liquor, Coffee, Tea, Soda.*
- **Artificial Colors** – *Blue 1, Blue 2, Green 3, Red 3, Red 40, Yellow 5, Yellow 6 (USA) Quinoline Yellow, Carmoisine, Ponceau 4R, Patent Blue V, Green S (Europe).*
- **GMOs** – *Genetically Modified Corn, Soy, Canola, Squash, Alfalfa, Sugar Beets, Milk.*

Important Vitamins, Minerals, and Nutrients

- **Bioflavonoids** – *Diindolylmethane, Quercetin, Resveratrol, Troxerutin.*
- **Carotenoids** – *Astaxanthin, Beta-Carotene, Lutein, Zeaxanthin, Lycopene.*
- **Super-Antioxidants** – *Alpha-Lipoic Acid, Glutathione, Solforaphane.*
- **Plant Nutrients** – *Agaricus, Curcumin, Gingko, Phytic Acid, St. John's Wort.*
- **Metals** – *Boron, Calcium, Chromium, Copper, Iron, Magnesium, Manganese, Potassium, Selenium, Zinc.*
- **Lettered Vitamins** – *A, B1, B2, B3, B6, B9, B12, C, D3, E, K.*
- **Amino Acids** – *Arginine, Carnitine, Lysine, Methionine, Proline, Taurine.*
- **Power Nutrients** – *CoQ10, Choline, SAMe.*
- **Essential Fatty Acids** – *Omega 3, DHA, EPA.*

Eye Supplements

- **Multivitamins** – *Vitamin A, B complex, C, D3, E, K, Trace Minerals and Metals.*
- **Eye Formulas** – *Lutein, Zeaxanthin, Beta Carotene, Selenium, Zinc, Bilberry, Bioflavanoids, Antioxidants, Amino Acids, N-acetyl cysteine, Alpha-lipoic acid.*
- **Adaptogens** – *Reishi, Cordyceps, Chaga, Rhodiola, Ashwaganda, Astragalus, Holy Basil, Ginseng, Ginkgo, Licorice, Schizandra.*
- **Plant Based Oils** – *Avocado, Coconut, Flax Seed, Olive, Sesame, Sunflower.*
- **Herbs and More** – *Eyebright, Cayenne, Coleus, Green Tea, Garlic, Turmeric, Marigold, Black Currant, Chlorella, Spirulina, Saffron.*
- **Homeopathic** – *Calcarea fluorica, Calendula officinalis, Cineraria maritime, Euphrasia officinalis, Kali muriaticum, Magnesia carbonica, Silicea.*

Neti Pot

Purpose:

- Cleanse the nasal cavities and sinuses.
- Lubricate the eyes.
- Improve the sense of smell.
- Decrease seasonal allergies.

Directions:

1) Fill a neti pot 1/3 to 1/2 full of warm filtered or distilled water *(not tap water).*
2) If desired, add a pinch of neti salt solution and stir to dissolve.
3) Insert spout of neti pot into right nostril, tilt your to the left and forward a bit.
4) Breathe through your open mouth, tip the pot, pour the water into your right nostril.
5) Breathe calmly as the water exits through your left nostril and into the sink or tub.
6) Once all the water has drained through, blow your nose.
7) Rinse and refill your neti pot, repeat on the other side, in the left nostril, out the right.

Description:

You can find either a plastic or ceramic neti pot at most health food stores or on my website. They look like little teapots with a long spout. Only use filtered or distilled water because tap water may introduce unintended chemicals and pollutants into your nasal passageway. For the greatest level of comfort use lukewarm water that is close to body temperature and not too cold or too hot. It is also optional to dissolve a little bit of neti salt solution in the water, which can help loosen up and clear out any hardened mucus.

If you've never done a neti pot before it may take a little practice to get used to the sensation of water going in one nostril and out the other. The two most important things to keep in mind while doing the neti pot are to breathe through your open mouth and to tilt your head slightly forward as you tip to one side. You want the water to go through your nose, not back and down your throat. It helps to have tissues handy to blow your nose with immediately after cleansing each side. Be aware that if your nasal passageway is clogged, the water may not make it through to your other nostril the first time. Regular use of the neti pot does wonders for your eyes and your nose.

Eye Bath

Have you ever taken an eye bath? It may sound strange, but your eyes need to be washed just like the rest of your body. Eye baths can help relieve eyestrain, reduce dryness and redness, and help keep your eyes lubricated and clean. The most efficient way to bathe your eyes is by using an eye cup. Before using your eye cup, wash or boil it to sterilize it. Only use filtered or distilled water for this practice, because tap water contains contaminants that could lead to eye infections.

As a beginner, you will probably want to use the simple dipping method. Fill your eye cup with warm water, tilt your head down, dip one eye into the water so it's totally submerged, blink a few times and look around in all directions. Pour out the used water, rise it out, refill it with new water and repeat with your other eye. Spend about 15 to 30 seconds on each eye. Once you get comfortable with that feeling you can try the tilt-back method. Fill your eye cup with warm water, tilt your head down, place the cup snugly against your eye orbit, then tilt your head back, blinking and looking around in all directions. Tilting your head back helps you wash all around and behind the eye, so make sure you look up, down, left, and right. Be warned though that some spillage may occur. You can either have a towel handy or just do it in the shower.

Once you are comfortable with washing your eyes with water, it's time to explore some even better eye baths. One that I recommend is Dr. Christopher's Herbal Eyebright solution, which contains extracts of bayberry bark, golden seal root, eyebright herb, red raspberry leaf, and cayenne. The cayenne greatly increases circulation, the astringent red raspberry leaf and bayberry bark reduce pain and shrink inflamed tissues, the golden seal root provides important trace minerals like cobalt, iron, magnesium, manganese, silicon and zinc, and the eyebright is an herb that has been used for over seven hundred years to treat eye problems. Start by diluting only one drop of Dr. Christopher's into your eye cup filled with warm water and slowly work your way up to seven drops as your tolerance increases for the nice tingle that the cayenne gives it. The eyebright solution can be taken internally as well in water or tea, but when taken externally in an eye bath the herbs absorb directly into the eye tissue and begin working immediately for invigorating results. The eyebright solution is especially effective for cataracts and glaucoma, so anyone who has those might want to try using this simple homeopathic remedy.

Energizing Your Vision

Many healing traditions refer to a vital life force energy that sustains all beings. Chinese Medicine refers to it as *qi*, which travels through a vast network of *meridian lines*. Yoga refers to it as *prana*, which travels through a vast network of *nadis* and *chakras*. In either framework, health problems are often viewed as energetic imbalances or blockages; a stagnation of qi or prana somewhere in the physical body. When these blockages get removed, the vital energy can flow freely through the system and more optimal health is achieved. If you wish to take the Chinese Medicine approach, you may want to consult an acupuncturist or reflexologist, or consider taking some qigong or tai chi instruction to accumulate and balance your qi. Over the next few pages you will learn the yogic framework for harnessing your prana and balancing your chakras with the specific intention of bringing more energy to your third eye chakra.

According to the ancient philosophy of yoga, humans have seven major chakras, or energy centers. Chakra is Sanskrit for 'wheel' and these energetic wheels rotate in opposite directions like gears running up the center of the body. You can think of them like pools that energy flows through from the first chakra at the bottom upwards to the seventh chakra at the top and beyond. The energy only flows freely when the chakras are balanced and there are no energetic blockages. However, the energy can get stuck in the lower chakras and not make it up to the higher chakras. Therefore, if the energy fails to rise all the way, the sixth chakra, or the third eye chakra that deals with inner vision and outer vision, may not be getting the energy it needs. Since the prana and chakras are parts of the subtle energy system, the blockages are not usually physical in nature, but rather mental, emotional, or spiritual.

As we go through each chakra one by one, reflect on the state of your own chakras and your own emotional past, present, and future, and how it relates specifically to your vision. Each chakra has a particular emotion or feeling associated with it when it is balanced and flowing. Each chakra also has an opposite emotion or feeling that can block it and prevent energy from flowing freely through it. By applying this ancient wisdom to your current life, you may gain insights into how to remove blockages and open up to more balance, energy, healing, and clarity.

Root Chakra

The first chakra, or root chakra, is located at the base of the spine. It represents your connection to the Earth and is associated with feelings of survival. The root chakra is blocked by fear. What are your fears? What were you afraid of in the past? What are you afraid of now? What are you afraid of in the future? Do any of your fears threaten your survival? Fear is the number one underlying root emotion beneath most vision problems. Think about the fears surrounding your eyes and vision. Are you afraid of not being able to see? What are you afraid to look at or think about? Write down some of your fears:

Past: ____

____

____

Present: ____

____

____

Future: ____

____

____

Identify and release your fears in order for the energy to flow fully into and through your first chakra to rise up to your second chakra and beyond. Since fear is the base emotion, see if you can trace all the following emotions that block the next six chakras back to the emotion of fear, and what you fear about those emotions or the consequences of those emotions.

Sacral Chakra

The second chakra, or sacral chakra, is located below your navel. It represents your creativity and sexuality and is associated with feelings of pleasure and desire. The sacral chakra is blocked by guilt. What do you feel guilty about? What things have you blamed yourself for in the past or present? Who have you hurt in the past? How does guilt prevent your pleasure? Write down some of your guilts:

Past: ____

____

____

Present: ____

____

____

Future: ____

____

____

Identify and release the blame and guilt within you and accept the fact that mistakes happen. Don't let these burdens or grudges cloud your perception or blur your vision. Clear vision is a birthright and is supposed to be a pleasurable experience. Once you forgive yourself, the energy will flow fully through your second chakra up to your third chakra and beyond.

Solar Plexus Chakra

The third chakra, or solar plexus chakra, is located above your navel. It represents your personal power and is associated with the choices you make and your willpower. The solar plexus chakra is blocked by shame. What do you feel ashamed of? What were you embarrassed about in the past? What have been your biggest disappointments in your self or in your life? Who has let you down? What do you feel angry about? What shames surround your eyes and vision? Does your vision problem make you feel like you have a handicap? Does the blur drain your vitality? Write down some of your shames or letdowns:

Past: ____

____

____

Present: ____

____

____

Future: ____

____

____

Identify and release your shames, embarrassments, letdowns, and disappointments and accept, embrace, and love all the aspects of who you are despite your flaws. You must also forgive others who have hurt you in the past to reclaim your own personal power. Once you accept yourself and others, the energy will flow fully through your third chakra up to your fourth chakra and beyond.

Heart Chakra

The fourth chakra, or heart chakra, is located in the center of your chest. It represents your relationships and connections to your self and to others and is associated with love. The heart chakra is blocked by grief. What pain, sadness, and loss has broken or closed your heart? What is your relationship with yourself like? How were your past relationships? Did you feel loved growing up? What is the current balance between the love you give and the love you receive? Have you experienced the loss of friends or family members? Do you feel like you fully grieved? Did your eyes release enough tears to process the pain? Are there any pains or losses that you anticipate or fear in the future? Write down some of your griefs:

Past: ____

____

____

Present: ____

____

____

Future: ____

____

____

Identify and release your pain, sorrow, and loss and realize that love is an infinite energy that is found within you and all around you. What fears were created in your mind in the midst of pain, sadness, and loss? Once you let the pain flow through you, it will be replaced by love, and the energy will flow fully through your fourth chakra up to your fifth chakra and beyond.

Throat Chakra

The fifth chakra, or throat chakra, is located at the base of your throat. It represents your communication and expression and is associated with truth. The throat chakra is blocked by lies. What lies are you telling yourself? What have other people lied to you about in the past? Do you feel like you are able to fully and freely express yourself through your words or actions? Can you explain yourself and your feelings easily? What is the status of your communication and conversation with your friends and loved ones? What things do you hold in or bottle up and do not tell anyone? What secrets are you keeping? What is your truth? Write down some of your secrets or lies:

Past: ____

____

____

Present: ____

____

____

Future: ____

____

Identify and release the denial and the lies you tell yourself. Your eye doctor may be lying to you if they tell you there is nothing you can do to make your eyes healthier or improve your vision. They may be lying if they say there is no nutritional connection to vision problems. You may be lying to yourself if you believe them. They may only be showing you partial truth. What fears are forcing you to lie? What are you afraid of happening if you do not lie? What are you hiding or protecting? Once you stop telling yourself lies and begin expressing your truth to yourself and those around you, the energy will flow fully through your fifth chakra up to your sixth chakra and beyond.

Third Eye Chakra

The sixth chakra, or third eye chakra, is located in the center of your forehead in between your eyebrows. It represents your inner and outer vision and is associated with insight and intuition. The third eye is often correlated with the pineal and pituitary glands in the center of your brain. These are the seats of consciousness that control all other endocrine glands in the body. The third eye chakra is blocked by illusion. What illusions have you encountered in your life? Maybe you thought one way about something and then came to a completely different realization of how it really is. What were some barriers or obstacles you thought were preventing you from achieving something that were actually false or irrational fears? What are some things you used to think about, dream about, or visualize when you were younger? What was your vision of your future or the future of the world? Which parts came to fruition and which parts turned out differently than expected? What do you think about or dream about right now? What is your current vision of your future or of the world? What illusions are within you regarding your eyes and vision? Write down some of your illusions:

Past: ____

Present: ____

Future: ____

Identify and see through all the illusions within you and around you. This entire process of going through your energies and emotions is exercising your third eye and your insight. You are looking within by analyzing your past, present, and future. Just by getting clear about your fears, your guilt, your shames, your griefs, your lies, and your illusions, you are activating and strengthening your third eye and your intuition. Once you release the illusions of limitations and separations and realize that everything is connected, the energy will flow fully through your sixth chakra up to your seventh chakra and beyond. Sometimes things are not always as they seem. You must lift the veil to expose clearer thinking and greater consciousness. This will enable you to begin seeing through illusions and seeing through the blur. Blurry vision is an illusion that you must dissipate by opening your third eye. If any fear, guilt, shame, grief, or untruth is blocking your energy flow, then your third eye may be shut and your inner and outer vision will remain unfocused.

Crown Chakra

The seventh chakra, or crown chakra, is located at the very top of the head. It represents your connection with the cosmos and is associated with pure cosmic energy and the feeling of peace and bliss. The seventh chakra is blocked by attachment. What attachments do you have to ideas, to people, or to material things? What attachments do you have to your vision? What expectations do you have about this holistic vision practice? Write down some of your attachments:

Past: ____

Present: ____

Future: ____

Identify and release all your earthly attachments and expectations of the fruits of your labor. It is quite a paradox that you may only receive something once you let go of your attachment to it. The path of the karma yogi is a path of selfless service, performing actions or serving others without expectation of receiving anything in return. Random acts of kindness, volunteering, and unconditional love are signs of a balanced crown chakra. When you apply this to your vision practice, you must try to loosen your grip on your expectations or anticipations of results. Only then will you begin to see clearly. If you only do the vision practice to get a specific result you may not succeed. If instead you do the vision practice without any expectations at all, simply for the sake of doing the practice, that is when the flashes of clarity multiply.

It may seem counterintuitive at first, but this is essentially just another form of a key principle you have been practicing this whole time: letting go. Although it is frightening, you must let go. The more you let go the more you receive. The harder you grasp on, the less you will receive. Once you realize that letting go of something does not necessarily mean that it truly disappears, you will understand how to absolve attachments. Without any attachments, the energy can flow fully through your seventh chakra and beyond, giving you a new sense of clarity and awareness amidst feelings of bliss, connectivity, and balance.

Mental Focus #8 and more...

Bar and Dots

The bar and dots is a great foundational mental focus practice that you can adapt into many others. You simply shift from one dot to the other, gently pivoting your head and observing that the bar in the middle appears to move in the opposite direction. When you look at the left dot with your central vision you see the left dot clearer than the bar and the right dot, which are both in your peripheral field. When you look at the right dot with your central vision you see the right dot clearer than the bar and the left dot, which are both in your peripheral field. Now rotate your bar and dots and repeat vertically and diagonally.

Do the bar and dots drill a few times with your eyes open so you can see what it looks and feels like and then practice it with your eyes closed or while palming. Even when you do this mental drill with your eyelids closed, your eyes ought to still be responding as if they were open and actually looking at it.

With your eyes closed it is important to picture the bar and the dots as perfectly black and clear. You can either picture them on a piece of white paper or you can have them floating in the air on a pleasing background. If you are nearsighted you can use the bar and the dots to stretch your imagination and visualization farther out. Begin by picturing the bar and dots at a comfortable clear distance then slowly move them farther out in increments until you are shifting from dot to dot at a distance of 20 feet or beyond. You can even imagine a huge bar and dots floating off in the horizon over the ocean or mountains. If you are farsighted you can use the bar and the dots to stretch your imagination and visualization closer in. Begin by picturing the bar and dots at a comfortable clear distance from you then slowly move them closer in and picture them smaller and smaller.

Dr. Bates taught that the shorter the shift, the greater the relaxation, so start big and slowly make it smaller and smaller.

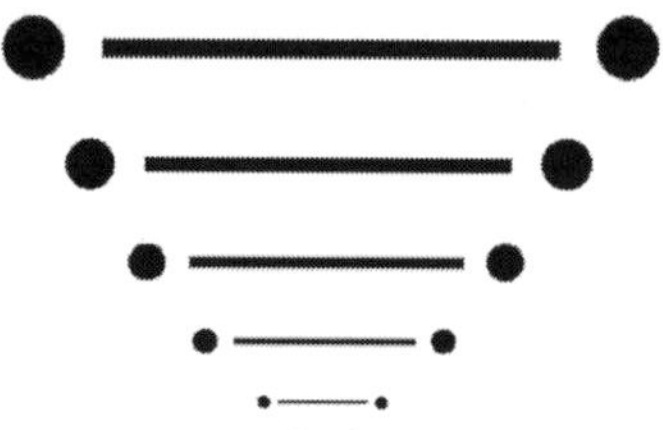

Ring of Life

While palming, picture a perfect circle floating in mid-air. If you are nearsighted imagine it far away and clear. If you are farsighted imagine it up close and clear.

First, apply imaginary pressure to the left and right sides of the circle to change the circle into a vertical egg shape. Hold it out of shape for a few seconds and, on a big exhale, release the imaginary pressure and watch it pop back to a perfect circle.

Next, apply imaginary pressure to the top and bottom to squash it into a horizontal egg shape. Hold it out of shape for a few seconds and, on a big exhale, release the imaginary pressure and watch it pop back into a perfect circle.

Now do the same thing in each diagonal direction, apply imaginary pressure, hold it out of shape for a few seconds, release the imaginary pressure on an exhale and watch it pop back into proper shape.

Not only does this represent your resiliency to the challenges of life in general, but it can specifically apply to your eyes too. Lots of vision problems are rooted in some sort of strain holding the eyeballs out of their correct shape. The ring of life is a mental version of the tense and release morning drill. Just by thinking about changing shapes of circles out in space you can influence the shape of your eyeballs to assume their proper and normal shape. This mental drill is especially beneficial for people with astigmatism.

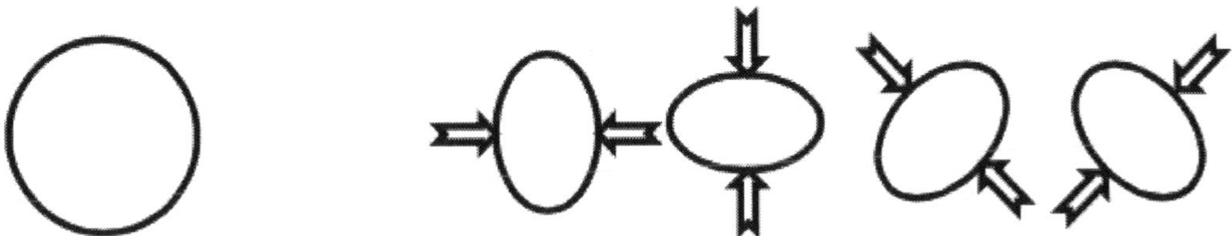

Spirals, Cones, and Floating Letters

With eyes closed, nose draw a flat, two-dimensional spiral from the outside in, and then from the inside out.

Now imagine you are looking into a deep, three-dimensional cone. For nearsightedness, start on the rim of the cone close to your face and spiral your way out to the point at the end of the cone. For farsightedness, start at the point at the end of the cone and spiral your way closer until you reach the rim up close to you.

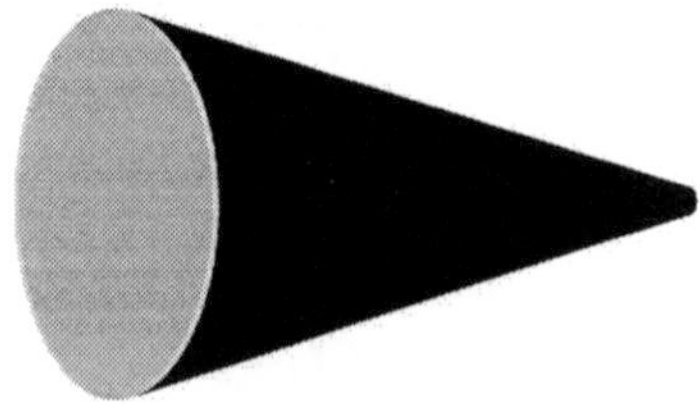

Imagine you are getting ready to read your eye chart and you are sitting or standing at a distance from a blank white chart. Imagine a big letter floating a few inches in front of your face. Visualize it perfectly clear and begin to watch it float away from you through the space in between you and the chart. Watch it land at the top of the chart and still see it perfectly clear. Now see a smaller letter floating in front of your face, watch it float out and land on the next line down on the chart. Repeat this with smaller and smaller letters until you have a completed chart and spend some time reading your mental chart perfectly clearly.

Stimulating Your Senses

To encourage longer palming sessions, put on something to listen to while you palm for 10 minutes, 20 minutes, 30 minutes, or longer. You can listen to music, nature sounds, an audiobook, a podcast, or a guided visualization or meditation. Picture what you hear through your ears. Conjure up your other senses. Imagine smells, tastes, and feelings.

Vision Work #8

Keep up with your daily holistic vision routine, cycling through any combination of relaxation, centralization, or fusion warm-ups for 5 to 15 minutes leading up to 10 to 30 minutes of vision building near with reading cards or far with eye charts or both. Keep cultivating flashes of external clarity with your eyesight and internal clarity with your insight, memory, imagination, and visualization. Gradually work your way down to smaller print over time at closer distances if you are farsighted and farther distances if you are nearsighted. Keep track of your progress by writing down your results once or twice a month. Make sure you are isolating one eye at a time using an eye patch and then working with both eyes together. Do not get overwhelmed by the amount of practices. Just fit in what you can and know that every little bit helps. Feel free to build a day or two off of your physical vision practices. Even if you skip the physical practices, you can still be doing mental practices and maintaining good vision habits.

In between your dedicated vision practice times of between 15 and 45 minutes once, twice, or three times a day, do your best to maintain good vision habits all day and night long. Breathe deeply, blink regularly, differentiate between your central and peripheral vision, sit and stand with proper posture, point with your nose and keep your eyes shifting as you nose draw, close or palm your eyes frequently, read between the lines on the white spaces, swing your focus from near to middle to far regularly, and sustain dynamic relaxation as much as possible.

Spend ample time looking within to clear your past, present, and future vision. Discover, acknowledge, and release suppressed emotions from the past. Transform your identity and personality in the present. Set goals and stick with them until completion in the future. If you take care of your eyes every single day with your daily vision routine and proper vision habits, one day holistic eye care will encompass your past, present, and future, and the period of your life where you neglected your eye health, and subsequently saw poorly, will be a distant memory.

Take this practice unto yourself. Become your own vision teacher. Keep yourself motivated and accountable. Stay on track and do not give up. If you struggle with this, please contact me and I will be more than happy to help you by becoming your personal vision coach.

Daily Practice Checklist Week 8

M	Tu	W	Th	F	S	Su			
☐	☐	☐	☐	☐	☐	☐	♥	Morning Relaxation Routine	3-6 minutes
☐	☐	☐	☐	☐	☐	☐		Swinging	2-6 minutes
☐	☐	☐	☐	☐	☐	☐		Sunning	1-4 minutes
☐	☐	☐	☐	☐	☐	☐		Palming & Mental Drill	2-8 minutes
☐	☐	☐	☐	☐	☐	☐		Picket Fence Shifter	1-4 minutes
☐	☐	☐	☐	☐	☐	☐		Centralization	2-4 minutes
☐	☐	☐	☐	☐	☐	☐		Brain Balancing	1-3 minutes
☐	☐	☐	☐	☐	☐	☐	VXA	Fusion Practices	2-10 minutes
☐	☐	☐	☐	☐	☐	☐		Vision Building	15-30 minutes
☐	☐	☐	☐	☐	☐	☐		TWL Reading	5-15 minutes
☐	☐	☐	☐	☐	☐	☐		Body/Eye Stretches	2-4 minutes
								Daily Target:	***20-60 mins***

Vision Journal: ____

____

____

____

____

____

"Vision is the art of seeing what is invisible to others." -Jonathan Swift

Conclusion

Phase ∞:
Continuing Your Vision Journey

"Learning to master what Aldous Huxley terms 'The Art of Seeing' is an exhilarating and a happy experience and the exercises and drills should be undertaken in a happy spirit. Boredom is a form of strain; do the exercises with an alert and interested mind, never with the martyred attitude of, 'Well, I've got to do my exercises now,' like a reluctant child being forced to practice tedious scales on the piano"

-Ralph MacFadyen

"The art of seeing is like the other fundamental or primary psycho-physical skills, such as talking, walking and using the hands. These fundamental skills are normally acquired in early infancy or childhood by a process of mainly unconscious self-instruction. It takes apparently several years for adequate seeing habits to be formed. Once formed, however, the habit of using the mental and physiological organs of vision correctly becomes automatic—in exactly the same way as does the habit of using the throat, tongue and palate for talking, or the legs for walking."

-Aldous Huxley

Continuing Your Vision Journey

Congratulations, you've made it to the end of this book! This is still just the beginning of your vision improvement journey though. Reading this book is not enough. You must apply what you have learned in the form of a daily vision practice routine that will eventually permanently replace bad vision habits with good vision habits. The next few pages will give you some insights of how to continue progressing toward clearer vision naturally using what you have learned in this book.

First you will learn a super simple way to dichotomize all the practices taught in this book into two main categories to make it easier for you to structure your daily routine: vision warm ups and vision building. Remember you are not expected to do every single practice every single day. Less is more. Spend more time doing fewer practices rather than spending less time doing more practices. Spending ten minutes repeating two practices for five minutes each is typically better than spending ten minutes doing ten different practices for one minute each. Both of the above scenarios exemplify a ten-minute practice routine, but the first example takes you into a deeper state of relaxation through repetition, whereas the second example keeps you on the surface and your eyes and mind may not get as deeply relaxed. In other words, quality over quantity.

After learning your typical two-part vision practice structure, you will see an example of a daily vision routine laid out in conjunction with the hours of the day. This is an example of an ideal vision routine on a totally free day but it might not be your everyday routine. Depending on your schedule, maybe you will only have time to fit this full day routine in once a week or once a month. When it comes to your more standard everyday routine when you're balancing school, work, family, or friends, your routine may be significantly shorter. As long as you do something every single day, you will maintain momentum and obtain improvements. It can take between 30 to 60 days to establish a new habit, so repetition and frequency are critical in order to ensure permanent changes and results.

On your busier days, it may be more realistic for you to use the ten-minute vision tune-ups instead, which adhere to a particular theme like relaxation, centralization, fusion, vision building, etc. Even on your busiest days, you ought to be able to carve out at least five or ten minutes to spend caring for your eyes in a relaxed and mindful way. And honestly, it is usually the hectic busy days when you need the physical and mental relaxation the most to make sure you are not stressing or straining too much.

Also remember that success hinges more on the mental practices and habits than the physical ones. Vision is nine-tenths mental and one-tenth physical. Therefore, even if you have a super busy day and you don't have time to do many physical practices, you can still be applying mental concepts like dynamic relaxation, centralization, shifting, blinking, breathing, etc. that can be performed while doing other tasks.

Success is about transforming your lifestyle and adopting relaxing vision habits, not about the most amount of time spent doing physical exercises. Success is also highly dependent on your ability to either wear weaker prescription glasses or spend time without any glasses. In either case, you must stay relaxed and avoid any form of strain. Squinting, staring, or straining while wearing training glasses or no glasses will only make your vision problem worse.

Set your bar low in order to accomplish daily small goals, rather than setting the bar too high and then you never reach it and feel like you're constantly failing.

Since vision training is a form of brain training, think about how neuroplasticity works. Consider how these seven tenets of neuroplasticity apply to your vision training process:

1. Change can only occur when the brain is in the mood.
2. Change strengthens the connections between neurons engaged at the same time.
3. Neurons that fire together, wire together. Repetition and frequency are key.
4. Strong emotions strengthen the connections.
5. Brain plasticity is a two-way street, can get better or worse.
6. Memory is crucial for learning.
7. Motivation is a key factor.

Not only do you need to be in the mood to do your vision practices and habits every day, but you need to make it fun. Mindlessly going through the motions of the eye exercises will not yield as many results. You must be engaged, interested, motivated, and excited about the process. Do not think of your vision improvement journey as a limited time thing. Consider it a lifelong journey. It may not take your entire life to achieve clearer vision, but as long as you have two eyes in your head, you need to be cognoscente of taking good care of them and maintaining their health and wellness through the simple means outlined in this book. The contents of this book are like tools that you have added to your tool belt. If, in the future your vision changes or declines in any way, you will know exactly what tools to pull back out of your tool belt to get your vision back in a state of health and equilibrium. Do you plan on stopping brushing or flossing your teeth anytime soon? If not, then you have no reason to plan on stopping your new holistic eye care routine anytime soon either.

Structuring Your Daily Vision Practice Routine

This book contains dozens of powerful vision improvement practices, and at times it can feel a little overwhelming. It is possible to overload yourself into a debilitating state of inaction, and then you won't end up doing anything. To avoid that, I want you to simplify your vision practice into a typical two-part structure: vision warm ups and vision building. Pick and choose one or two practices from each list to complete a single vision routine.

1. **Vision Warm Ups:** 5 to 15 mins	2. **Vision Building:** 5 to 30 mins
• **Sunning & Palming** (Light Therapy, Dark Therapy, Mental Focus, Visualization) • **Shifting & Swinging** (Long Swing, Medium Swing, Short Swing, Picket Fence Shifter) • **Centralizing** (Nose Drawing, One Thing Best, Counting, Reverse Blinking) • **Fusing** (Brain Balancing, Gateposts, Near to Far Shifting, Lens Flexor, Rope Fusion, Convergence, Divergence) • **Eye Yoga** (Eye Movements, Asanas, Pranayamas, Meditations)	• **Reading Warm Ups** (Sunning, Palming, Microprint, Crowding, Space Riding) • **Convergence/Divergence** (Stimulating Accommodation) • **Relaxed White Line Reading** (Left + Right + Both) • **6 Step Chart Formula Near** (Left + Right + Both) • **6 Step Chart Formula Far** (Left + Right + Both) • **Inner Vision & Insight** (Memory, Imagination, Visualization, Mental Focus, Emotional Root Causes, Clearing Past, Present, Future Vision)

Whenever preparing to begin your vision practice in the morning, afternoon, evening, or night, just remind yourself that all you must do is start with some vision warm ups and then finish with some vision building. It's just two steps: warming up & relaxed reading.

The warm ups include everything from Chapters 3, 4, 5, 6, and 8. Vision building includes everything from Chapter 7. Simply spend five to fifteen minutes warming your eyes and mind up, and then follow your warm up with five to thirty minutes of vision building near or far. Just pick one or two practices from the left column and fill five to fifteen minutes with repeating them until you feel nice and relaxed and ready for vision building. If you are nearsighted, spend between five and thirty minutes repeating your vision building techniques for the distance. If you are farsighted, spend between five and thirty minutes repeating your vision building techniques for the near point.

Ideal Daily Vision Routine

5:00 am ***6:00 am*** ***7:00 am*** ***8:00 am*** ***9:00 am***	**Morning Relaxation Routine** *Stretch & Yawn, Tapping, Acupressure, Eyebrow Raises / Tense & Release* *Yoga / Breathing / Meditation* *Sunning, Palming + Mental Focus of your choice* *Body Swing / Head Swing / Optical Swing*
10:00 am ***11:00 am*** ***12:00 pm*** ***1:00 pm*** ***2:00 pm***	**Afternoon Fusion Routine** *Swinging, Picket Fence Shifter* *Gateposts, Near to Far Shifting, Lens Flexor, Rope Fusion* *Convergence/Divergence Games* *Palming + Mental Focus of your choice*
3:00 pm ***4:00 pm*** ***5:00 pm*** ***6:00 pm*** ***7:00 pm***	**Evening Vision Building Routine** *Swinging, Sunning, Palming, Vision Stretching / Distance Gazing* *Vision Building Near and/or Far with Eye Patch* *6 Step Chart Formula, Chart Techniques, Relaxed Reading* *Palming + Mental Focus of your choice*
8:00 pm ***9:00 pm*** ***10:00 pm*** ***11:00 pm***	**Night Pre-Sleep Routine** *No Screens 1-2 hours before bed* *Night Vision Walk, Slow Swinging, Yoga, Breathing, Meditation* *Palming + Mental Focus of your choice*

10 Minute Vision Tune-Ups

1) **RELAXATION**
Stretching/Yawning, Tapping, Acupressure, Eyebrow Raises/ Tense Release, Nose Drawing (5 mins)
Palming & Happy Memory (5 mins)

2) **THE TRIFECTA**
Long / Head Swinging (3 mins)
Sunning (3 mins)
Palming + Picturing Black (4 mins)

3) **BRAIN BALANCING**
Cross Marching (2 mins)
Brain Buttons (1 mins)
Hook Ups (2 mins)
Palming + Teeter Totter (5 mins)

4) **EYE YOGA**
Eye Movements (1 mins)
Asanas (3 mins)
Pranayamas (2 mins)
Palming + 3rd Eye Meditation (4 mins)

5) **CENTRALIZING**
One Thing Best (2 mins)
Nose Drawing / Outlining (2 mins)
Reverse Blinking (2 mins)
Palming + ABC Categories (4 mins)

6) **SHIFTING**
Picket Fence Shifter (2 mins)
Near to Far Shifting (2 mins)
Optical Swing (2 mins)
Palming + Bar and Dots (4 mins)

7) **FUSION 1**
Gatepost Swinging (2 mins)
Lens Flexor w/ Eye Patch (4 mins)
Palming + Mental Flexing (4 mins)

8) **FUSION 2**
Rope Fusion (3 mins)
Converge/Diverge (3 mins)
Palming + Nose Drawing (4 mins)

9) **VISION BUILDING NEAR**
Crowding & Space Riding (2 mins)
Thin White Line Reading (2 mins)
Chart Clearing Techniques (4 mins)
Palming + Picturing White (2 mins)

10) **VISION BUILDING FAR**
Relaxation Warm Up (1 min)
Fusion Warm Up (1 min)
Chart Clearing Techniques (5 mins)
Palming + Letter Classification (3 min)

Review: Ten Goals of Vision Training

- **Replace Bad Vision Habits with Good Vision Habits** – It can be very difficult to drop bad habits. It is much easier to introduce good habits because they push out the bad habits automatically. You must have something better (good vision habits) to take the mind off the bad vision habits.

- **Stop Staring -** Get your eyes in motion and the world to move. Normal eyes vibrate dozens of times per second. Eyes with good vision move more and eyes with poor vision move less. These saccadic eye movements are referred to as 'shifting.' Many of the practices in this book help to get the eyes shifting more rapidly and subtly. Staring is the opposite of shifting and is a bad vision habit that leads to more strain, cuts off circulation, slows down the speed of the eyes, and decreases vision overall.

- **Establish Deep & Rhythmic Breathing** – The eyes need sufficient oxygen to function properly. Shallow breathing leads to shallow vision. The breath is the best vehicle to relaxation so regular deep breaths where you contract your abdomen on the exhale and expand your abdomen on the inhale will ultimately help your eyes. The best breath for vision is the 'sigh.' When you take a big sigh exhale out of your mouth, not only do your eyes relax, but your entire mind and nervous system gets relieved of stress and strain. Try it now, breathe deeply, sigh out loud, and see clear.

- **Address Eye Muscles** – Eye muscles must be trained and toned for coordinating and focusing (accommodating) both near and far. Strained eye muscles can lead to nearsightedness, farsightedness, astigmatism, glaucoma, amblyopia, strabismus, and more. Many of the practices in this book help to loosen tight eye muscles and get them to work harmoniously.

- **Normalize the Weaker Eye** – Discover and normalize your weaker eye and bring the two into balance. You may need to spend more time working with your weaker eye at first until it strengthens. This can be assisted by wearing an eye patch over your stronger eye while performing the vision practices or while relaxing at home. The weaker eye is actually more strained than the stronger eye, so make sure you give your weaker eye even more rest than you give your stronger eye.

- **Achieve Dynamic Relaxation** – There are two types of relaxation: passive and dynamic. Passive relaxation is when you totally relax your body and mind inactively. Dynamic relaxation is when you remain relaxed while in action or in motion. You must learn how to keep your eyes relaxed while in use. When you remove your lenses and begin doing vision practices, you must avoid ever straining your eyes. Can you keep your eyes relaxed while using them without wearing glasses, without squinting, and without straining? What about when you feel stressed?

- **Cultivate Clear Flashes** - Once dynamic relaxation is achieved, your eyes and mind harmonize and you experience a 'clear flash.' For an instant, you will experience perfect or near-perfect clarity without glasses. At first the flashes are only temporary. However, these flashes are precisely what you are working toward and provide a glimpse of what is to come as you continue practicing. Learn what practices bring about flashes and try to stay relaxed when they come. Notice how your eyes feel and how your mind feels when they appear. Experiment ways to encourage them to last longer. The goal is to achieve a flash that does not go away.

- **Achieve Fusion** – Encourage teamwork between the eyes so they work together to focus on the same point at the same time at the same rate, fusing the two images of both eyes into one clear image. Fusion can be developed through repetition of the practices in Chapter 6.

- **Develop Eye-Mind Coordination** – The eyes are extensions of the brain and are made of brain tissue. The Bates Method reestablishes any lost or weak connections between the eyes (body) and brain (mind). The plasticity of your brain allows for new neural pathways to be carved out through learning new psychophysical skills like vision. Perfect vision occurs when the eyes and mind are both focused on the same thing at the same time. Centralize your eyes and mind.

- **Banish Fear** – Fear causes refractive error and defeats relaxation. Most vision problems are deeply rooted in fear, whether it's fear of the unknown, fear of the future, fear of the present, fear of the past, or fear of not being able to see near or far. Trust yourself and the process. Be brave and nobly explore this unchartered territory with confidence and curiosity.

Modern Day Bates Method

The year this book was published is just two years shy of the 100-year anniversary of Dr. Bates' book *Perfect Sight Without Glasses* being published back in 1920. His original book was a pioneering work that paved the way for the development of Holistic Eye Care. As an ophthalmologist and scientist, Dr. Bates' book isn't the most compelling read. It is a little dry, full of jargon, run-on sentences, and complex explanations that sometimes go over the reader's head. While technically designed for the layperson, Dr. Bates was also tasked with attempting to convince other ophthalmologists of his research and findings. In trying to do so, he sometimes loses the layperson along the way, making his method a little less accessible. Especially when you fast forward to the present day and take into account the evolution of language. At times Bates' language and communication styles seem outdated and hard to grasp or apply to our modern, hyper-civilized world. However, this does not mean that his original work doesn't still contain some very important concepts that are just as applicable today as they were a century ago.

What I wish to address here are a few points where my interpretation and teaching of the Bates Method differs slightly from how Dr. Bates presented them in his original work.

Theory of Accommodation

Dr. Bates made the discovery that the six extraocular muscles (four recti muscles and two oblique muscles) play a part in accommodation, or your eye's ability to focus light correctly from the outside world onto the retina on the inside back of the eye. When the eye fails to do so, it is called a 'refractive error,' nearsightedness being when the light focuses in front of the retina because the eyeball is too long, farsightedness being when the light focuses behind the retina because the eyeball is too short, and astigmatism being when the light focuses on multiple points on the retina instead of one because the eyeball is too unevenly shaped.

Six years before Bates was born, Helmholtz put forth his theory of accommodation in 1855 that stated that the lens inside the eye is the sole factor of accommodation. The ciliary muscles contract and relax to thicken the lens to focus near and to thin the lens to focus far. The six muscles around the eyes had no role to play, other than to turn the eyes in different directions. Once Bates became an authority in the ophthalmological community and began retesting Helmholtz's theory of accommodation, he kept finding exceptions to that rule.

Most notably, he performed a cataract surgery on a patient and removed both of his lenses. According to the Helmholtz theory, this man should not have been able to accommodate, yet he was still able to focus on fine print up close and focus on the eye chart in the distance. This got Bates scratching his head and wondering what else could be contributing to the power of accommodation.

He proceeded to perform dozens of experiments on different types of animal eyes in the lab, applying electrical currents to the extraocular muscles when they were continuous and severed. He was surprised to find that when an electrical current was applied to the oblique eye muscles it elongated the eye organ to focus near, and when an electrical current was applied to the recti eye muscles it shortened the eye organ to focus far. He then cut the eye muscles and applied the electrical current to the back portion of the cut eye muscle, and no accommodation would take place. When he sewed the eye muscles back together and reapplied the electrical current, accommodation would occur yet again. This led him to the discovery that the six muscles around the eye are not just for turning the eyes, but also for accommodating the eyes by changing the shape of the entire eye organ slightly. Thinking back on the story of his patient who could accommodate without lenses in his eyes, he went as far as to claim that the lens had no accommodative role, and it was 100% the extraocular muscles.

This is one of the main contention points that orthodox ophthalmologists have with Dr. Bates, because they believe accommodation to be the other way around, 100% in the lens and 0% in the extraocular muscles. In my personal opinion, my understanding of the matter falls somewhere in between. I believe both the lens and the extraocular muscles have accommodative power, not just one or the other. And not only that, I believe they influence each other. When the four recti muscles contract to shorten the eye, it initiates the thinning of the lens by the ciliary muscles to focus far. Then, when the two oblique muscles contract to lengthen the eye, it initiates the thickening of the lens by the ciliary muscles to focus near. And going beyond the lens and the extraocular muscles, I believe there is even more to accommodation than just those two factors. There are so many moving parts of the eye organs, plus the whole mental perception element. To focus, the cornea must bend the light, the iris must contract to make the pupil the perfect size, the lens must assume the perfect shape, the extraocular muscles must get the eyeball into the perfect focal length, the retina must be able to receive the light in the relaxed way, the optic nerves must transmit the signals instantly, and the visual cortex in the brain must perceive the signals perfectly. Why would you want to limit this extremely complex process to just one or two parts of such a multifaceted and interdependent system?

So instead of fighting back and forth over who is right - the lens camp or the eye muscle camp - why not focus our attention and energy on balancing all the different muscles of the eyes to relearn automatic and effortless accommodation? I try not to get too hung up on the mechanics of focusing, and instead try to focus on the art of focusing itself.

The Role of Glasses

Dr. Bates was one of the first eye doctors to question the role of glasses as being the absolute best solution for treating vision problems. He quickly noticed the trend, as all eye doctors eventually do, that his patients kept needing continually stronger and stronger prescription lenses the more they wore the original prescription lenses he gave them on their prior visit. In other words, he put two and two together that the glasses were actually making the underlying vision problem worse and worse over time, because they were leaving the root cause untreated. They were simply treating the symptoms of the vision problems.

In his book, Bates stated that in order to improve your vision naturally you must discard your glasses permanently. He was fairly strict about this and warned that if you wear glasses it will retard your progress. Later in his career he did say that glasses can still be worn while in treatment if your vocation depends on it, or you need them to be safe in certain situations, but he still remained steadfast that it would really slow the process down and even lead to relapses.

I personally believe that gradually weaning down to weaker prescription glasses as stepping-stones is a more realistic approach in this day and age than quitting cold turkey.

Eye Floaters

In Dr. Bates' book he says that floaters are a product of the mind and are not actually there. We now know that not to be true. Floaters actually are physical things that appear when the vitreous body begins to break down and particles get suspended in the fluid inside the eye, casting shadows on the retina. However, Dr. Bates was definitely onto something when he said the mind has the ability to see through them or to tune them out, especially in light of the fact that floaters are more noticeable when the mind is strained and stressed, and less noticeable when the mind is at ease and the vision is clearer.

Telescopic Vision

When introducing and explaining the concept of central fixation in his book, Dr. Bates gives the example of people who have 'telescopic vision', who could actually see the moons of Jupiter with the naked eye.

"The limits of vision depend upon the degree of central fixation. A person may be able to read a sign half a mile away when he sees the letters all alike, but when taught to see one letter best he will be able to read smaller letters that he didn't know were there. The remarkable vision of savages, who can see with the naked eye objects for which most civilized persons require a telescope, is a matter of central fixation. Some people can see the moons of Jupiter, with the naked eye. It is not because of any superiority in the structure of their eyes, but because they have attained a higher degree of central fixation than most civilized persons do."

-Dr. William H. Bates

At first this may seem hard to believe, but one must consider the fact that in the early 1900s Earth's atmosphere was likely less polluted than it is today and there was certainly less light pollution, meaning that the complete night sky was more visible back then.

Also consider the fact that tribal groups of people had already mapped the cosmos well before the invention of telescopes. Although I have not met anyone presently who can see the moons of Jupiter with the naked eye, I don't necessarily discount it as being impossible or unachievable. Therefore, the main thing I disagree with Bates on this topic is his use of the word 'savages', which is much more of a 20th century way to describe tribal and indigenous groups of people. As an anthropologist, I cringe when I hear the word 'savages' used to describe human beings.

Instantaneous Cures

If you have read Dr. Bates' book, you know that it includes many success stories to demonstrate the power, potential, and efficacy of the Bates Method. Many of the examples of the cure of imperfect sight by treatment without glasses are seemingly instantaneous, with some of his patients achieving perfect vision in a matter of days, hours, or even minutes. Sometimes when he would get his patients to demonstrate the truth of central fixation to themselves, it would secure an immediate and permanent cure. Bates shares the now well-known story of his patient who palmed his eyes for 20 hours straight, which led to his permanent cure.

These case histories are meant to instill inspiration in the reader, but to be honest there were times when those stories actually frustrated me because they did not reflect my own experience. From start to finish, it took me between 3 and 4 years to achieve sustainably clear vision without using my glasses, which seemed really long compared to the examples Bates gave in his book. If I had only used these instant cures as a standard to hold myself against, I probably wouldn't have held my faith and stuck with it for the long run.

Luckily, I also read other books about the Bates Method and met other people using the method in the present day who shared different types of success stories that seemed more realistic and seemed to match my progress. I'm afraid that one of the main reasons people don't succeed with the Bates Method is because they don't stick with it long enough, which is understandable because if you're not seeing improvements after a couple weeks or months of practicing it may make you lose hope or think it's not working. In my own experience, I had to get through those initial periods of doubt in order to begin experiencing improvements in my vision. I also hired a vision coach to help me get more improvements, which is definitely something you should consider if you have not been seeing as many improvements as you had hoped.

I'm not saying it's impossible to achieve a seemingly miraculous reversal of your vision problem, and I've even met people in my career that have woken up one day and not needed their contacts or glasses anymore because they could all of a sudden see clearly without them. What I am saying is that if you're not one of those select few who get instant improvement, don't let that discourage you and don't give up. If you don't achieve an instant permanent cure, maybe you can at least experience some instant temporary cures, or 'clear flashes'. These 'clear flashes' or moments of improved or perfect vision without glasses, are like little previews of what is possible with continued practice. These flashes are possible to attain very early on in the vision reeducation process, even just by trying some of the suggestions on *Pages 12 and 13,* but they are often temporary cures, not permanent ones.

The majority of people who practice the Bates Method experience more gradual improvements, and the total time it takes to achieve permanent improvement is more like several months or sometimes even several years, which at first may sound like a long time, but remember to ask yourself this: how long have you already been wearing glasses? I had already been wearing glasses for 15 years by the time I learned about the Bates Method, so 3 to 4 years spent working on improving my vision paled in comparison to the amount of time I had already been misusing and mistreating my eyes.

Dr. Bates worked with thousands of patients in his lifetime and witnessed countless reversals of vision problems. So I'm sure that when it came time to write his book he could only include a limited number of examples and case histories (for more case histories, check out *Stories From The Clinic* by Dr. Bates' wife, Emily Lierman). I guarantee that there were many cases which took longer to heal or improve, but maybe Bates wanted to share the 'best of' case histories or a selection of the most impressive ones to really get people's attention and show the reader what is possible through this simple and natural method.

Like the last point about telescopic vision being potentially more possible 100 years ago with a more conducive environment, maybe instantaneous cures were also more possible back then because of different lifestyles. Maybe people in the early 20th century had more liberty to go without glasses for longer periods of time. People didn't have to worry so much about driving cars, staring at computer screens, or existing in a globally connected and increasingly stressful world. Even if permanently improving your vision naturally takes longer in the 21st century than it did in the 20th century, don't let that dissuade you from trying it, or continuing to work on achieving healthier eyes and mind using the method that Bates pioneered a century ago because it is still just as powerful and potent today as it was then.

I did not only use the Bates Method to improve my vision. I knew about Yoga, Meditation, and Breathwork before I knew about the Bates Method, so naturally I felt inclined to incorporate additional alternative healing practices into my vision healing process. Since other approaches assisted my own healing journey, I also like to incorporate elements of yoga into my teaching of the Bates Method, as you got a glimpse of in this book.

Despite these slight disagreements and differences in the way that Dr. Bates taught 100 years ago and the way I teach his method today, I still view the Bates Method as one of the most specific and viable ways to prevent and reverse nearly all types of vision problems in a simple, natural, and holistic way. If you disagree with some elements of Dr. Bates' original teachings, I encourage you not to toss the baby out with the bathwater.

At the end of my yoga teacher training, we were shown a video of Swami Satchidananda sending off graduates of a teacher training program in the past. He said that over the past month we have all been cows grazing in a field and chewing on grass. The grass represented all the new knowledge we obtained about yoga, meditation, breathing practices, yoga philosophy and lifestyle, diet and nutrition, and more. He said as we left the ashram and went back home to our communities; we would continue to chew this 'cud' and assimilate what we experienced. He said that before we swallow it and digest it to make our own version of the yoga practice, we need to feel around for little twigs and pebbles, which represented things that we disagreed with, or didn't fully accept, and to spit them out. He was not forcing us to accept every single thing that he said or taught. He said to take what we needed, and to leave the rest.

That is what you can do with the Bates Method. I absolutely love the Bates Method, and consider it to be the primary way that I reversed my myopia and astigmatism gradually over time with practice and repetition. But I do not consider myself to be a die-hard Bates Method follower, because I have the consciousness to pick and choose what I know to be true and recognize the things that have been updated since Bates' time. I pride myself in teaching the original Bates-Corbett Method as was taught by Dr. Bates, handed down to Margaret Corbett, to my teacher Dr. Jerriann Taber, and then to me. But I am not so bull-headed to claim that every single thing Bates said was absolutely true or correct, and those slight discrepancies like the ones listed above did not prevent me from still giving the Bates Method my whole-hearted attempt... and I'm so glad I didn't let my skeptical mind prevent me from doing so, because if I had then I would probably still be wearing glasses!

Afterword

My goal with this book is to show you how easy and fun it can be to make this a part of your everyday life. Vision improvement is an exciting, relaxing process and the regular practice of it will lead to some serious changes and shifts in your existence. Vision is the most important sense that you rely on every day. Better vision leads to a better life.

Succeeding is simply a matter of actually performing the practices, having them become a part of your everyday life, and remaining a good long-term vision student. You will not see improvements if you only do the practices a few times and then give up. Devoting yourself to the practice long-term and learning the new habits leads to success. Do your vision improvement practices every day with determination until you start seeing clearer.

A note on forming new habits: new habits can only form with repetition and frequency. A tip to build a new habit is to set an alarm to beep on every hour. Set tiny and easily achievable goals throughout the day. Every time the watch beeps, do one minute of vision practices, whether palming, swinging, sunning, shifting, flexing, fusing, centralizing, gazing off in the distance, closing your eyes, conscious deep breathing, or any of the morning relaxation practices to help you relax your eyes and mind. At the minimum, you will have accomplished at least 15 minutes of vision practices for the day. Most likely though, once you start one of the practices, you will want to keep going for more than a minute. That way, you didn't just achieve the minimum goal, but you exceeded it by accomplishing 30 minutes or even an hour of vision practices for the day simply by spacing them out and doing two or three minutes every hour.

This was a critical part of the process for me - being able to incorporate the vision practice into my preexisting daily routines. Start small, cultivate your practice, and it will grow on its own. If you don't like to be as rigid with set time frames, simply tack your daily vision practice onto something else that you already do every day. Right after you eat your breakfast or brush your teeth or walk your dog, do your vision practices. You probably don't eat breakfast, brush your teeth, or walk your dog at the same exact time every day so there is a little more wiggle room. After a week straight of adding a new habit right onto a pre-existing one, the new habit quickly gets embedded into your day-to-day routine.

As the title of this book suggests, permanent success is dependent upon giving up your glasses for good. The Bates Method gives you lots to do without your glasses on. The more time a day you spend without your glasses on the better. If your mind says, "But I can't do anything without my glasses on." remind yourself that everything in this book can be done without glasses. If you keep up with your daily practice checklists, you will be spending at least an hour, if not more, without your glasses on every day. Slowly but surely, your eyes will turn back on and your confidence will grow. Before you know it, you will be able to do all kinds of things without your glasses; things you never thought you could do without their help. The less you wear them the less you will want to wear them. The more improvements you see, the more you will want to keep training.

The Bates Method rewires your brain. The basic foundations in **Chapters 3, 4, and 5** set the stage for the process of vision improvement through relaxation. The vision warm ups in **Chapter 6** begin the process of carving new neural pathways through repetitive and relaxed visual stimuli. The vision building habits and practices from **Chapter 7** fills in those new neural pathways and solidifies new neural connections. **Chapters 2 and 8** give you tools to rewrite your vision past, present, and future. **Chapter 1** shows you how it all ties together and how to customize this vision improvement practice to fit your specific vision.

Remember, the only way to learn new skills, to learn new habits, and to rewire the brain is through repetition, frequency, and genuine enjoyment of the practice. Stick with this program and you will see results. As taught by Dr. Bates, vision is 90% mental and only 10% physical. While continuing your vision practice it is important to remember that it is not all about the physical effort you put into it; it is more about the level of mental relaxation you can attain and how well you can keep your eyes relaxed while in use.

Reading this book and beginning your own home vision practice is just the first step. You can go pretty far on your own using this book alone, but working with a Certified Bates Method Teacher in person locally or with me online will take your vision practice to the next level. I am constantly offering various vision-related services. I teach private vision training lessons to students in person as well as at a distance online. So no matter where in the world you live, you can access one-on-one vision coaching with me. Another option is to set up a personal vision improvement retreat that can span over a weekend or even a full week. I also regularly offer one-day workshops and seminars in various locations. Due to the great need for more Bates Method teachers and vision educators in the world, I also offer teacher training programs to dedicated students who wish to make teaching vision improvement into a part-time or full-time career option. If any of the above interests you, please visit www.integraleyesight.com for more information.

I wish you luck and encourage you to reach out to me with any questions or to arrange an online or in-person vision consultation or vision training lessons to take your vision improvement practice to the next level. Thank you so much for reading my book and thank yourself for taking your eye health back into your own hands.

-Nathan T. Oxenfeld

👁 *Are you still following the 13 Rules of Relaxed Reading from Page 12-13?* 👁

How is your posture? How are the muscles in your face, eyes, and brow? How is your breathing? How is your blinking? Are you stopping at the end of every few sentences to close your eyes and picture the last word you read clearly? Are you looking off into the distance every so often? Can you see an imaginary bright white line underlining the sentences as you read? Can you imagine a bright white line underlining these words with your eyes closed?

Make sure you continue to apply these relaxed reading techniques in the next book you read.

Holistic Vision Program

The *Holistic Vision Program* is my six-week online course that takes this book to the next level. It is an individual, self-guided program that you can begin whenever you want and go through entirely at your own pace. It brings this book to life with follow-along videos and audios.

There are two main types of videos contained in the Holistic Vision Program: vision training videos and vision education videos. There are six vision training videos (Week 1, Week 2, Week 3, Week 4, Week 5, and Week 6) and four vision education videos (Introduction, Class 1, Class 2, and Class 3). The vision training videos are more experientially based because I filmed myself demonstrating the practices and you are meant to follow along with me in real time. The vision education videos are more explanation based because I lead you through a PowerPoint presentation where I get a chance to explain more about the practices, principles, habits, and application into your everyday life. The introduction provides an orientation, class 1 reviews weeks 1 and 2, class 2 reviews weeks 3 and 4, and class 3 reviews weeks 5 and 6. The combination of the weekly vision training videos and the biweekly vision education videos fully cover the practical side and the principle side of the practice.

Along with the videos, there are also vision practice audio guides that you can download and listen to with headphones or over speakers and follow along as my voice guides you through various twenty-minute vision practice routines.

The *Holistic Vision Program* comes with a bonus one-hour private session with me online that you can use either during the program or after you complete the program to go over your vision history and vision practice experience to help customize the material to fit your current visual state, lifestyle, and schedule. There is also an option to add three more private one-on-one online sessions in addition to the *Holistic Vision Program* to get even more customization and accountability from me as your coach throughout your vision improvement process.

To get more information and enroll, please visit:

www.integraleyesight.com/program

Resources

Holistic Vision Program – www.integraleyesight.com/program

Bates Method 101 Videos – www.youtube.com/c/nathanoxenfeld

The Naked Eye Podcast – www.integraleyesight.com/podcast or search on iTunes

Association of Vision Educators – www.naturalvisionteachers.com

Bates Method International – www.seeing.org

Bates Association for Vision Education - www.batesvisioneducation.org

Natural Vision Improvement Blog – www.iblindness.org

Bates Method Online Library – www.central-fixation.com

Recommended Readings

Perfect Sight Without Glasses and Better Eyesight Magazine by Dr. William H. Bates

Help Yourself To Better Sight by Margaret Corbett

The Art of Seeing by Aldous Huxley

See Without Glasses by Ralph MacFadyen

The Bates Method by Peter Mansfield

Healthy Vision by Dr. Neal Adams

Greater Vision and Magic Eye Beyond 3D by Dr. Marc Grossman

Health and Light by Dr. John Ott

How To Improve Your Child's Eyesight Naturally by Janet Goodrich

Take Off Your Glasses and See and Light: Medicine of the Future by Dr. Jacob Liberman

Better Vision Now by Clara Hackett

Cataracts, Glaucoma, and Other Eye Conditions by John Tobe

Find A Vision Teacher Near You

Dr. Jerriann Taber – San Diego, CA - www.eyerobics.net

Esther Joy Van Der Werf – Ojai, CA – www.visionsofjoy.com

Claudia Muehlenweg – Los Angeles, CA – www.myholisticvision.com

Meir Schneider – San Francisco, CA – www.self-healing.org

Marybetts Sinclair – Corvallis, OR – www.marybettssinclair.com

Greg Marsh – Fort Collins, CO – www.bettereyesightnow.com

Dr. Marc Grossman – New Paltz, NY – www.naturaleyecare.com

Rosemary Gaddum Gordon – Eliot, ME – www.visioneducators.com

Kate Keilman – Hawaii – www.keilman.org/eyeballs

Cassandra Arnold – Canada – www.naturalvisioneducator.com

Anna Bambridge – Scotland - www.indivisual.org.uk

Charlotte Schuman – England - www.seenaturally.co.uk

Wolfgang Hätscher-Rosenbauer – Germany – www.institut-fuer-sehtraining.de

Nina Hutchings – France - www.methodebates.fr

Maurizio Cagnoli – Italy - www.metodobates.it

Tony Helinsky – Sweden – www.tonyhelinsky.com

Barry Auchettl – Australia – www.barryauchettl.com

Loy Chye Bin – Singapore - www.makeithappen.sg

Acknowledgements

I wish to express gratitude to my parents, Thomas and Jeanne Oxenfeld, for their guidance and support, Emily Gamble for her inspiration and her huge heart, Ben Kamens for first introducing me to the Bates Method, Roberta Binder for her compassionate editing skills, Dr. William H. Bates for developing the method that has helped thousands of people give up their glasses for good, Margaret Corbett for her continuation of and contribution to the Bates Method, Sri Swami Satchidananda for showing me the depth and breadth of a true yoga practice, Brian and Jenny Lumb for helping me bloom, Dr. Jerriann Taber for being my vision teacher and training me to become a certified Bates Method teacher, all of my brave vision students for giving me such valuable teaching experience, and to all the vision educators who have carved this path before me. Thank you.

References

1. Maino, Dominick. “Neuroplasticity: Teaching an Old Brain New Tricks” (Jan. 2009)

2. Barry, Susan. “Evidence-Based Peer-reviewed Scientific Research Shows that Amblyopia or Lazy Eye Can be Successfully Treated in Older Children and Adults” (Jun. 2009)

3. Mohamed, Samia A. Abdel Rahman. "Vision Therapy-Based Program for Myopia Control in Adolescents."*Middle-East Journal of Scientific Research* (2013): Pgs 390-96.. .

4. Sabel BA, Gudlin J. “Vision restoration training for glaucoma: a randomized clinical trial.” *JAMA Ophthahlmology* (2014): Pgs 381-389.

5. Murphy, Kate. “Vision Training to Boost Sports Performance” *The New York Times* (2014)

6. Bates, William. "Medical Articles” Central Fixation Publishing Company. (1886-1923)

7. Bates, William. The Cure of Imperfect Sight by Treatment Without Glasses, Central Fixation Publishing Company (1920)

8. Lee V, Rekhi E, Hoh Kam J, Jefferey G, “Vitamin D rejuvenates ageing eyes by reducing inflammation, clearing amyloid beta and improving visual function” (Oct. 2012)

9. Mutti Donald, Marks AR. “Blood levels of vitamin D in teens and young adults with myopia” (Mar. 2011) and “Scientists study effects of sunlight to reduce number of nearsighted kids” (Nov. 2014)

10. Rosenfield, Mark. “Computer Vision Syndrome: a review of ocular causes and potential treatments” (Sep. 2011) Ophthalmic and Physiological Optics, Volume 31, Issue 5, pages 502-515

Vision Tools

The following pages contain a collection of Vision Tools like eye charts and reading cards that you can either remove or scan and reprint. If you do not want to take them out of the book, you can also visit *www.integraleyesight.com/visiontools* to download the PDF versions of all the vision tools and print them out on your own.

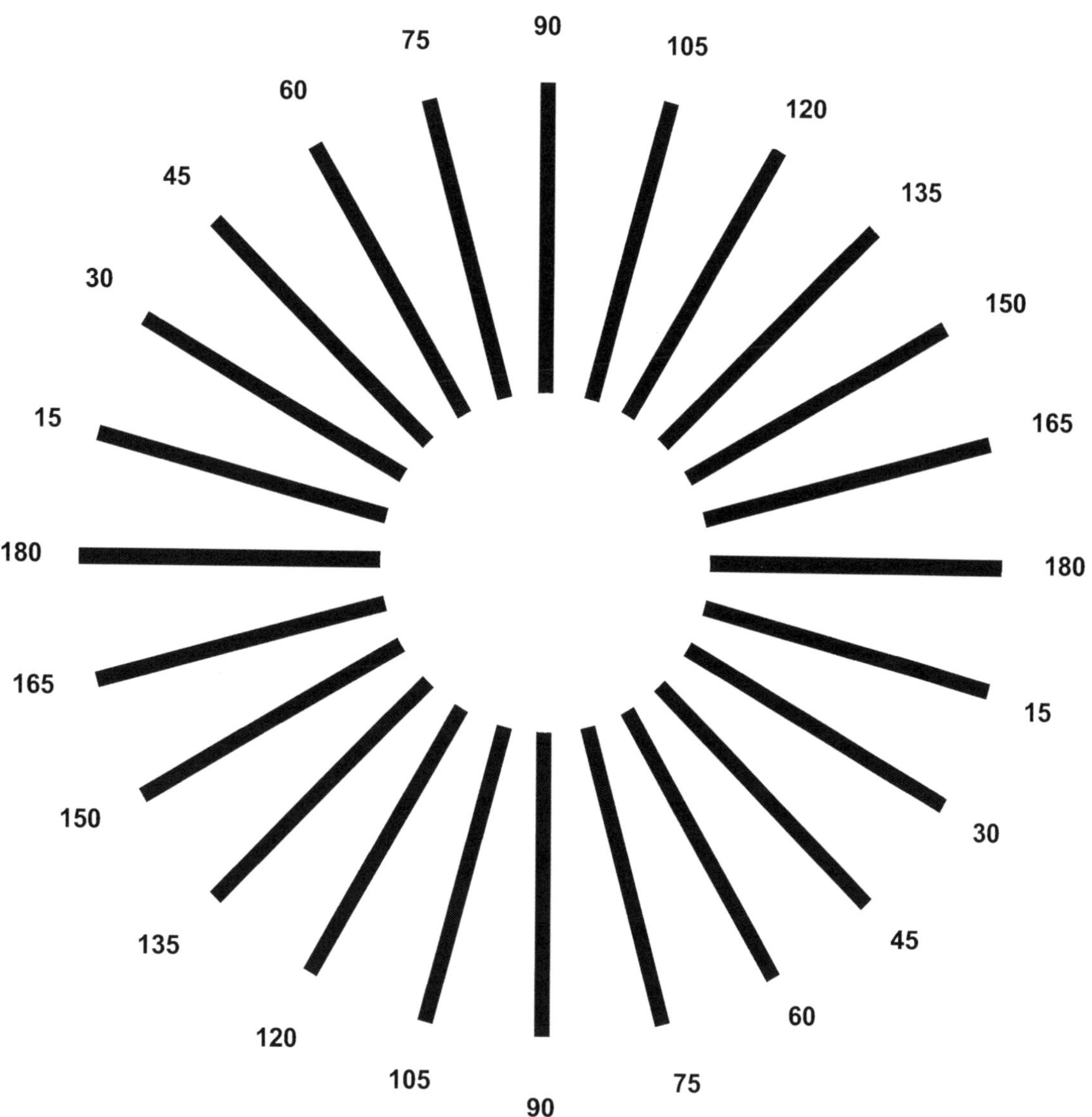
90
105
120
135
150
165
180
15
30
45
60
75
90
105
120
135
150
165
180
15
30
45
60
75

Astigmatism Wheel

Instructions on *Page 80.*

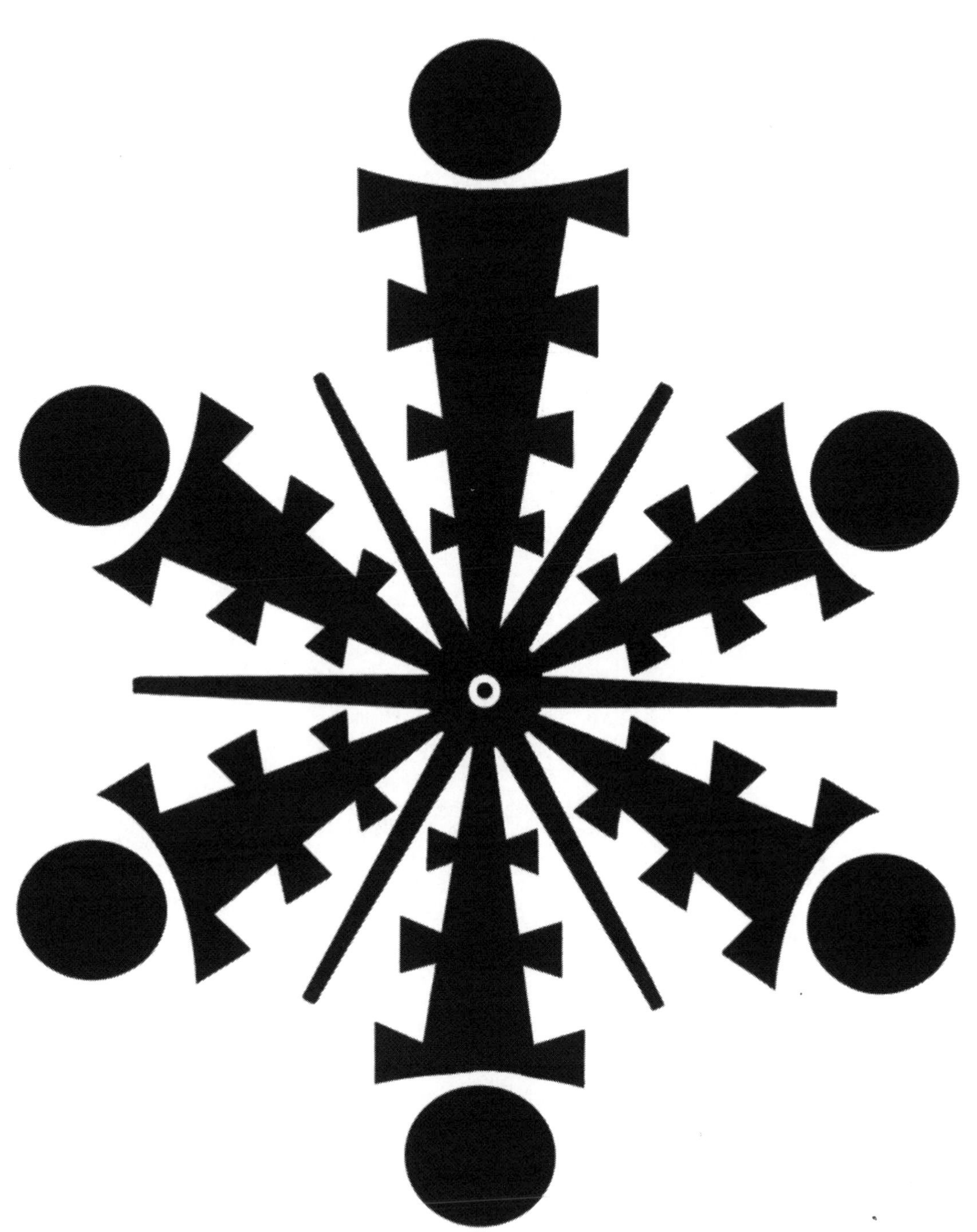

Tibetan Wheel

Instructions on *Page 251.*

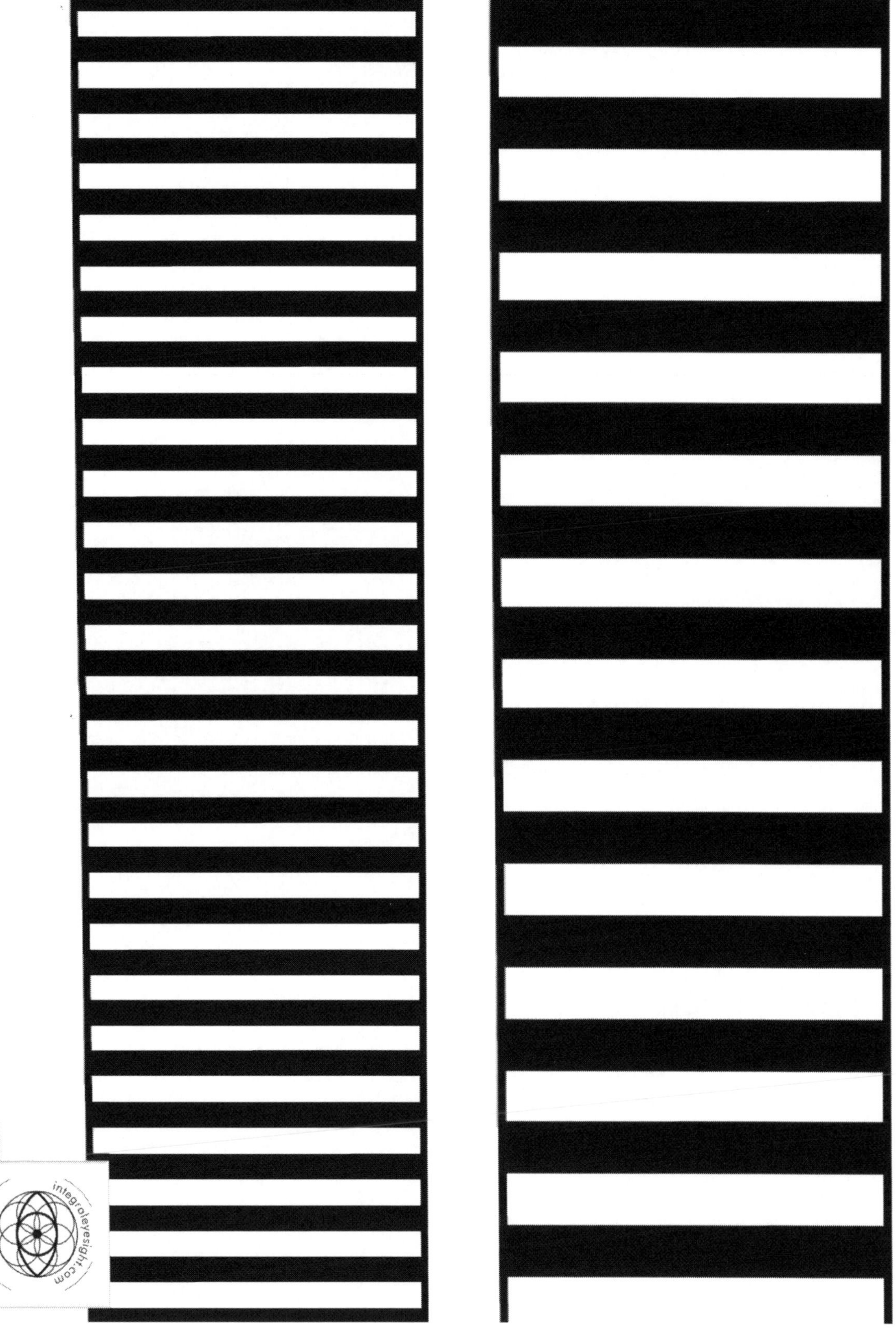
integraleyesight.com

Picket Fence Shifter

Instructions on *Pages 140-141.*

The Fundamental Principle

Instructions on *Pages 161-162.*

THE FUNDAMENTAL PRINCIPLE

1. **Do you see imperfectly?**

2. Can you observe then that when you look at the first word, or the first letter, of a sentence you do not see best where you are looking; that you see other words, or other letters, just as well as or better than the one you are looking at?

3. **Do you observe also that the harder you try to see the worse you see?**

4. Now close your eyes and rest them, remembering some color, like black or white, that you can remember perfectly.

5. Keep them closed until they feel rested, or until the feeling of strain has been completely relieved. Now open them and look at the first word or letter of a sentence for a fraction of a second. If you have been able to relax, partially or completely,

6. **you will have a flash of improved or clear vision, and the area seen best will be smaller.**

7. After opening the eyes for this fraction of a second, close them again quickly, still remembering the color, and keep them closed until they again feel rested.

8. Then again open them for a fraction of a second.

9. **Continue this alternate resting of the eyes and flashing of the letters for a time, and you may soon find that you can keep your eyes open longer than a fraction of a second without losing the improved vision.**

10. **If your trouble is with distant instead of near vision, use the same method with distant letters.**

11. In this way you can demonstrate for yourself the fundamental principle of the cure of imperfect sight by treatment without glasses.

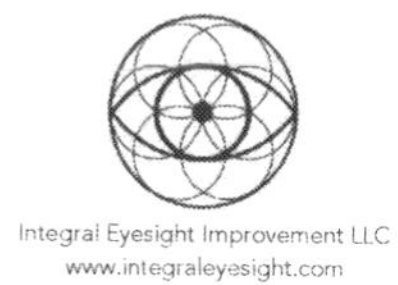

Integral Eyesight Improvement LLC
www.integraleyesight.com

THE FUNDAMENTAL PRINCIPLE

1. **Do you see imperfectly?**

2. Can you observe then that when you look at the first word, or the first letter, of a sentence you do not see best where you are looking; that you see other words, or other letters, just as well as or better than the one you are looking at?

3. **Do you observe also that the harder you try to see the worse you see?**

4. Now close your eyes and rest them, remembering some color, like black or white, that you can remember perfectly.

5. Keep them closed until they feel rested, or until the feeling of strain has been completely relieved. Now open them and look at the first word or letter of a sentence for a fraction of a second. If you have been able to relax, partially or completely,

6. **you will have a flash of improved or clear vision, and the area seen best will be smaller.**

7. After opening the eyes for this fraction of a second, close them again quickly, still remembering the color, and keep them closed until they again feel rested.

8. Then again open them for a fraction of a second.

9. Continue this alternate reading of the eyes and flashing of the letters for a time, and you may soon find that you can keep your eyes open longer than a fraction of a second without losing the improved vision.

10. **If your trouble is with distant instead of near vision, use the same method with distant letters.**

11. In this way you can demonstrate for yourself the fundamental principle of the cure of imperfect sight by treatment without glasses.

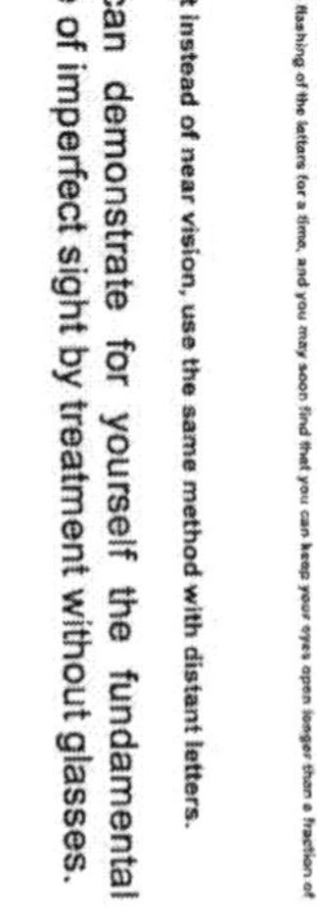

1. **Do you see imperfectly?**

2. Can you observe then that when you look at the first word, or the first letter, of a sentence you do not see best where you are looking; that you see other words, or other letters, just as well as or better than the one you are looking at?

3. **Do you observe also that the harder you try to see the worse you see?**

4. Now close your eyes and rest them, remembering some color, like black or white, that you can remember perfectly.

5. Keep them closed until they feel rested, or until the feeling of strain has been completely relieved. Now open them and look at the first word or letter of a sentence for a fraction of a second. If you have been able to relax, partially or completely,

6. **you will have a flash of improved or clear vision, and the area seen best will be smaller.**

7. After opening the eyes for this fraction of a second, close them again quickly, still remembering the color, and keep them closed until they again feel rested.

8. Then again open them for a fraction of a second.

9. Continue this alternate reading of the eyes and flashing of the letters for a time, and you may soon find that you can keep your eyes open longer than a fraction of a second without losing the improved vision.

10. **If your trouble is with distant instead of near vision, use the same method with distant letters.**

11. In this way you can demonstrate for yourself the fundamental principle of the cure of imperfect sight by treatment without glasses.

THE FUNDAMENTAL PRINCIPLE

1. **Do you see imperfectly?**

2. Can you observe then that when you look at the first word, or the first letter, of a sentence you do not see best where you are looking; that you see other words, or other letters, just as well as or better than the one you are looking at?

3. **Do you observe also that the harder you try to see the worse you see?**

4. Now close your eyes and rest them, remembering some color, like black or white, that you can remember perfectly.

5. Keep them closed until they feel rested, or until the feeling of strain has been completely relieved. Now open them and look at the first word or letter of a sentence for a fraction of a second. If you have been able to relax, partially or completely,

6. **you will have a flash of improved or clear vision, and the area seen best will be smaller.**

7. After opening the eyes for this fraction of a second, close them again quickly, still remembering the color, and keep them closed until they again feel rested.

8. Then again open them for a fraction of a second.

9. Continue this alternate reading of the eyes and flashing of the letters for a time, and you may soon find that you can keep your eyes open longer than a fraction of a second without losing the improved vision.

10. **If your trouble is with distant instead of near vision, use the same method with distant letters.**

11. In this way you can demonstrate for yourself the fundamental principle of the cure of imperfect sight by treatment without glasses.

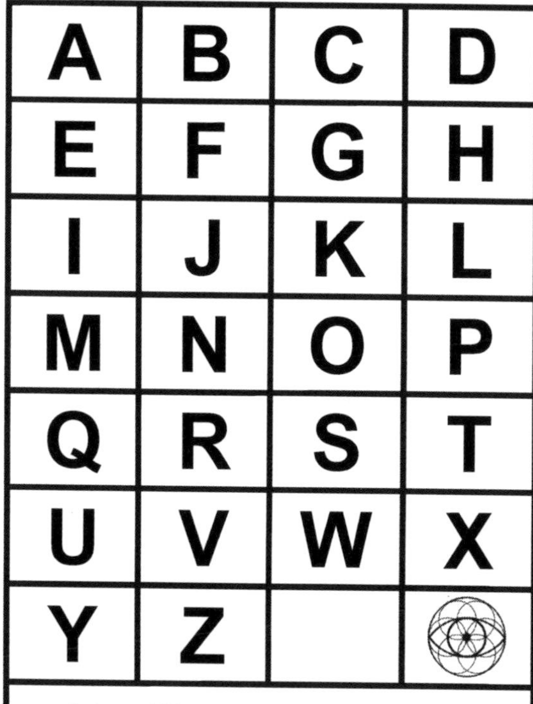

A	B	C	D
E	F	G	H
I	J	K	L
M	N	O	P
Q	R	S	T
U	V	W	X
Y	Z		

Integral Eyesight Improvement LLC
www.integraleyesight.com

A	B	C	D
E	F	G	H
I	J	K	L
M	N	O	P
Q	R	S	T
U	V	W	X
Y	Z		

Integral Eyesight Improvement LLC
www.integraleyesight.com

A	B	C	D
E	F	G	H
I	J	K	L
M	N	O	P
Q	R	S	T
U	V	W	X
Y	Z		

Integral Eyesight Improvement LLC
www.integraleyesight.com

A	B	C	D
E	F	G	H
I	J	K	L
M	N	O	P
Q	R	S	T
U	V	W	X
Y	Z		

Integral Eyesight Improvement LLC
www.integraleyesight.com

Alphabet Cards

Instructions on *Pages 180-182 & Chapter 7.*

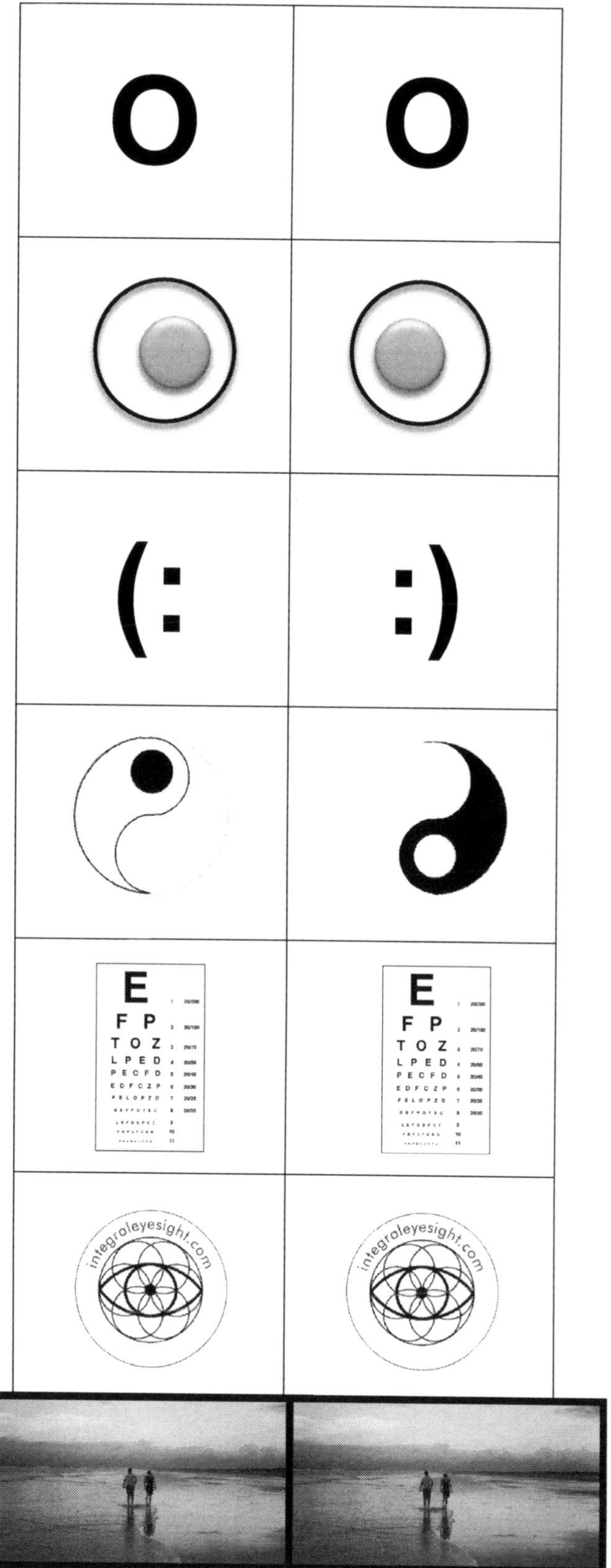

O O
(: :)
E
F P
T O Z
L P E D
integraleyesight.com
integraleyesight.com

Fusion Cards

Instructions on *Pages 186-188.*

"The

memory,

or imagination,

is best when one thing is imagined

better than all other things, Central Fixation,

but constant shifting is necessary to maintain Central Fixation."

-Dr. William H. Bates

"The

memory,

or imagination,

is best when one thing is imagined

better than all other things, Central Fixation,

but constant shifting is necessary to maintain Central Fixation."

-Dr. William H. Bates

Convergence Dots

Instructions on *Page 204.*

"The memory, or imagination, is best when one thing is imagined better than all other things,

Central Fixation, but constant shifting is necessary to maintain Central Fixation." -Dr. William H. Bates

"The memory, or imagination, is best when one thing is imagined better than all other things,

Central Fixation, but constant shifting is necessary to maintain Central Fixation." -Dr. William H. Bates

"The memory, or imagination, is best when one thing is imagined better than all other things,

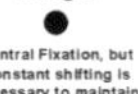

Central Fixation, but constant shifting is necessary to maintain Central Fixation." -Dr. William H. Bates

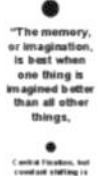

"The memory, or imagination, is best when one thing is imagined better than all other things,

Central Fixation, but constant shifting is necessary to maintain Central Fixation." -Dr. William H. Bates

"The memory, or imagination, is best when one thing is imagined better than all other things,

Central Fixation, but constant shifting is necessary to maintain Central Fixation." -Dr. William H. Bates

"The memory, or imagination, is best when one thing is imagined better than all other things,

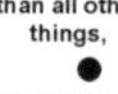

Central Fixation, but constant shifting is necessary to maintain Central Fixation." -Dr. William H. Bates

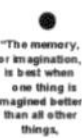

Divergence Dots

Instructions on *Page 204.*

The Art of Reading

Instructions on *Pages 220-222.*

The Art of Reading

"When reading, you should look at the white spaces between the lines and not directly at the lines themselves. The reason for this is that it is no effort to sweep the eyes over a plain background. Fixing the eyes on individual words and letters involves strain, and strain impairs vision.

When a person with normal sight regards the white spaces with a sweeping shift across the page from margin to margin, he can read easily, rapidly and without fatigue. If the same person looks at the letters, the eyes grow tired and the vision becomes poor.

People who cannot read well at the near point always tend to fix their attention on the print. Consequently they see worse. Improvement cannot take place until they learn to look at the white spaces between the lines.

Reading can be improved by improving the power to remember or imagine whiteness. This improvement can be achieved in the following way. Close your eyes and imagine something even whiter than the page before you – white snow, white starch, white linen. Then open your eyes again. If your mental images of whiteness have been clear and intense, you will find that the white spaces between the lines will appear for a few moments to be whiter than they really are.

Repeat this process as a regular drill. When your imagination of whiteness has become so good that you can constantly see the spaces between lines as whiter than they really are, the print will seem blacker by contrast and the eye will find itself reading easily and without effort or fatigue.

When the imagination of whiteness has reached its maximum intensity, it often happens that one can see a thin white line much whiter than the rest of the white space. This white line may be compared to a neon light moving swiftly from one margin to the other immediately under the letters.

The consciousness of this thin white line is a great help in reading, increasing as it does the speed both of the eyes and of the mind. Once this illusion of the white line is seen, imagined or remembered, unlimited reading without fatigue becomes possible."

-Dr. William H. Bates

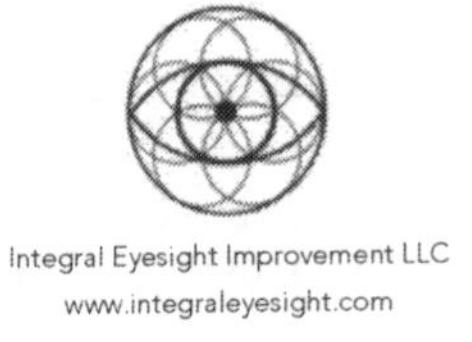

Integral Eyesight Improvement LLC
www.integraleyesight.com

“MORE than thirty years ago, not knowing any better and being guided by the practice of other eye doctors, I recommended patients with imperfect sight to throw away their eyes and see with their glasses. Since that time I have made some valuable discoveries, which have enabled me to cure people without glasses. The slogan now is: "Throw away your glasses and see with your eyes."

“MORE than thirty years ago, not knowing any better and being guided by the practice of other eye doctors, I recommended patients with imperfect sight to throw away their eyes and see with their glasses. Since that time I have made some valuable discoveries, which have enabled me to cure people without glasses. The slogan now is: "Throw away your glasses and see with your eyes."

“MORE than thirty years ago, not knowing any better and being guided by the practice of other eye doctors, I recommended patients with imperfect sight to throw away their eyes and see with their glasses. Since that time I have made some valuable discoveries, which have enabled me to cure people without glasses. The slogan now is: "Throw away your glasses and see with your eyes."

“MORE than thirty years ago, not knowing any better and being guided by the practice of other eye doctors, I recommended patients with imperfect sight to throw away their eyes and see with their glasses. Since that time I have made some valuable discoveries, which have enabled me to cure people without glasses. The slogan now is: "Throw away your glasses and see with your eyes."

“MORE than thirty years ago, not knowing any better and being guided by the practice of other eye doctors, I recommended patients with imperfect sight to throw away their eyes and see with their glasses. Since that time I have made some valuable discoveries, which have enabled me to cure people without glasses. The slogan now is: "Throw away your glasses and see with your eyes."

“MORE than thirty years ago, not knowing any better and being guided by the practice of other eye doctors, I recommended patients with imperfect sight to throw away their eyes and see with their glasses. Since that time I have made some valuable discoveries, which have enabled me to cure people without glasses. The slogan now is: "Throw away your glasses and see with your eyes."

“MORE than thirty years ago, not knowing any better and being guided by the practice of other eye doctors, I recommended patients with imperfect sight to throw away their eyes and see with their glasses. Since that time I have made some valuable discoveries, which have enabled me to cure people without glasses. The slogan now is: "Throw away your glasses and see with your eyes."

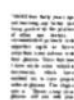

Microprint Reading Card

Instructions on *Pages 193-196, 212-222.*

FUNDAMENTALS OF EYE TRAINING

Reading Card by Dr. William H. Bates

1. Vision can be improved by natural methods.

2. Tension causes eyestrain and impairs vision. Relaxation relieves tension.

3. Relaxed eyes are normal eyes. When eyes lose their relaxation and become tense, they strain and stare and the vision becomes poor.

4. Vision can be improved only by education in proper seeing. Proper seeing is relaxed seeing. Normal eyes shift rapidly and continuously. Eyes with defective vision are fixed and staring. When staring eyes learn to shift, vision is improved.

5. The eyeball is like the camera, and changes in focal length. To focus the camera, you must adjust the distance from the negative to the front of the camera.

6. To focus the eye, the distance between the retina at the back and the cornea in the front must be increased for close vision and decreased for the distant view.

7. Six muscles on the outside of the eyeball control its shape; four, reaching from front to back, flatten the eye; two, belting it around the middle, squeeze it long from front to back.

8. When the eyes are relaxed, these six muscles are flexible and cooperate automatically, adjusting the focal length so eyes may see both near and far.

9. Just as dependence on crutches weakens leg muscles, so dependence on glasses weakens eye muscles by relieving them of responsibility. But muscles can be reeducated to do their duties.

10. Relaxation of the eyes and mind brings relaxation of the entire body. This general relaxation increases circulation and brings improved physical, visual and mental health.

11. Relaxation is a sensation.

THOU SHALT NOT STRAIN
The eye records images, the mind interprets and sees. When the mind is tense, the eye is tense; when the mind is relaxed, the eye is relaxed. Perfect memory of any object increases mental relaxation. Mental relaxation results in relaxation of the eyes, and both together result in better vision.

1 2 3 4 5 6 7 8 9 10

Fundamentals of Eye Training Reading Card

Instructions on *Pages 28-30, 193-196, 212-222.*

YES

I CAN

L E A R N

T O   S E E

Distance Eye Chart - Letters

Instructions on *Pages 28-30, 193-196, 198-208.*

Line 1 ~ 20/150

Line 2 ~ 20/100

Line 3 ~ 20/70

Line 4 ~ 20/50

Line 5 ~ 20/40

Line 6 ~ 20/30

Line 7 ~ 20/25

Line 8 ~ 20/20

Line 9 ~ 20/15

Line 10 ~ 20/10

C L E A R L Y

A G A I N C L E A R

F O C U S D E P E N D S

O N A C L E A R M I N D

R E L A X A N D B R E A T H E

I A M S E E I N G C L E A R L Y

0

1 2

3 4 5

6 7 8 9

0 1 2 3 4

5 6 7 8 9 0

1 2 3 4 5 6 7 8

9 0 1 2 3 4 5 6 7 8

Distance Eye Chart - Numbers

Instructions on *Pages 209-211.*

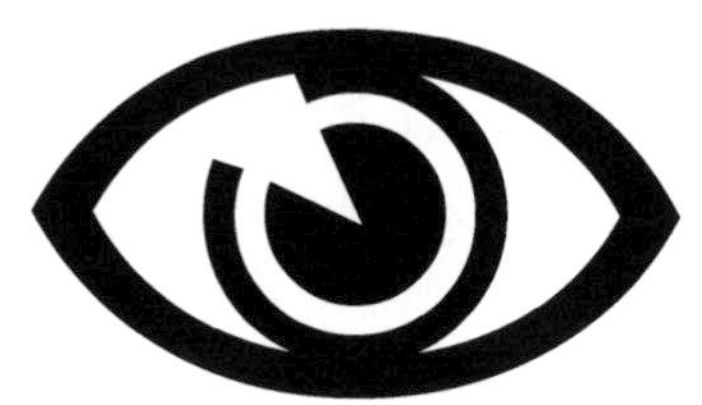

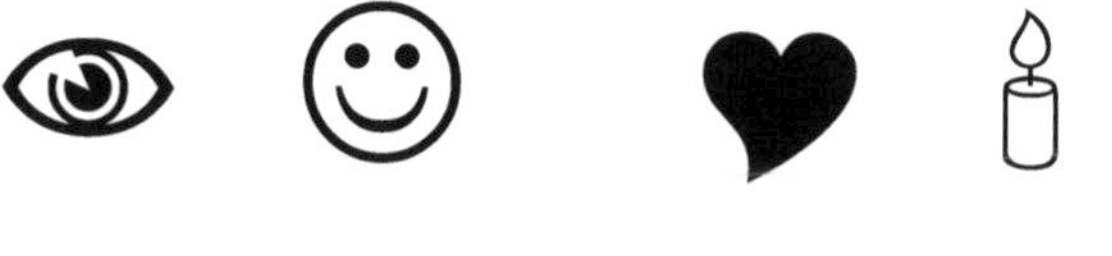

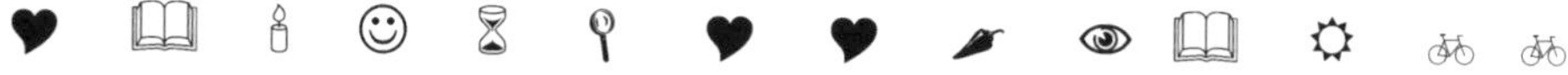

Distance Eye Chart - Pictures

Instructions on *Pages 209-211.*

0

1 2

3 4 5

6 7 8 9

0 1 2 3 4

5 6 7 8 9 0

1 2 3 4 5 6 7 8

9 0 1 2 3 4 5 6 7 8

Number and Picture Matching Cards

Instructions on *Pages 209-211.*

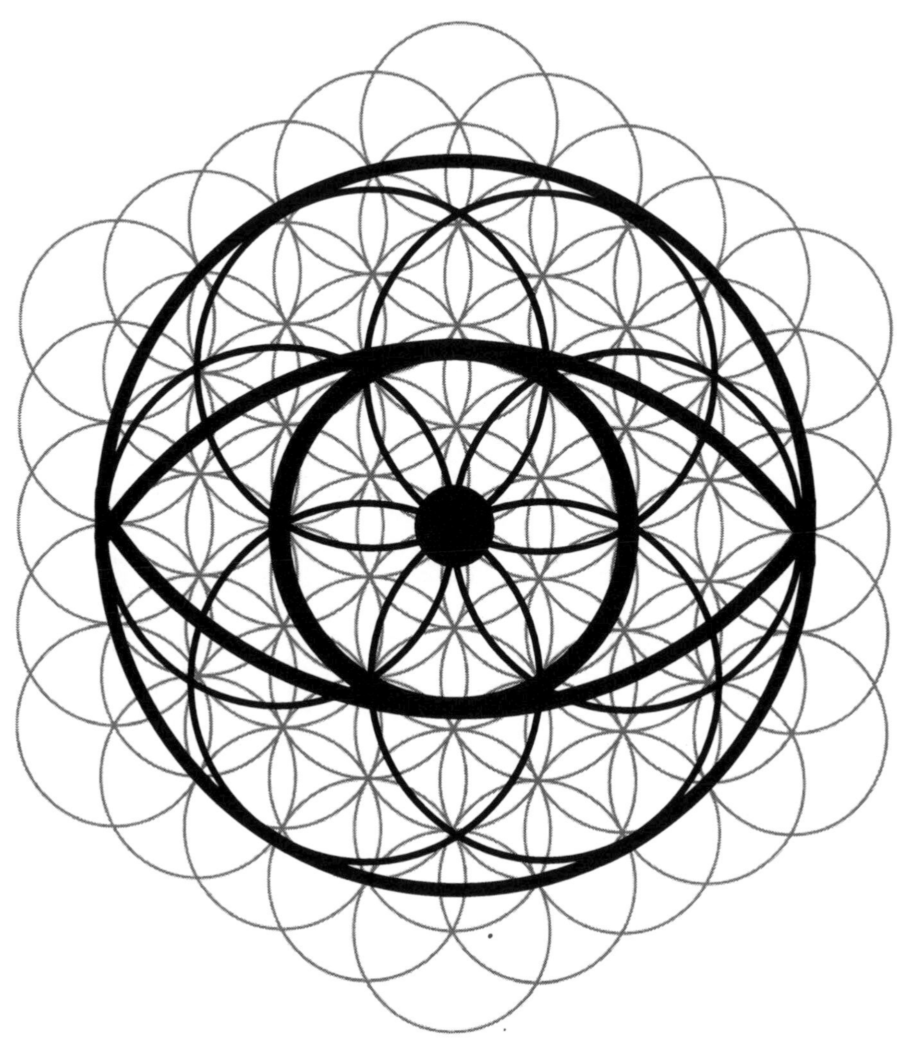

www.integraleyesight.com

Made in the USA
Middletown, DE
08 February 2020

84431704R00188